TACHYCARDIA

Edited by **Takumi Yamada**

Tachycardia
Edited by Takumi Yamada

Published by InTech
Janeza Trdine 9, 51000 Rijeka, Croatia

Publishing Process Manager Molly Kaliman

Technical Editor Teodora Smiljanic

Cover Designer InTech Design Team

Additional hard copies can be obtained from orders@intechopen.com

Tachycardia, Edited by Takumi Yamada
p. cm.
ISBN 978-953-51-0413-1

For EU product safety concerns:
IN TECH d.o.o., Prolaz Marije Krucifikse Kozulić 3, 51000 Rijeka, Croatia,
info@intechopen.com or visit our website at intechopen.com.

Meet the editor

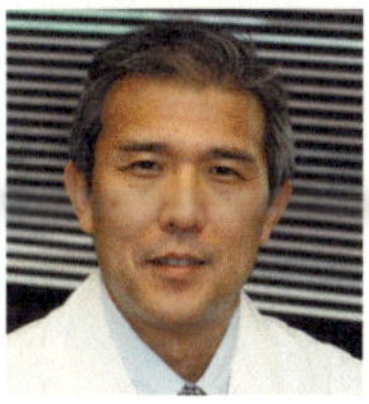

Dr Takumi Yamada is currently Assistant Professor of Medicine at the University of Alabama at Birmingham in the United States of America. He was born in Tottori, Japan. He graduated from Faculty of Medicine, Nagoya University and was trained in Japan. His specialty is pharmacological and non-pharmacological treatments of cardiac arrhythmias. He has more than 150 scientific publications including book chapters. He is an internationally recognized authority in the treatment of ventricular arrhythmias. He is a regular lecturer at several international cardiology and electrophysiology meetings. He has served as a book editor, and an associate editor and reviewer for 20 major international cardiology and electrophysiology journals.

Contents

Preface

Tachycardia is defined as a faster heart rhythm than normal sinus rhythm (with a rate of greater than 100 beats per minute in humans). Tachycardias can occur from different clinical backgrounds including congenital or acquired heart diseases, electrophysiological mechanisms and origins. The diagnosis of tachycardias is made by surface electrocardiograms and electrophysiological testing. The management and treatment of tachycardias including pharmacological and non-pharmacological approaches are determined based on these factors. These concerns have been studied and the details have been increasingly recognized. In this book, internationally renowned authors have contributed chapters detailing these concerns of tachycardias from basic and clinical points of view and the chapters will lead to a further understanding and improvement in the clinical outcomes of tachycardias.

Dr. Takumi Yamada
Distinguished Professor of Medicine,
Division of Cardiovascular Disease, University of Alabama at Birmingham,
USA

1

Accurate Detection of Paediatric Ventricular Tachycardia in AED

U. Irusta, E. Aramendi, J. Ruiz and S. Ruiz de Gauna
University of the Basque Country
Spain

1. Introduction

Sudden cardiac death (SCD) is the single most important cause of death in the adult population of the industrialized world (Jacobs et al., 2004). SCD accounts for 100–200 deaths per 100 000 adults over 35 years of age annually (Myerburg, 2001). The most frequent cause of SCD is fatal ventricular arrhythmias: ventricular fibrillation (VF) and ventricular tachycardia (VT) (de Luna et al., 1989). In fact, degenerating VT to VF appears to be the mechanism for a large majority of cardiac arrests (Luu et al., 1989).

Most sudden cardiac arrests occur out of hospital, and the annual incidence of out-of-hospital cardiac arrest (OHCA) treated by emergency medical services in the USA is 55 per 100 000 of the population (Myerburg, 2001). Survival rates in untreated cardiac arrest decrease by 7–10 % per minute (Larsen et al., 1993; Valenzuela et al., 1997), as the heart function deteriorates rapidly. Consequently, early intervention is critical for the survival of OHCA victims. The sequence of actions to treat OHCA includes rapid access to emergency services, early cardiopulmonary resuscitation, early defibrillation and advanced cardiac life support as soon as possible. These four links constitute what the American Heart Association (AHA) calls the chain of survival. Compressions and ventilations during cardiopulmonary resuscitation maintain a minimum blood flow until defibrillation is available. The only effective way to terminate lethal ventricular arrhythmias and to restore a normal cardiac rhythm is defibrillation, through the delivery of an electric shock to the heart.

Automated external defibrillators (AED) are key elements in the chain of survival. An AED is a portable, user-friendly device that analyzes the rhythm acquired through two electrode pads and delivers an electric shock if pulseless VT or VF is detected. The shock advice algorithm (SAA) of an AED analyzes the electrocardiogram (ECG) to discriminate between shockable and nonshockable rhythms. Given a database of classified ECG records, the performance of the SAA is evaluated in terms of the proportion of correctly identified shockable—*sensitivity*—and nonshockable—*specificity*—rhythms, which must exceed the minimum values set by the AHA (Kerber et al., 1997).

SCD is 10 times less frequent in children than in adults. However, the social and emotional impact of the death of a child is enormous. In the USA alone, an estimated 16 000 children die each year from sudden cardiac arrest (Sirbaugh et al., 1999). The most common cause of cardiac arrest in children is respiratory arrest, although the incidence of cardiac arrest caused by ventricular arrhythmias increases with age (Appleton et al., 1995; Atkins et al.,

1998). Initially two independent studies provided evidence for the use of AED in paediatric patients (Atkinson et al., 2003; Cecchin et al., 2001). Based on that evidence, in 2003, the International Liaison Committee on Resuscitation (ILCOR) recommended the use of AED in children aged 1–8 years (Samson et al., 2003). Since 2005, the resuscitation guidelines[1] have incorporated this recommendation, which indicates the need to adapt AED for paediatric use. This adaptation involves adjusting the defibrillation pads and energy dose, and, furthermore, demonstrating that SAA accurately detect paediatric arrhythmias.

SAA of commercial AED were originally developed for adult patients. Adapting these algorithms for paediatric use requires the compilation of shockable and nonshockable rhythms from paediatric patients in order to assess their SAA performance. The first studies on the use of AED in children showed that two adult SAAs from commercial AED accurately identified many paediatric rhythms (Atkinson et al., 2003; Cecchin et al., 2001). The specificity for nonshockable rhythms and the sensitivity for VF were above the values recommended by the AHA. However, those studies failed to meet AHA criteria for shockable paediatric VT. In 2008, a third study showed that a SAA designed for adult patients did not meet AHA criteria for nonshockable paediatric supraventricular tachycardia (SVT) (Atkins et al., 2008). This study suggested that the specificity of SAA originally designed for adult patients could fail to meet AHA performance goals for paediatric SVT.

The SAA first extracts a set of discrimination parameters or features from the surface ECG recorded by the AED, and then combines those features to classify the rhythm as shockable or nonshockable. There are important differences in heart rate, amplitude and ECG wave morphology between paediatric and adult rhythms (Cecchin et al., 2001; Rustwick et al., 2007). The faster heart rates and shorter QRS durations of paediatric rhythms produce differences in the values of the discrimination parameters which may affect the performance of SAA designed for adult use. Some of these differences have been previously assessed, and the discrimination power of several parameters has been evaluated for adult and paediatric arrhythmias (Aramendi et al., 2006; 2010; 2007; Irusta et al., 2008; Ruiz de Gauna et al., 2008). These studies underlined the inadequacy of many parameters and discrimination thresholds for discriminating VT from SVT safely when adult and paediatric rhythms were considered. A reliable SVT/VT discrimination algorithm is therefore a key requirement for adapting or developing SAA for paediatric use.

This chapter comprises five sections. Section 2 describes the database compiled to develop and test a SVT/VT discrimination algorithm in the context of AED arrhythmia classification. More than 1900 records from adult and paediatric patients were compiled, and a thorough description of the sources and rhythm classification process is given. Special attention is paid to the SVT/VT subset, which contains more than 650 records. The criteria for classification are reported, and heart rate analysis for both adult and paediatric populations is detailed. In section 3, we conduct the spectral analysis of SVT and VT rhythms and define a number of spectral parameters that discriminate between VT and SVT. Emphasis is placed on the influence of the age group and the heart rate on the values of the parameters. Based on these spectral parameters, a SVT/VT discrimination algorithm is designed in section 4. The discriminative power of the algorithm is assessed through the receiver operating characteristic (ROC) curve and the sensitivity/specificity values. The algorithm accurately discriminates between SVT and VT in both adults and children, and it could safely be incorporated into

[1] The latest version of the guidelines was released in 2010 (Biarent et al., 2010).

SAA. Section 5 discusses the main conclusions of this work and analyzes what issues need to be addressed when using adult SAA with children. Several strategies to adapt SAA for paediatric use are discussed, and an overall scheme to adapt adult SAA for paediatric use, integrating the SVT/VT discrimination algorithm described in section 4, is proposed.

2. Adult and paediatric data collection

The accurate identification of VT and SVT by an AED is well described in the 1997 AHA statement on the performance and safety of AED SAA (Kerber et al., 1997). The AHA statement describes the composition of the databases used to develop and test SAA, including the types of rhythms and the minimum number of records per rhythm type. It divides the rhythm types into three categories: shockable, nonshockable and intermediate[2]. It also specifies that within a rhythm type, all records must be obtained from different patients. Finally, the statement defines the performance goals of the SAA for shockable and non-shockable rhythms, i.e. the minimum sensitivity and specificity of the SAA per rhythm type. These values are exhibited in table 1.

Rhythms	Minimun no. of records	Performance goal	Observed performance	90 % One-sided CI
Shockable				
Coarse VF [a]	200	> 90 % Sens	> 90 %	87 %
Rapid VT	50	> 75 % Sens	> 75 %	67 %
Nonshockable	**300 total**			
NSR	100	> 99 % Spec	> 99 %	97 %
Other	30	> 95 % Spec	> 95 %	88 %
Asystole	100	> 95 % Spec	> 95 %	92 %
Intermediate				
Fine VF	25	Report only	–	–
Other VT	25	Report only	–	–

[a] Peak-to-peak amplitude above 200µV.
[b] Specified by the manufacturer, because tolerance to VT varies widely among patients.

Table 1. Definition of the databases used to validate SAA, adapted from the AHA statement (Kerber et al., 1997). The other nonshockable rhythms include supraventricular tachycardia (SVT), atrial fibrillation, premature ventricular contractions, heart blocks, sinus bradycardia and idioventricular rhythms. The 90 % one-sided confidence intervals (CI) are computed for the observed performance goals. no.=number; NSR=normal sinus rhythm; Sens=sensitivity; Spec=specificity; VF=ventricular fibrillation; VT=ventricular tachycardia.

Currently, there exists no public database of ECG records compliant with the AHA statement. Each AED manufacturer compiles its own data, which must include paediatric rhythms if the AED will be used to treat children. However, the studies describing paediatric databases (Atkins et al., 2008; Atkinson et al., 2003; Cecchin et al., 2001) report fewer shockable rhythms than those specified in the AHA statement because paediatric ventricular arrhythmias are scarce.

[2] Rhythms for which the benefits of defibrillation are uncertain.

An adult and a paediatric database were compiled using ECG records collected from in- and out-of-hospital sources. Three cardiologists assigned a rhythm type and a shock/no-shock recommendation to each record. For potentially shockable rhythms, the criteria by which to determine the shock/no-shock recommendation were: the patient was unresponsive, had no palpable pulse, and was of unknown age (Cecchin et al., 2001). Diagnostic discrepancies among the reviewers were further discussed, and a consensus decision for the shock/no-shock recommendation was agreed upon after the assessment of the risks. Most of the reviewer disagreements in diagnosis occurred between SVT and VT rhythms.

The database contains shockable rhythms (VF and rapid VT) and the most representative nonshockable rhythms: normal sinus rhythm (NSR) and SVT. Although the AHA includes SVT among the other nonshockable rhythms (see table 1), we have added an individual SVT category because adult SAA may fail to detect high-rate paediatric SVT (Atkins et al., 2008) accurately. Although the complete database is initially described, the SVT/VT subset was extracted to study VT discrimination. We considered VT shockable for heart rates above 150 bpm in adults and 20 bpm above the age-matched normal rate in children (Atkinson et al., 2003), which amounts to 180 bpm in infants (under 1 year) and 150 bpm in children older than 1 year. Table 2 presents a summary of the database, where the paediatric data are divided into three age groups: under 1 year, 1–8 years (ILCOR recommendation) and above 8 years. All records were stored with a common format and sampling frequency of $f_s = 250$ Hz.

	Paediatric					
Rhythms	<1y	1y–8y	>8y	**Total**	**Adult**	**Minimum** [a]
Shockable						
Coarse VF	3 (1)	18 (11)	37 (10)	58 (22)	374 (374)	200
Rapid VT	8 (4)	39 (19)	19 (13)	**66 (33)**	**200 (200)**	50
Nonshockable						
NSR	14 (13)	312 (280)	214 (161)	540 (454)	292 (292)	100
SVT	38 (29)	147 (103)	137 (104)	**322 (236)**	**89 (89)**	30
Total	**63 (39)**	**516 (357)**	**407 (216)**	**986 (612)**	**955 (820)**	–

[a] As specified in the AHA statement for adult records, see table 1.

Table 2. Number of records per rhythm class in the adult and paediatric databases. The number of patients is indicated in parentheses. Asystole and intermediate rhythms were excluded from the analysis, and the others category is composed of SVT. The SVT/VT subset is highlighted.

2.1 Adult records

The adult database contains 955 records from 820 patients: 574 shockable records from 541 patients and 381 nonshockable records from 351 patients. The mean duration of the records was 13.0 ± 5.3 s overall, with 15.4 ± 4.2 s for the nonshockable and 11.4 ± 5.4 s for the shockable records. The adult database was compiled following the AHA statement; hence, all records within a rhythm type come from different patients.

The adult records were obtained from three sources. Two hundred fifty-one nonshockable and 63 shockable records were extracted from public ECG databases[3]. The adult data also include 127 nonshockable and 325 shockable records from in-hospital electrophysiology (EP) studies and intensive care units at two Spanish hospitals (Basurto and Donostia hospitals). Finally, the database contains three nonshockable and 186 shockable out-of-hospital records recorded by two Spanish emergency services in Madrid and in the Basque Country.

Public databases are available in digital format with different sampling rates and storage formats. In-hospital data were gathered in digital format (Prucka Cardiolab and EP-Tracer systems) or as printed ECG paper strips. All out-of-hospital data came in paper format from AED printouts.

2.2 Paediatric records

The paediatric database contains 986 records from 612 paediatric and adolescent patients aged between 1 day and 20 years (mean age, 7.1 ± 4.5 years). There are 862 nonshockable records from 579 patients and 124 shockable records from 49 patients. The mean duration of the records was 13.7 ± 9.0 s, with 14.1 ± 9.3 s for the nonshockable and 10.9 ± 4.9 s for the shockable records.

Shockable paediatric rhythms were difficult to obtain because lethal ventricular arrhythmias are rare in children. Furthermore, their occurrence increases with age, and this is reflected in our database, in which most VF rhythms were collected from patients aged 9 years or older. Several records from the same patient were included in the same rhythm type when the morphology of the arrhythmias was different. This procedure is contrary to the AHA statement; however, all studies on the use of SAA in children have allowed rhythm repetition because paediatric ventricular arrhythmias are scarce (Atkins et al., 2008; Atkinson et al., 2003; Cecchin et al., 2001; Irusta & Ruiz, 2009).

All the paediatric records were collected in hospitals, from archived paper and digital EP studies (Prucka Cardiolab and EP-Tracer systems). The records were retrospectively obtained from five Spanish hospitals: Cruces, Donostia, La Paz, Gregorio Marañón and San Joan de Deu.

2.3 Analysis of the SVT/VT subset

Accurate discrimination between SVT and VT is crucial in order to adapt adult SAA for paediatric use (Atkins et al., 2008; Irusta & Ruiz, 2009). Consequently, the SVT/VT subset was extracted from the collected data in order to analyze the accurate detection of VT in the context of a SAA. We will use this subset to compare the characteristic features of each rhythm and to define a set of parameters that discriminate between SVT and VT in adult and paediatric patients.

The SVT/VT database consists of 677 rhythms distributed as described in table 2. There are 89 adult and 322 paediatric SVT records, and 200 adult and 66 paediatric VT records. The subset includes a large number of paediatric SVT, which is, in the context of SAA, the most challenging rhythm type for accurate detection of VT (Aramendi et al., 2010; Atkins et al., 2008; Irusta & Ruiz, 2009).

---

[3] The MIT-BIH arrhythmia, the AHA and Creighton University ventricular tachyarrhythmia databases.

Several records from the SVT/VT database were the most difficult to agree on for the cardiologists who classified the records in our databases. Based on a single-lead recording of a duration of approximately 10 s, consensus was not always easy. Fig. 1 shows four paediatric examples in which similar heart rates correspond to different rhythms. The cases shown in Figs 1(a) and 1(d) have the same 255 bpm heart rate, but there is atrial activity in the former and exclusively ventricular activity the latter. In general, disagreements were resolved by adopting the original interpretation of the physician aware of the clinical history of the patient. This interpretation is more reliable, but it is only available when records are obtained from documented EP studies. For out-of-hospital records, forced consensus was used to integrate the record in the database.

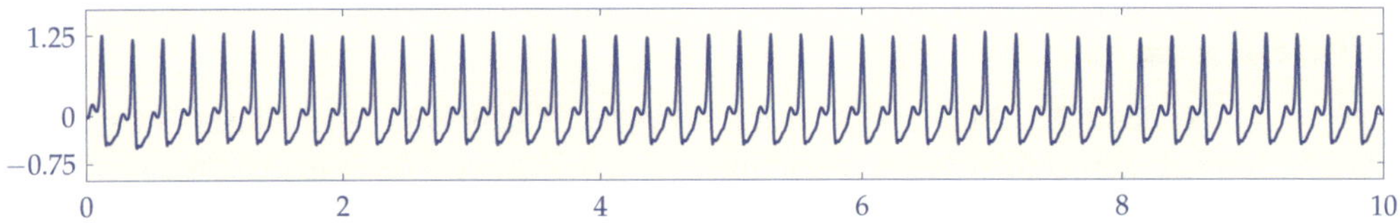

(a) Paediatric SVT with disagreements in diagnosis (heart rate 255 bpm).

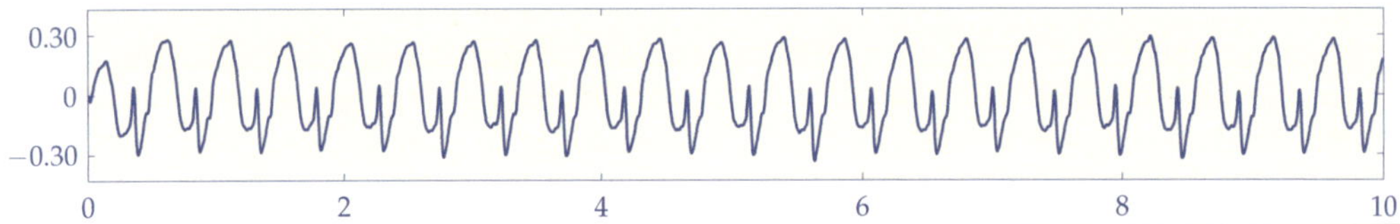

(b) Paediatric SVT with disagreements in diagnosis (heart rate 125 bpm).

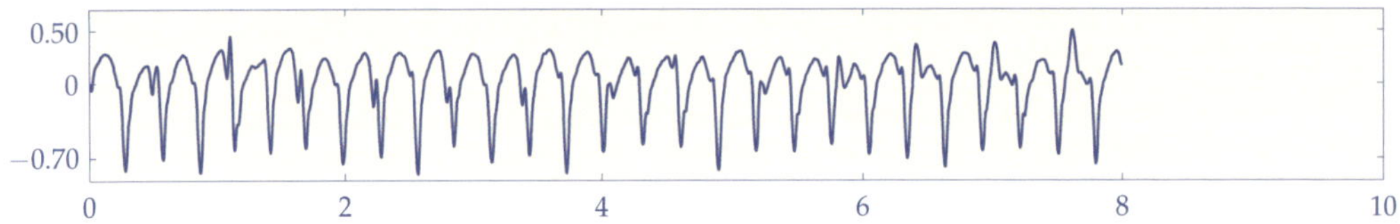

(c) Paediatric VT with disagreements in diagnosis (heart rate 210 bpm).

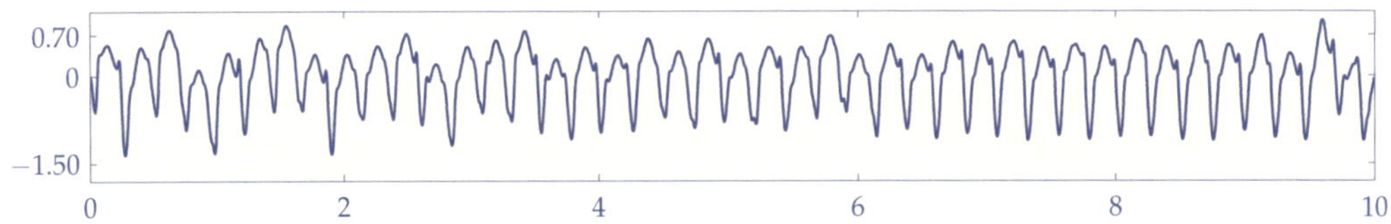

(d) Paediatric VT with disagreements in diagnosis (heart rate 255 bpm).

Fig. 1. Paediatric supraventricular tachycardia (SVT) and ventricular tachycardia(VT) records that required a forced consensus between cardiologists for the rhythm classification.

For an accurate SVT/VT diagnosis, attention should be paid to the differences in the ECG between adults and children. It is well known that to maintain cardiac output, children present higher heart rates to compensate for smaller stroke volumes (Rustwick et al., 2007). With age, stroke volume increases and contributes more significantly to overall cardiac output. The duration of the QRS complex is shorter in children than in adults because of the smaller cardiac muscle mass in children (Chan et al., 2008), while the QT interval is similar in children and adults. The QT interval, however, depends on and is normally adjusted to the heart rate.

SVT is the most common paediatric tachydysrhythmia. SVT heart rates are typically above 220 bpm in infants and above 180 bpm in children (Manole & Saladino, 2007). SVT is usually associated with an accessory atrioventricular pathway in neonates and young children. In adolescents and adults, the most common cause of SVT is an atrioventricular nodal reentry tachycardia (Chan et al., 2008).

Although SVT is more common in children, tachycardias of ventricular origin do occur in paediatric patients (Chan et al., 2008). As the normal QRS complex is of shorter duration in children than in adults, VT is more difficult to diagnose in young children. What appears as a slightly prolonged QRS complex in the ECG may, in fact, represent a significantly prolonged or wide complex tachycardia in infants and children. Consequently morphology features rather than rate information should be considered by the SVT/VT discrimination algorithm.

2.4 Analysis of the heart rate

Heart rate (HR) calculations are inherent to many SAA because fatal ventricular arrhythmias are associated with very high ventricular rates. We have analyzed the HR for the SVT/VT database in order to assess the effect of patient age on the HR for SVT and VT rhythms. QRS complexes were automatically detected, and results were visually inspected and corrected when necessary. The value of the HR for each record was computed as the inverse of the mean RR interval, and the result is given in beats per minute (bpm)[4]:

$$\text{HR}\,(\text{bpm}) = 60 \cdot \frac{1}{\overline{RR}\,(s)}\,, \tag{1}$$

where $\overline{RR}$ is the mean RR interval expressed in seconds.

Table 3 shows the mean HR of the nonshockable SVT and the shockable VT records for all age groups—adult and paediatric. The mean values of the HR were compared using the unequal variance t-test and a value of $p < 0.001$ was considered significant. The HR for paediatric SVT (187 bpm) was significantly higher than for adult SVT (131 bpm) ($p < 0.001$). Furthermore, the database contains 19 SVT values from infants with HR values above 180 bpm and 222 SVT values from children aged 1 year or older with HR values above 150 bpm; i.e., with rates above the threshold for shockable VT. The mean HR values did not differ significantly between adult VT (241 bpm) and paediatric VT (232 bpm) ($p = 0.39$).

The high rate of paediatric SVT largely overlaps with paediatric and adult VT rates. This fact is clearly shown in Fig. 2, in which the normalized histograms of the HR values for the SVT and VT records are plotted for the different populations. The overlap between the HR histograms of SVT and VT records is larger in the paediatric population (Fig. 2(b)) than in the adult population (Fig. 2(a)). When both population groups are aggregated (Fig. 2(c)), the overlap remains because the HR of paediatric SVT overlaps with that of adult and paediatric VT. This overlap precludes poor SVT/VT discrimination based exclusively on the HR.

[4] All the signal processing algorithms and calculations described in this chapter were carried out using MATLAB (MathWorks, Natick, MA), version 7.10.0.

Rhythms	Paediatric <1y	1y–8y	>8y	Total	Adult	p value
SVT	186 ± 45	194 ± 39	180 ± 39	187 ± 40	131 ± 32	<0.001
VT	226 ± 31	247 ± 57	206 ± 46	232 ± 54	241 ± 58	0.3857

Table 3. Mean heart rate (HR) (mean ± standard deviation) expressed in bpm for the SVT/VT database. The difference in mean HR between adult and paediatric patients is significant for SVT but not for VT.

Fig. 3 shows the results of the analysis of the HR for the complete database, including NSR, VT and SVT rhythms[5]. The HR distribution shows a clearer separation between VT and the nonshockable rhythms (NSR and SVT), particularly for the adult patients (Fig. 3(a)). Although a SAA based on HR dependent parameters might be reliable enough for adults, such an approach will fail when high-rate paediatric SVT is considered, compromising both paediatric SVT specificity and the overall VT sensitivity.

Many SAAs base their shock/no-shock decisions on heart rate calculations. Discrimination parameters of adult SAA that strongly depend on the heart rate fail to diagnose paediatric SVT accurately as nonshockable (Aramendi et al., 2010; Atkins et al., 2008), compromising the specificity of the SAA. The addition of high-rate paediatric SVT to a database to test SAA may compromise not only SVT specificity, but also VT sensitivity. It is therefore necessary to develop safe SVT/VT discrimination algorithms based on heart rate independent features.

3. Spectral analysis

As shown in Fig. 2, the HR of paediatric SVT presents a large overlap with the HR of adult and paediatric VT. The accurate discrimination of VT by an AED SAA must therefore rely on ECG features not affected by the HR. Power spectral analysis of the ECG, which quantifies the power distribution of the ECG as a function of frequency, is an adequate and simple tool for the definition of HR-independent features.

3.1 Power spectral distribution

Following standard AED practice, the ECG was first preprocessed with an order 6 Butterworth band-pass filter (0.7–35 Hz) to suppress baseline wander and power line interferences. The preprocessed ECG, x_{ecg}, was analyzed using nonoverlapping segments of 3.2 s duration, and a maximum of three segments per record were used. Each segment was windowed using a Hamming window, and the power spectral density (PSD) of the segment was estimated as the square of the amplitude of the fast Fourier transform (FFT), zero padded to 4096 points.

Some frequency components of the ECG segment were made zero: frequency components outside the 0.7–35 Hz analysis band; and insignificant components, defined as those with amplitudes below 5 % of the maximum amplitude of the FFT (Barro et al., 1989). The PSD

[5] VF records were excluded from the analysis because VF is an irregular ventricular rhythm characterized by the absence of QRS complexes and a well-defined heart rate.

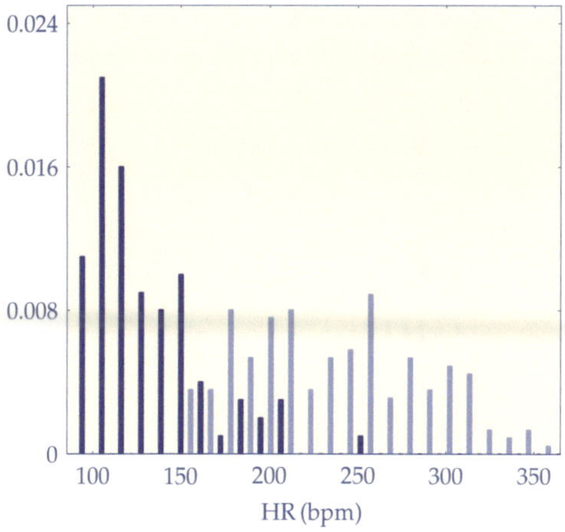

(a) HR distribution of the adult SVT and VT records.

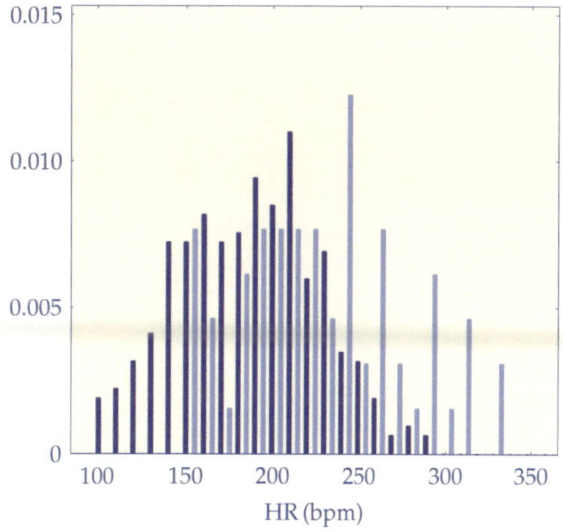

(b) HR distribution of the paediatric SVT and VT records.

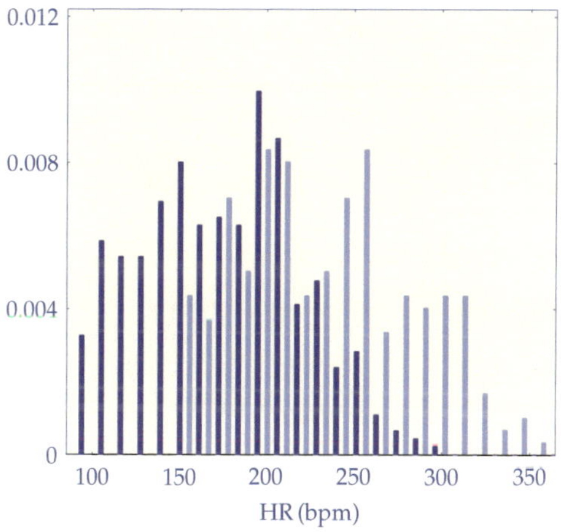

(c) HR distribution of SVT and VT records, for the adult and paediatric populations.

Fig. 2. Heart rate (HR) distributions for each population group for the SVT records (■) and VT records (■).

normalized to a unit area under the curve, $P_{xx}(f)$, was then estimated as:

$$P_{xx}(f) = \frac{|X_{\text{ecg}}(f)|^2}{\sum_{f=0.7\,Hz}^{35\,Hz} |X_{\text{ecg}}(f)|^2}, \tag{2}$$

where $X_{\text{ecg}}(f)$ is the FFT of the 3.2 s segment after zeroing the components mentioned above. $P_{xx}(f)$ was then used to define a set of spectral features that capture the morphological differences between the PSD of VT and SVT rhythms.

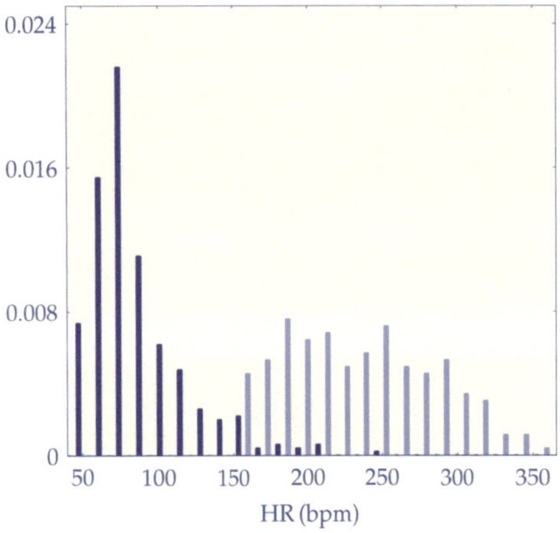

(a) HR distribution of the adult records in the complete database.

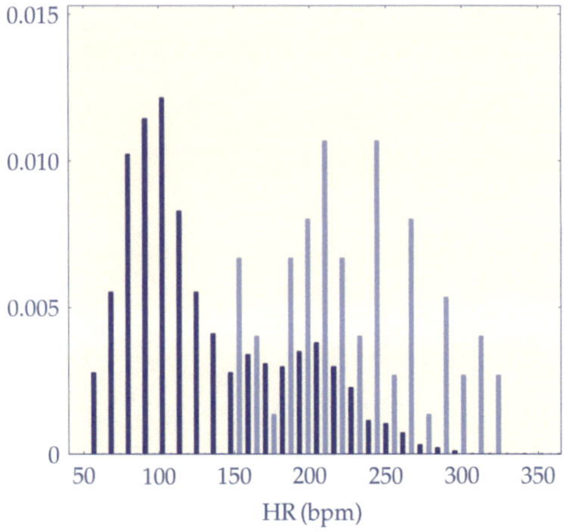

(b) HR distribution of the paediatric records in the complete database.

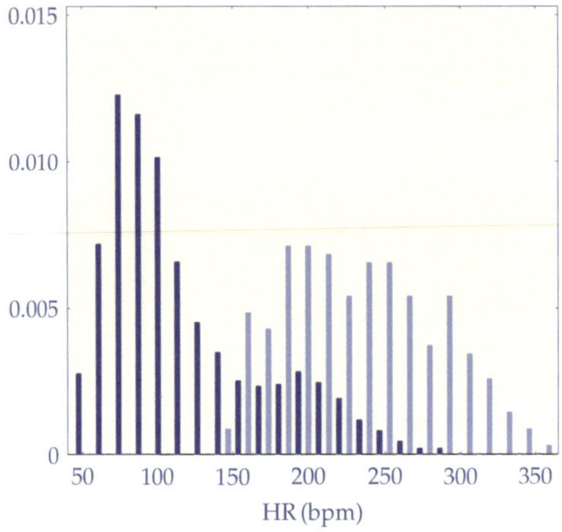

(c) HR distribution of the records in the complete database, adult and paediatric combined.

Fig. 3. HR distributions for each population group for the complete database: nonshockable records (■) and VT records (■).

Both monomorphic VT and SVT are regular rhythms. The morphology of the QRS complex changes slowly from beat to beat, and beats occur at very regular intervals. These rhythms can therefore be regarded as quasiperiodic, and their power spectrum concentrates around the harmonics of the fundamental frequency. The beat repetition period is the mean RR interval, $\overline{RR}$, so the fundamental frequency is the cardiac frequency:

$$f_c\,(Hz) = \frac{1}{\overline{RR}\,(s)}. \tag{3}$$

The harmonics are located at the integer multiples of the cardiac frequency:

$$f_k = k \cdot f_c. \tag{4}$$

Although SVT and VT distribute their power around the harmonic frequencies, f_k, the relative power content of each harmonic is very different in SVT and VT. The examples in Fig. 4, which represent a typical $P_{xx}(f)$ for a VT and a SVT, illustrate such differences.

Monomorphic VT presents wide QRS complexes that frequently resemble a sinus-like waveform. In the frequency domain, most of the power of the ECG is concentrated in a narrow frequency band around f_c, which corresponds to the ventricular rate of the VT (see Fig. 4(a) for an example). Rather than using the RR intervals computed in the time domain, the ventricular rate can easily be estimated in the frequency domain as the frequency at which $P_{xx}(f)$ is at its maximum:

$$f_d\,(Hz) = \underset{f \in (0.7-35)}{\arg\max}\,\{P_{xx}(f)\}. \tag{5}$$

This frequency is called the dominant frequency and has been extensively used to characterize ventricular arrhythmias and to estimate the effectiveness of defibrillation shocks (Strohmenger et al., 1996).

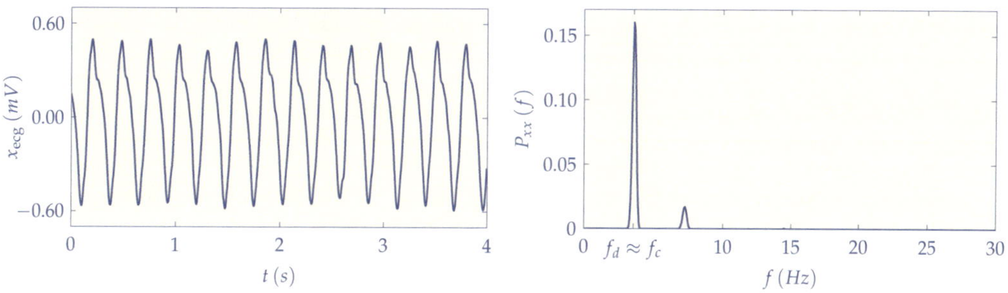

(a) A VT with a ventricular rate of 214 bpm (3.6 Hz) in the time and frequency domains. For VT most of the power is concentrated around the dominant frequency, $f_d \approx f_c = 4\,Hz$, which corresponds to the ventricular rate.

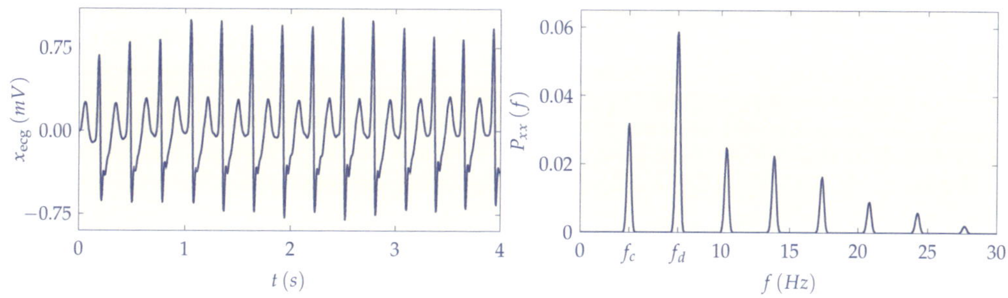

(b) A SVT with a heart rate of 208 bpm (3.5 Hz) in the time and frequency domains. In this case, the dominant frequency appears in the second harmonic, $f_d \approx 2f_c = 7\,Hz$, which corresponds to twice the heart rate. Most of the power is distributed among the higher harmonics.

Fig. 4. Examples of a SVT and VT in the time and frequency domains. Although in both cases power is distributed among the harmonics of f_c, the power content of the harmonics is very different.

During SVT, the ECG changes more abruptly; QRS complexes are narrower, and the signal power is distributed among several harmonics of the cardiac frequency. The number of harmonics can be large because of the rapid variations in the QRS complexes, and the power

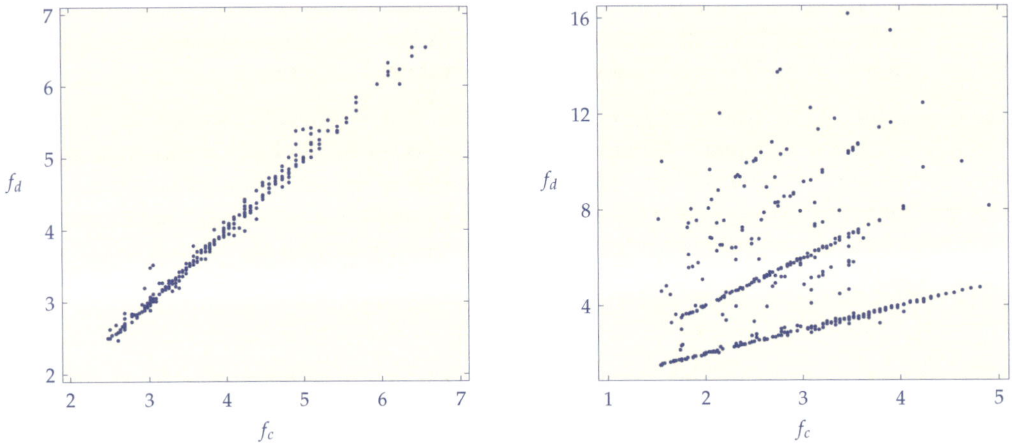

(a) VT. The dominant frequency accurately represents the ventricular rate.

(b) SVT. The dominant frequency frequently appears in higher harmonics as shown by lines of increasing slope.

Fig. 5. Relation between f_d computed in the frequency domain and f_c computed in the time domain for SVT and VT.

is therefore distributed in a larger frequency band than for VT, as shown in the example in Fig. 4(b). Frequently, $P_{xx}(f)$ is at its maximum at a high harmonic ($k > 1$), so the dominant frequency is a multiple of the cardiac frequency rather than the cardiac frequency itself ($k = 1$).

3.2 Relation between f_d and f_c in SVT and VT

We conducted a standard Pearson correlation analysis in order to investigate further the relation between f_c and f_d in our database of SVT and VT. We used the first 3.2 s segment to estimate f_d. In this way, we compared the cardiac frequency obtained from the identification of the QRS complexes in the time domain f_c, equation (3), to the dominant frequency obtained from the spectral analysis of the ECG, f_d.

Fig. 5 shows the relation between f_d and f_c for all the SVT and the VT records in the database. As shown in Fig. 5(a), $f_d \approx f_c$ for all VT instances in our database; there are no outliers, and the correlation coefficient is almost one ($r = 0.998$). The relation is more complex for SVT, however, as shown in Fig. 5(b). There are four lines of increasing slope corresponding to $f_d = k \cdot f_c$ for $k = 1, .., 4$, and the correlation coefficient is low ($r = 0.134$). Furthermore, these lines cover cardiac frequencies in the $2 - 4\,Hz$ range, indicating that the dominant frequency may fall in a higher harmonic for a large range of SVT heart rates (120–240 bpm). When the cardiac frequency of SVT is above $4\,Hz$, the dominant frequency corresponds to the cardiac frequency.

The mean values for f_d, f_c and the correlation coefficient between these two variables $r(f_d, f_c)$ are compiled in Table 4. This table presents the results for both types of rhythms and also for adult and paediatric patients. The differences in the values of the frequencies between adult and paediatric rhythms are not significant for VT, while paediatric SVT presents significantly higher dominant and cardiac frequencies, as expected from the HR analysis described in section 2.3. The relative difference between the dominant and the cardiac frequency is smaller in the paediatric population because paediatric SVT with heart rates above 240 bpm are frequent in our database, and in those cases, $f_d \approx f_c$.

In summary, the dominant frequency of VT rhythms has a clear physiological interpretation as the ventricular rate of the arrhythmia, which can therefore be easily estimated in the frequency domain. For SVT, the dominant frequency customarily falls in one of the first four harmonic frequencies and only when the heart rate is very high (above 240 bpm) can it be interpreted as the heart rate.

3.3 Distribution of the power content

In this section we analyze how the power of the ECG is distributed among the different harmonics of the cardiac frequency. VT rhythms will concentrate most of their power around the fundamental component ($f_c \approx f_d$). For SVT, the signal power will be distributed among several harmonics of f_c. These differences are caused by the morphology of the arrhythmias—wide sinus-like QRS complexes in VT and narrower QRS complexes in SVT—and are, for the most part, independent of the heart rate.

Let P_k stand for the power content percentage of the kth harmonic. We estimated this value by adding all power components in a $f_c\,(Hz)$ frequency band centered in $k \cdot f_c$:

$$P_k(\%) = 100 \cdot \sum_{kf_c-0.5f_c}^{kf_c+0.5f_c} P_{xx}(f) \qquad k = 1, \ldots, 10. \tag{6}$$

A graphical example of the computation of the power of the harmonics is shown in Fig. 6 for a SVT and a VT.

Table 5 compares the values of P_k between SVT and VT for all age groups in our database: paediatric, adult and all patients. VT rhythms present small differences in harmonic content between adults and children. On average, P_1 accounts for over 80 % of the total power, and it always has the largest power content—as we already know from the analysis of the dominant frequency. The value of P_1 slightly increases as the heart rate increases, but the dependence is very weak ($r = 0.28$), as shown in Fig. 7. Although the difference is not large, P_1 is smaller in paediatric VT than in adult VT; in fact, children may have VT with narrower QRS complexes with durations under 90 ms (Schwartz et al., 2002). The total power content of the first three harmonics accounts for over 95 % of the total power in VT, both in children and in adults.

	paediatric		Adult		Total	
Parameter	SVT	VT	SVT	VT	SVT	VT
$f_c\,(Hz)$	3.1 ± 0.7	3.9 ± 0.9	2.2 ± 0.5	4.0 ± 1.0	2.9 ± 0.8	4.0 ± 1.0
$f_d\,(Hz)$	5.2 ± 2.8	3.9 ± 0.9	4.3 ± 2.6	4.0 ± 1.0	5.0 ± 2.8	4.0 ± 1.0
$r(f_d, f_c)$	0.06 (-0.05-0.17)	1.00 (1.00-1.00)	0.19 (-0.02-0.38)	1.00 (1.00-1.00)	0.13 (0.04-0.23)	1.00 (1.00-1.00)

Table 4. Mean value (mean ± standard deviation) of f_c and f_d by rhythm type and population group. The correlation coefficient $r(f_d, f_c)$ between these variables and its corresponding 95 % CI are also reported.

On average, SVT presents up to six significant harmonics[6], although some adult SVT have over 10 significant harmonics. When the heart rate is low, SVT may present a larger number of significant harmonics. This explains why the power content of the lower harmonics is smaller in adult than in paediatric SVT. On average, the higher SVT harmonics ($k \geq 4$) contain 40 % of the total power: 47 % in adults and 37 % in children. In this study, we define P_H, the

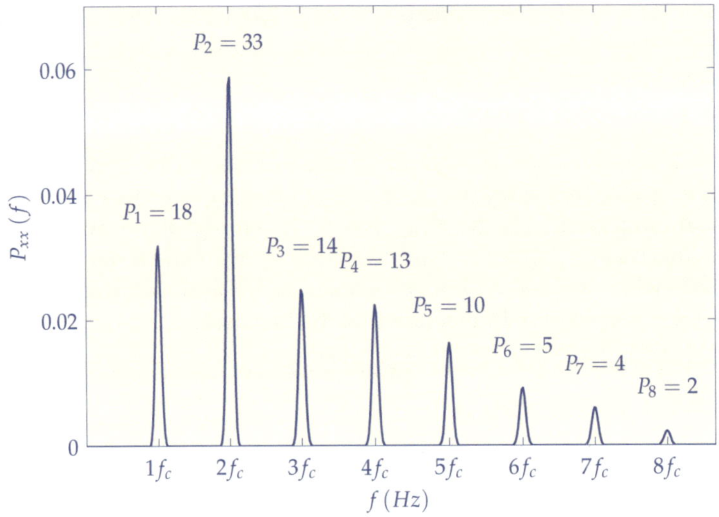

(a) Power is distributed among several harmonics in SVT, with up to six significant harmonics.

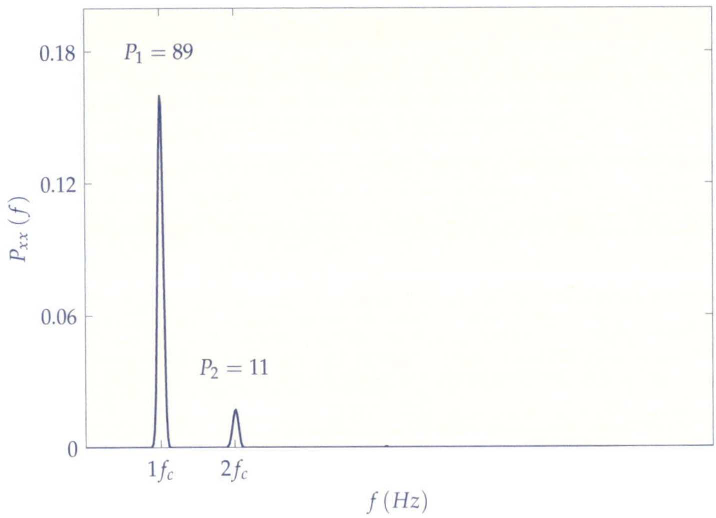

(b) Most power is concentrated around the fundamental component in VT ($f_c = f_d$).

Fig. 6. Computation of the power content of the harmonics, for the examples shown in Fig.4.

[6] Harmonics that contribute at least 5 % of the total power.

	paediatric		Adult		Total	
P_k	SVT	VT	SVT	VT	SVT	VT
$k = 1$	28 (6 − 56)	83 (71 − 92)	23 (3 − 51)	88 (76 − 96)	27 (5 − 55)	86 (75 − 96)
$k = 2$	19 (8 − 31)	10 (3 − 18)	18 (7 − 33)	8 (2 − 17)	19 (8 − 32)	9 (2 − 18)
$k = 3$	16 (8 − 23)	3 (1 − 8)	12 (6 − 19)	2 (0 − 4)	15 (7 − 22)	2 (0 − 6)
$k = 4$	12 (6 − 17)	2 (0 − 4)	11 (5 − 17)	1 (0 − 2)	12 (6 − 17)	1 (0 − 3)
$k = 5$	8 (3 − 13)	1 (0 − 2)	9 (4 − 12)	0 (0 − 1)	9 (3 − 13)	0 (0 − 1)
$k \geq 6$	17 (3 − 36)	1 (0 − 1)	25 (5 − 48)	0 (0 − 1)	18 (3 − 40)	0 (0 − 1)

Table 5. Mean content of the harmonics by rhythm type and population group. The range in parentheses represents the 10-90 percentile range.

power content of the higher harmonics ($k \geq 4$), in the following way:

$$P_H = \sum_{k \geq 4} P_k. \tag{7}$$

The values of P_H slowly decrease as the heart rate increases, as shown in Fig. 8, which explains the differences in power distribution between adult and paediatric SVT. These differences are not large, however, because P_H depends very weakly on the heart rate ($r = -0.37$).

In summary, the differences in spectral content between SVT and VT are large, regardless of the age group. VT concentrates its power around the fundamental component: on average, P_1 contains over 80 % of the total power, and P_H less than 5 %. The small differences between adult and paediatric VT are caused by the narrower QRS complexes in paediatric VT, since the heart rates of adult and paediatric VT in our database are not significantly different. SVT distributes its power among many harmonics: on average, P_1 contains less than 30 % of the total power, and P_H more than 35 %. The power content of the higher harmonics is smaller in paediatric SVT than in adult SVT because the heart rate in paediatric SVT is larger; however, the differences are not large.

4. An accurate SVT/VT discrimination algorithm

The spectral differences between SVT and VT described in the previous section are, for the most part, independent of the heart rate. An accurate SVT/VT discrimination algorithm valid for adult and paediatric patients can therefore be designed based on those differences. In this work, we propose the use of two spectral features described in the preceding section: P_1 and P_H.

Fig. 9(a) and Fig. 9(b) show the histograms of the two spectral parameters for the SVT and VT records, both in adult and paediatric cases. Both parameters show a clear separation, which is independent of the age group, between the types of arrhythmias. This confirms their adequacy for discriminating between VT and SVT accurately in children and adults.

4.1 Classification algorithm

The adult and paediatric databases were randomly split into two groups containing equal numbers of patients. The first database was used to develop the SVT/VT algorithm, and the

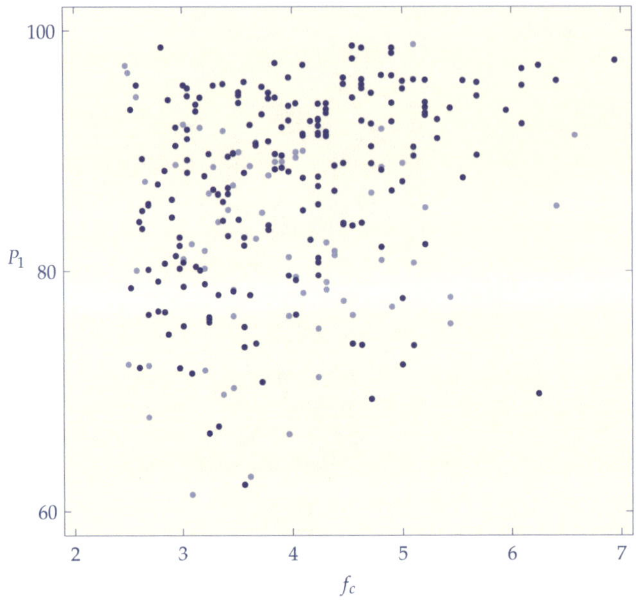

Fig. 7. Relationship between f_c and P_1 for adult VT (•) and paediatric VT (•). There is a weak increase in P_1 as the heart rate increases. The correlation coefficient is $r = 0.28$.

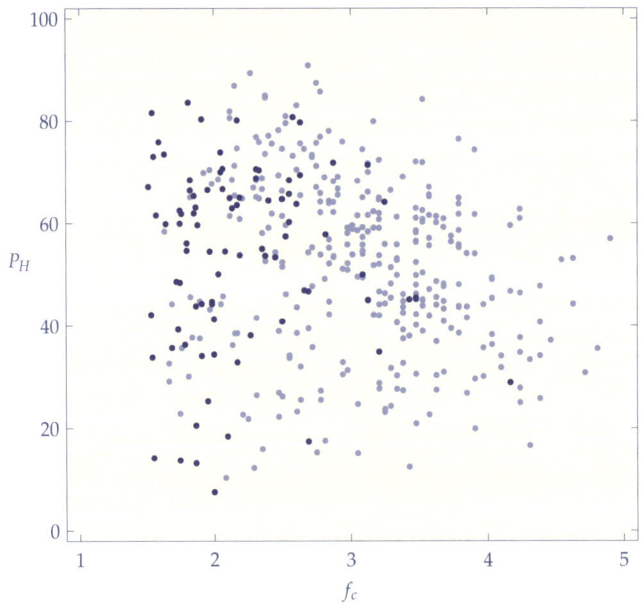

Fig. 8. Relationship between f_c and P_H for adult SVT (•) and paediatric SVT (•). There is a weak decrease in P_H as the heart rate increases. The correlation coefficient is $r = -0.37$.

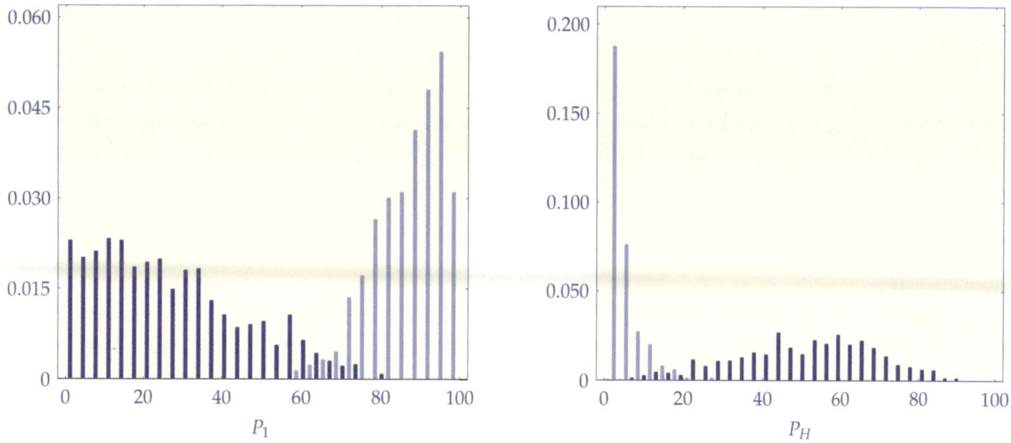

(a) Normalized histogram of the P_1 parameter. (b) Normalized histogram of the P_H parameter.

Fig. 9. Normalized histograms of the discrimination parameters for the SVT records (■) and VT records (■) in the database.

second to test and report the results. All patients within a rhythm type are different in the development database. The test database contains all rhythm repetition from the paediatric database[7].

The discrimination features were computed for all the 3.2 s ECG segments of the development database and were linearly combined to fit a logistic regression model. For each segment, we defined the following feature vector:

$$\boldsymbol{x} = \{1, P_1, P_H\}. \tag{8}$$

Then, the logistic regression model assigned the following probability of being VT to the segment:

$$P_{VT} = \frac{1}{1+e^{-Y}} = \frac{1}{1+e^{-\boldsymbol{\beta x}^T}}, \tag{9}$$

$$Y = \boldsymbol{\beta x}^T = \beta_o + \beta_1 P_1 + \beta_2 P_H, \tag{10}$$

where β_i are the regression coefficients. The decision threshold was set at $P_{VT} = 0.5$; i.e., the segment was classified as VT for $P_{VT} > 0.5$ or as SVT for $P_{VT} \leq 0.5$[8].

Each feature vector was assigned a weight so that all records within a rhythm class contributed equally in the algorithm optimization process, regardless of the number of 3.2 s segments[9]. The AHA recommendation is more demanding for SVT specificity than for VT sensitivity, so we therefore tripled the total weight of the SVT rhythm category. The weights assigned to a register with ℓ segments were:

$$\omega_{VT,\ell} = \frac{1}{N_{VT} \cdot \ell} \quad \text{and} \quad \omega_{SVT,\ell} = \frac{3}{N_{SVT} \cdot \ell}, \tag{11}$$

[7] When a paediatric patient contributed more than one record per rhythm type, the morphologies of the arrhythmias in those records were different; see section 2.2.

[8] This is equivalent to VT for $Y > 0$ and SVT for $Y \leq 0$.

[9] Records may have one to three segments, depending on their duration.

where N_{VT} and N_{SVT} are the numbers of VT and SVT records in the development database, respectively.

The weighted instances from the development database were used to determine the regression coefficients using Waikato Environment for Knowledge Analysis (WEKA) software(Hall et al., 2009). The regression coefficients, adjusted using 460 SVT segments from 163 records and 303 VT segments from 119 records in the development database, were:

$$\beta_o = -6.000 \qquad \beta_1 = 0.145 \qquad \beta_2 = -0.245. \tag{12}$$

Fig. 10 shows the ROC curve of the SVT/VT algorithm for the adult and paediatric records in the test database. The ROC curve depicts the proportion of correctly classified VT segments (sensitivity) against the proportion of wrongly classified SVT segments (1-specificity) as the classification threshold (the value of Y) varies. The area under the curve (AUC) was 0.999 for the adult database and 0.998 for the paediatric database, which proves the goodness of the classification algorithm for both patient groups.

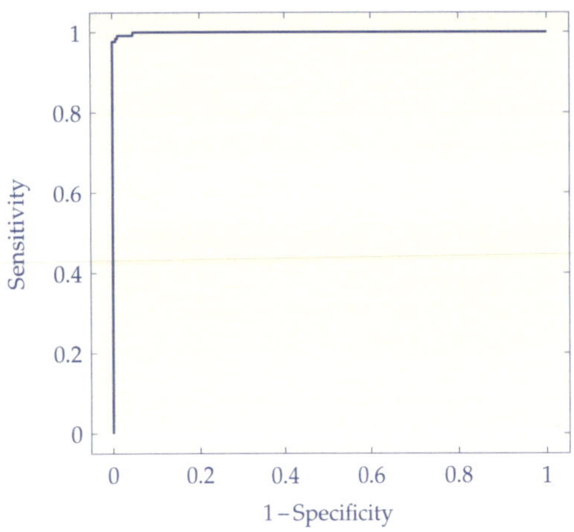

(a) ROC curve for the adult records, AUC=0.999.

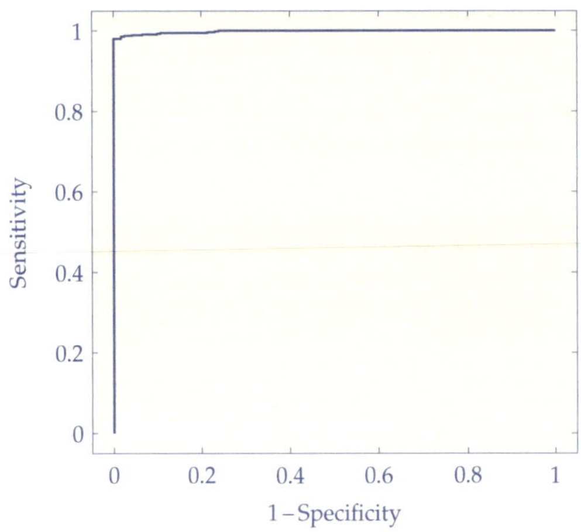

(b) ROC curve for the paediatric records, AUC=0.998.

Fig. 10. Receiver operating charactesistic (ROC) curves for the SVT/VT algorithm for the adult and paediatric records in the test database. AUC=area under the curve.

4.2 Classification results

Table 6 shows the classification results for the test database and the corresponding 90 % one-sided CI, estimated using the adjusted Wald interval for binomial proportions. The results for the development database are given per segment and per record. The classification of the record reflects the predominant diagnosis of its segments; when the diagnoses of the segments were balanced, the record was classified as SVT. As shown in table 6, the algorithm meets AHA criteria for SVT and VT classification in both adults and children.

Furthermore, the results are similar when computed per segment and per record. This demonstrates that changes in the dynamics of the arrhythmias in a 9.6 s analysis interval (record) have very little influence on the spectral features and the classification algorithm.

SVT and VT can be accurately discriminated using simply a 3.2 s ECG segment, i.e. a high-time-resolution algorithm.

	Segment		Record		
Rhythms	number [a]	Sens/Spec	number [a]	Sens/Spec [b]	AHA goal
Adult					
SVT	132 (44)	97.0	44 (44)	97.7 (92.3)	95
VT	253 (99)	100	99 (99)	100 (98.0)	75
Paediatric					
SVT	560 (155)	98.8	204 (155)	98.5 (96.9)	95
VT	121 (24)	97.5	48 (24)	97.9 (92.9)	75
Total					
SVT	692 (199)	98.4	248 (199)	98.4 (97.0)	95
VT	374 (123)	99.2	147 (123)	99.3 (97.6)	75

[a] Number of patients in parenthesis.
[b] 90 % one-sided lower confidence interval in parentheses.

Table 6. Classification results per 3.2 s ECG segment and per record for the test database. The SVT/VT algorithm meets American Heart Association (AHA) classification criteria for SVT and VT in both children and adults.

Fig. 11 shows examples of correctly classified high-rate VT and paediatric SVT. SVT with no abnormalities in conduction exhibit narrow QRS complexes, and SVT and VT are accurately discriminated, despite the high rate of the paediatric SVT shown in the examples. When SVT presents abnormalities in conduction leading to wider QRS complexes, or when paediatric VT presents narrow QRS complexes, the discrimination might fail, even for low-rate SVT, as illustrated in the examples shown in Fig. 12.

5. Discussion and conclusions

SCD in children is less common than among adults; however, it is less tolerable to families and health care providers. Fatal ventricular arrhythmias have been underappreciated as paediatric problems (Samson et al., 2003). Recent studies show that their incidence varies depending on setting and age (Berg, 2000), and that their presence has been increasingly recognized in both out-of-hospital and in-hospital cardiac arrest (Mogayzel et al., 1995; Nadkarni et al., 2006).

The use of AED in children aged 1–8 years has been recommended since 2003 (Samson et al., 2003), and the European Resuscitation Council Guidelines for Resuscitation integrate the AED in paediatric cardiopulmonary resuscitation (Biarent et al., 2010). The guidelines assume that AED are safe and accurate when used in children older than 1 year and mention that AED are extremely unlikely to advise a shock inappropriately. Nevertheless, the guidelines urge AED purchasers to check that the performance of the AED to be used in children has been tested against paediatric arrhythmias. The 2003 ILCOR recommendation was based on published evidence reporting that AED rhythm analysis algorithms generally satisfied AHA criteria for paediatric rhythms. Two studies (Atkinson et al., 2003; Cecchin et al., 2001) had shown that SAA from adult AED met AHA criteria for VF sensitivity and overall specificity for paediatric rhythms. Their results for paediatric VT were, however, below AHA performance

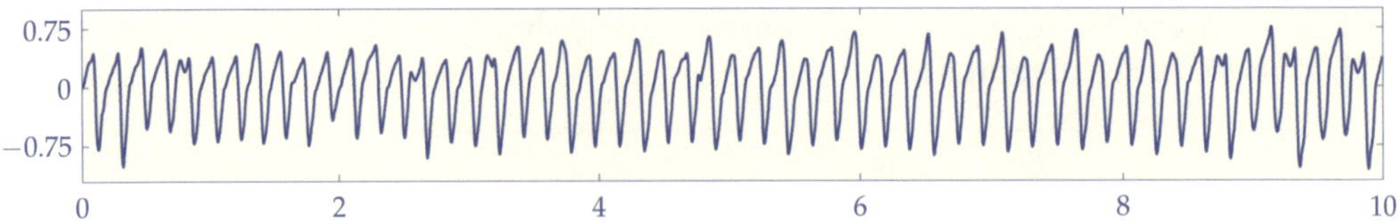

(a) Paediatric VT (heart rate, 326 bpm).

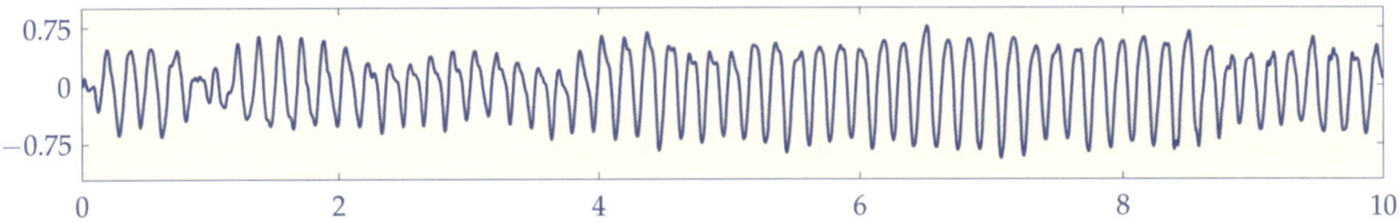

(b) Adult VT (heart rate, 357 bpm).

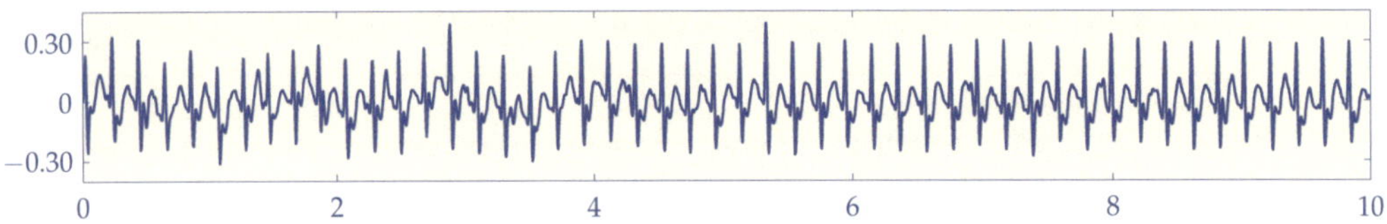

(c) Paediatric SVT (heart rate, 294 bpm).

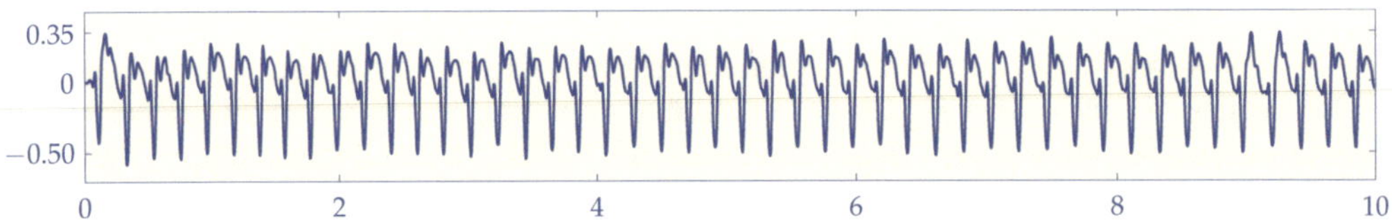

(d) Paediatric SVT (heart rate, 288 bpm).

Fig. 11. Examples of correctly classified high-rate SVT and VT from the test database. Although rates are high in both cases, VT presents wide QRS complexes

goals in one instance (Cecchin et al., 2001), and tested on only three paediatric VT records in the other instance (Atkinson et al., 2003), so the accurate discrimination of paediatric VT was not addressed. A later study that used a comprehensive database of paediatric SVT and VT demonstrated that an adult SAA failed to identify high-rate paediatric SVT as nonshockable accurately (Atkins et al., 2008). This study proposed the use of specific detection criteria adapted for paediatric use and encouraged adult algorithm verification with paediatric rhythm databases.

Adapting AED SAA to discriminate VF and rapid VT from nonshockable rhythms accurately in children involves two fundamental steps: first, a comprehensive database of paediatric arrhythmias must be compiled to test the algorithm; and second, a reliable SAA for adult and paediatric patients must be developed. Lethal ventricular arrhythmias are rare in children; consequently, the creation of a paediatric database is difficult, particularly for shockable rhythms. In fact, none of the studies in this field has reported an AHA-compliant database for paediatric shockable rhythms (Atkins et al., 2008; Atkinson et al., 2003; Cecchin et al., 2001), and all studies included more than one rhythm per patient and rhythm type. However, adult SAAs accurately detect paediatric VF (Aramendi et al., 2007; Atkins et al., 2008; Atkinson

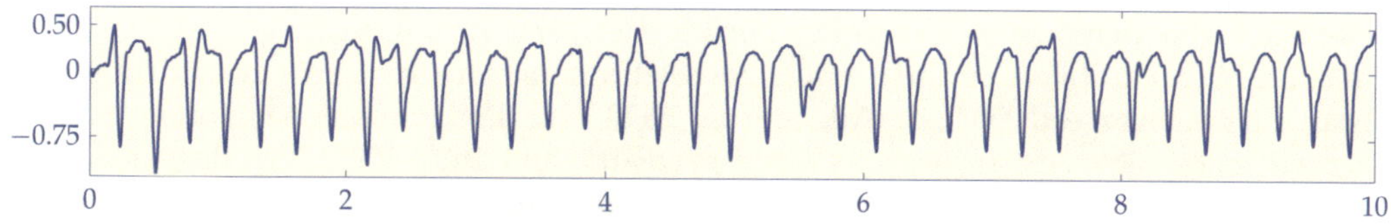

(a) Paediatric VT (heart rate, 217 bpm).

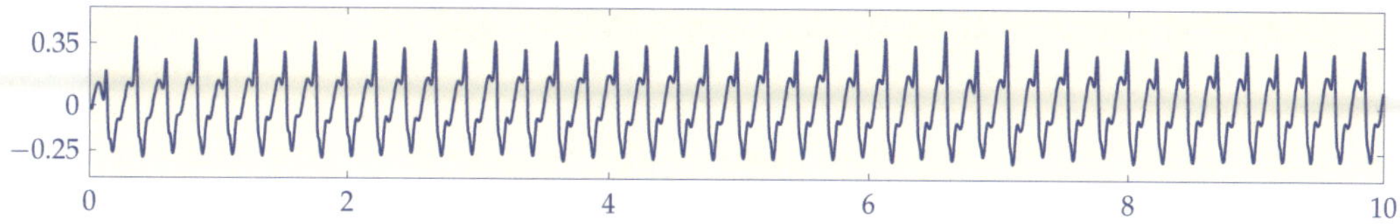

(b) Paediatric SVT (heart rate, 259 bpm).

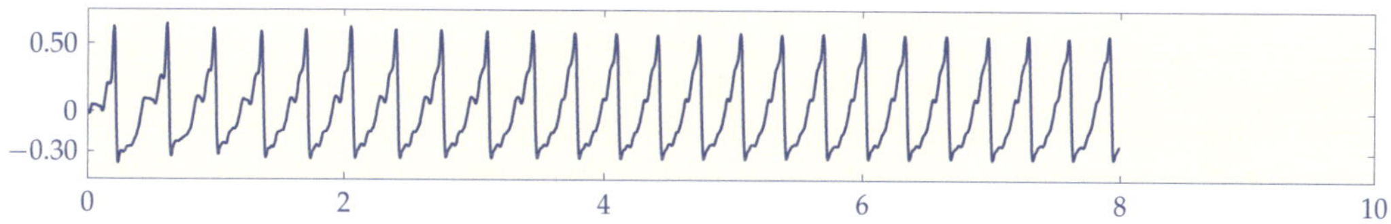

(c) Paediatric SVT (heart rate, 169 bpm).

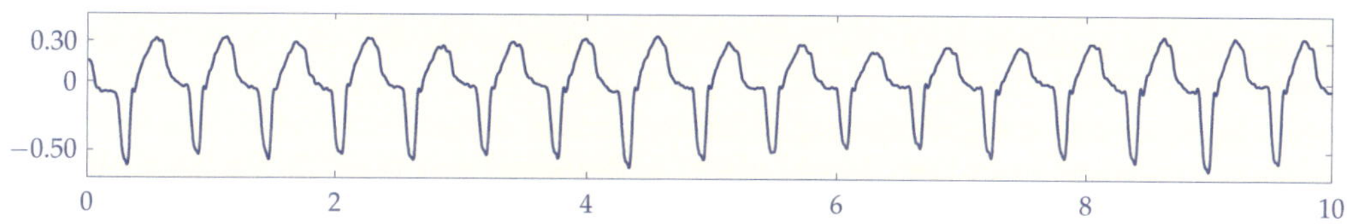

(d) Adult SVT (heart rate, 105 bpm).

Fig. 12. Examples of misclassified records from the test database.

et al., 2003; Cecchin et al., 2001). The sensitivity for VT and the specificity for SVT of adult SAAs are compromised when high-rate paediatric SVT are included in the databases (Atkins et al., 2008). Consequently, when compiling paediatric rhythms, emphasis should be placed on including a large number of high-rate paediatric SVT and a representative number of paediatric VT. Furthermore, the criteria for the definition of rapid VT depend on the study: 250 bpm in (Cecchin et al., 2001), 200 bpm in (Atkins et al., 2008) and 20 bpm above the age-matched normal rate in (Atkinson et al., 2003). The latter is the most inclusive criterion[10] and also the most demanding from a SVT/VT discrimination standpoint because lower-rate VTs are included in the databases. The criteria adopted for the definition of rapid VT determine the amount of VT included in the database, and may seriously affect the VT sensitivity and SVT specificity results of the SAA.

SAAs efficiently combine several discrimination parameters obtained from the surface ECG to classify a rhythm as shockable or nonshockable. There exist well-known electrophysiological differences between adult and paediatric rhythms (Chan et al., 2008; Rustwick et al., 2007). Differences between children and adults in both the rate and conduction of VF have been

[10] It amounts to 180 bpm in infants and 150 bpm in children.

identified, although these differences do not affect VF sensitivity (Cecchin et al., 2001). Heart rates are higher in children than in adults, and SVT occurs more frequently in children whose heart rates often exceed 250 bpm (Atkins et al., 2008). Our data confirm an important overlap in heart rates between paediatric SVT and paediatric and adult VT, which does not occur with adult SVT. Paediatric SVT had significantly higher mean heart rates than did adult SVT (187 bpm vs 131 bpm, $p < 0.001$). This demonstrates that SAA based on heart rate could either misclassify paediatric SVT or fail to identify paediatric and adult VT accurately, as suggested by Atkins et al. (Atkins et al., 2008). An accurate SVT/VT discrimination must be based on ECG features unaffected by the heart rate. In particular, the distribution of ECG power among the harmonic frequencies is independent of the heart rate, as shown in section 3. We have designed a robust SVT/VT algorithm based on these features that accurately discriminates between SVT and VT in paediatric and adult patients. Furthermore, the algorithm needs only 3.2 s of the ECG to discriminate between the arrhythmias.

An accurate SVT/VT discrimination algorithm can be integrated in current adult SAA to address the classification problems posed by high-rate paediatric SVT. Other strategies, ranging from the use of unmodified adult SAA (Atkinson et al., 2003; Cecchin et al., 2001) to the definition of paediatric-specific thresholds Atkins et al. (2008), have also been proposed [11]. Using the strategy proposed in this study, the same AED algorithm can be applied to paediatric and adult patients. The SVT/VT algorithm would be integrated in the SAA as indicated in Fig. 13, which shows the block diagram for a general SAA design. Rhythm identification can be structured in three stages. First, asystole is detected based on the amplitude or energy of the ECG. Then, nonshockable and shockable rhythms are discriminated. Finally, a VF/VT discrimination algorithm is needed, for two reasons: VT can be better treated using cardioversion therapy rather than a defibrillation shock, and VT is shocked based on heart rate. It is precisely at this stage that the SVT/VT discrimination algorithm described in section 4 should be incorporated.

To conclude, we have shown how a SVT/VT discrimination algorithm based on spectral features can be designed and incorporated into an adult SAA to make its use safe for children.

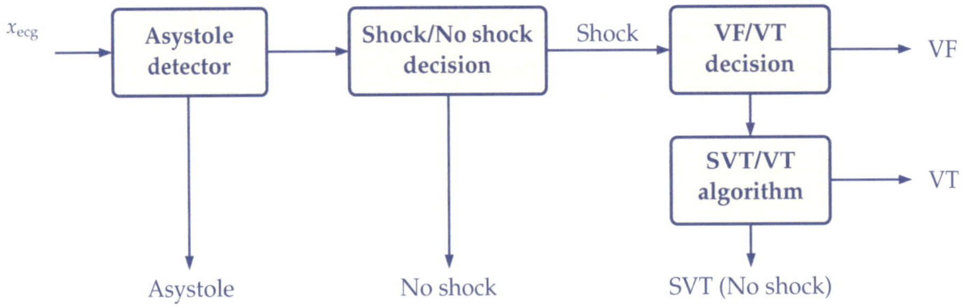

Fig. 13. General block diagram of a shock advice algorithm (SAA). The addition of the SVT/VT algorithm addresses the problem of the accurate detection of high-rate paediatric SVT, and the SAA can therefore be safely used both in adults and children.

[11] Paediatric and adult thresholds can be independently set in an AED because the AED must be aware of the type of patient in order to adjust the defibrillation energy dose.

6. References

Appleton, G. O., Cummins, R. O., Larson, M. P. & Graves, J. R. (1995). CPR and the single rescuer: at what age should you "call first" rather than "call fast"?, *Annals of Emergency Medicine* 25(4): 492–494.

Aramendi, E., Irusta, U., de Gauna, S. et al. (2006). Comparative analysis of the parameters affecting aed specificity: Pediatric vs. adult patients, *Computers in Cardiology, 2006*, pp. 445–448.

Aramendi, E., Irusta, U., Pastor, E. et al. (2010). ECG spectral and morphological parameters reviewed and updated to detect adult and paediatric life-threatening arrhythmia., *Physiological Measurement* 31(6): 749–761.

Aramendi, E., Irusta, U., Ruiz de Gauna, S. & Ruiz, J. (2007). Comparative analysis of the parameters affecting AED rhythm analysis algorithm applied to pediatric and adult ventricular tachycardia, *Computers in Cardiology, 2007*, pp. 419–422.

Atkins, D. L., Hartley, L. L. & York, D. K. (1998). Accurate recognition and effective treatment of ventricular fibrillation by automated external defibrillators in adolescents, *Pediatrics* 101(3 Pt 1): 393–397.

Atkins, D. L., Scott, W. A., Blaufox, A. D. et al. (2008). Sensitivity and specificity of an automated external defibrillator algorithm designed for pediatric patients., *Resuscitation* 76(2): 168–174.

Atkinson, E., Mikysa, B., Conway, J. A. et al. (2003). Specificity and sensitivity of automated external defibrillator rhythm analysis in infants and children., *Ann Emerg Med* 42(2): 185–196.

Barro, S., Ruiz, R., Cabello, D. & Mira, J. (1989). Algorithmic sequential decision-making in the frequency domain for life threatening ventricular arrhythmias and imitative artefacts: a diagnostic system., *J Biomed Eng* 11(4): 320–328.

Berg, R. A. (2000). Paediatric sudden death, *Best Practice & Research Clinical Anaesthesiology* 14(3): 611–624.

Biarent, D., Bingham, R., Eich, C. et al. (2010). European Resuscitation Council Guidelines for Resuscitation 2010 Section 6. Paediatric life support., *Resuscitation* 81(10): 1364–1388.

Cecchin, F., Jorgenson, D. B., Berul, C. I. et al. (2001). Is arrhythmia detection by automatic external defibrillator accurate for children?: Sensitivity and specificity of an automatic external defibrillator algorithm in 696 pediatric arrhythmias., *Circulation* 103(20): 2483–2488.

Chan, T. C., Sharieff, G. Q. & Brady, W. J. (2008). Electrocardiographic manifestations: pediatric ECG., *J Emerg Med* 35(4): 421–430.

de Luna, A. B., Coumel, P. & Leclercq, J. F. (1989). Ambulatory sudden cardiac death: Mechanisms of production of fatal arrhythmia on the basis of data from 157 cases, *American Heart Journal* 117(1): 151–159.

Hall, M., Frank, E., Holmes, G. et al. (2009). The weka data mining software: An update, *ACM SIGKDD Explorations Newsletter* 11(1): 10–18.

Irusta, U. & Ruiz, J. (2009). An algorithm to discriminate supraventricular from ventricular tachycardia in automated external defibrillators valid for adult and paediatric patients., *Resuscitation* 80(11): 1229–1233.

Irusta, U., Ruiz, J., Aramendi, E. & de Gauna, S. R. (2008). Amplitude, frequency and complexity features in paediatric and adult ventricular fibrillation., *Resuscitation* 77: S53–S53.

Jacobs, I., Nadkarni, V., Bahr, J. et al. (2004). Cardiac arrest and cardiopulmonary resuscitation outcome reports: update and simplification of the Utstein templates for resuscitation registries., *Circulation* 110(21): 3385–3397.

Kerber, R. E., Becker, L. B., Bourland, J. D. et al. (1997). Automatic external defibrillators for public access defibrillation: recommendations for specifying and reporting arrhythmia analysis algorithm performance, incorporating new waveforms, and enhancing safety. A statement for health professionals from the American Heart Association Task Force on Automatic External Defibrillation, Subcommittee on AED Safety and Efficacy., *Circulation* 95(6): 1677–1682.

Larsen, M. P., Eisenberg, M. S., Cummins, R. O. & Hallstrom, A. P. (1993). Predicting survival from out-of-hospital cardiac arrest: a graphic model., *Ann Emerg Med* 22(11): 1652–1658.

Luu, M., Stevenson, W., Stevenson, L., Baron, K. & Walden, J. (1989). Diverse mechanisms of unexpected cardiac arrest in advanced heart failure, *Circulation* 80(6): 1675–1680.

Manole, M. D. & Saladino, R. A. (2007). Emergency department management of the pediatric patient with supraventricular tachycardia, *Pediatric Emergency Care* 23(3): 176–185.

Mogayzel, C., Quan, L., Graves, J. R. et al. (1995). Out-of-hospital ventricular fibrillation in children and adolescents: causes and outcomes, *Annals of Emergency Medicine* 25(4): 484–491. PMID: 7710153.

Myerburg, R. J. (2001). Sudden cardiac death: exploring the limits of our knowledge., *J Cardiovasc Electrophysiol* 12(3): 369–381.

Nadkarni, V. M., Larkin, G. L., Peberdy, M. A. et al. (2006). First documented rhythm and clinical outcome from in-hospital cardiac arrest among children and adults, *JAMA: The Journal of the American Medical Association* 295(1): 50–57.

Ruiz de Gauna, S., Ruiz, J., Irusta, U. & Aramendi, E. (2008). Parameters affecting shock decision in pediatric automated defibrillation., *Proc. Computers in Cardiology*, pp. 929–932.

Rustwick, B., Geheb, F., Brewer, J. & Atkins, D. (2007). Electrocardiographic characteristics for automated external defibrillator algorithms are different between children and adults., *Circulation* 116.

Samson, R. A., Berg, R. A., Bingham, R. et al. (2003). Use of automated external defibrillators for children: an update: an advisory statement from the pediatric advanced life support task force, International Liaison Committee on Resuscitation., *Circulation* 107(25): 3250–3255.

Schwartz, P. J., Garson, A., Paul, T. et al. (2002). Guidelines for the interpretation of the neonatal electrocardiogram. A task force of the European Society of Cardiology., *Eur Heart J* 23(17): 1329–1344.

Sirbaugh, P. E., Pepe, P. E., Shook, J. E. et al. (1999). A prospective, population-based study of the demographics, epidemiology, management, and outcome of out-of-hospital pediatric cardiopulmonary arrest., *Ann Emerg Med* 33(2): 174–184.

Strohmenger, H. U., Lindner, K. H., Keller, A. et al. (1996). Spectral analysis of ventricular fibrillation and closed-chest cardiopulmonary resuscitation., *Resuscitation* 33(2): 155–161.

Valenzuela, T. D., Roe, D. J., Cretin, S. et al. (1997). Estimating effectiveness of cardiac arrest interventions: a logistic regression survival model., *Circulation* 96(10): 3308–3313.

2

Surgical Maze Procedures for Atrial Arrhythmias in Univentricular Hearts, from Maze History to Conversion–Fontan

Charles Kik and Ad J.J.C. Bogers
Department of Cardiothoracic Surgery, Thoraxcentre, Erasmus MC
The Netherlands

1. Introduction

Atrial fibrillation is a common cardiac arrhythmia and occurs in up to 2% of the general population, but may be present in more than half of the patients late after Fontan surgery for single ventricle physiology (Chugh et al., 2001, Freedom et al., 2003; Steinberg, 2004).

Atrial fibrillation is often considered to be a mild arrhythmia. However, even in patients with a structurally normal heart atrial fibrillation may result in significant symptoms, systemic and pulmonary thrombo-embolism and tachycardia-induced cardiomyopathy leading to a diminished quality of life with increased morbidity and mortality (Ad, 2007).

In patients with a Fontan repair often atrial dilatation occurs and consequently atrial arrhythmias develop that are not only frequent, but easily evolve into life threatening events as well (Ad, 2007).

In general, symptoms of atrial fibrillation are an indication for intervention, the most important being the elevated risk for thrombo-embolism. While pharmaco-medical treatment for atrial fibrillation is aimed at either rate or rhythm control (van Gelder et al., 2002), invasive treatment for atrial fibrillation is aimed at rhythm control. An invasive approach may consist of percutaneous catheter techniques, various surgical approaches or hybrid approaches. With regard to the Fontan circulation, the lateral tunnel has been introduced as primary surgical technique to reduce later atrial enlargement and Fontan constructions with an atrio-pulmonary or atrio-ventricular connection are changed into a Fontan with a lateral tunnel or with an extra-cardiac conduit (Fontan & Baudet, 1971; de Leval et al., 1998; Mavroudis et al., 1998). This chapter concentrates on surgical maze procedures for atrial fibrillation occurring late after Fontan surgery.

2. Definitions

The most widely used classification for atrial fibrillation is published jointly by the American Heart Association, the American College of Cardiology, and the Heart Rhythm Society (American Heart Association, American College of Cardiology & Heart Rhythm Society, 2002; Cox, 2003). Atrial fibrillation is defined as either paroxysmal, persistent, or permanent. Atrial fibrillation is considered recurrent when two or more episodes have occurred. If recurrent atrial fibrillation terminates by itself, it is defined paroxysmal; if not, it is defined persistent. Termination by pharmacologic therapy or electrical cardioversion before expected spontaneous termination does not change the designation of paroxysmal. Permanent atrial fibrillation includes cases of long-standing atrial fibrillation (>1 year), in which cardioversion has not been indicated or has failed to convert the arrhythmia. This terminology applies to episodes of atrial fibrillation that last more than 30 seconds and that are unrelated to a reversible cause.

3. A history of Fontan constructions

In patients with one of the many variations of a univentricular heart, surgical palliation can be accomplished to construct a Fontan circulation. In a Fontan circulation essentially the systemic circulation is supported by the single ventricle and all systemic venous return is directed directly to the pulmonary circulation in the absence of a subpulmonary ventricle. At the introduction of the Fontan circulation, the awareness that sinus rhythm was important was already appreciated. However, at that time this was because brady-arrhythmic atrioventricular conduction disturbances turned out to be related to adverse outcome after these procedures (Fontan & Baudet, 1971). Only in later years, atrial fibrillation was explicitly described in the failing Fontan circulation and attempts at surgical treatment in the conversion-Fontan were initiated (Mavroudis et al., 1998).

3.1 Implementation of a concept

The concept of a separated systemic and pulmonary circulation without a subpulmonary ventricle for the palliation of patients with a univentricular heart was first described by Fontan and Baudet (Fontan & Baudet, 1971). Successful application of this complete right heart bypass was soon confirmed by others (Kreutzer et al., 1973)

The fact that the circulation could be maintained in the absence of the pulmonary ventricle was one of the most important contributions to the field of congenital heart disease and allowed survival of many patients with a univentricular heart into adulthood. However, the original procedures turned out to be not at all free from complications and events at follow up, with early reoperation rates of over 40 percent. Although the basic concept of diverting the systemic venous return directly to the pulmonary circulation is still essential, the Fontan procedure has been extensively modified since its original description, each modification being an attempt to address a specific problem (Davies et al., 2011).

3.2 Fontan physiology

The goal of the Fontan procedure was to treat cyanosis. Indeed, the separation of the pulmonary and systemic circulations resulted in improved peripheral oxygen saturation, up to a nearly normal level. However, this was accomplished with a definitely palliative and abnormal hemodynamic arrangement. The most obvious clinical observations included an elevated systemic venous pressure. Combined with intrinsic abnormalities of the single ventricle systolic and diastolic dysfunction can be found. These dysfunctions, together with the obligatory passive circulation of the venous return through the pulmonary vascular bed before filling the systemic ventricle, limit ventricular preload, stroke volume, and ultimately cardiac output. The result is a relative reduction in systemic cardiac output.

Over the years, it became clear that the success factors for a Fontan circulation are defined by an adequate pulmonary blood flow at an acceptable systemic venous pressures, requiring a low left atrial pressure and a low trans-pulmonary gradient (Hosein et al., 2007). In the absence of a propulsive pump, there is little tolerance for energy loss or inefficiency in the system (Gewillig, 2005).

3.3 Work in progress

With the observation that a hypertrophied right atrium was often found in tricuspid atresia and other univentricular hearts, in the early experience of Fontan operations valves were used at various locations in the circuit. The idea was that this right atrial contraction was able to provide some pressure up stream of the implanted valve or valves. In case of a hypoplastic, but approachable right ventricle, this was often incorporated as well. In this regard modifications with valve implants at cavo-atrial level, atrioventricular level (in the situation of a hypoplastic subpulmonary ventricle) and atrio-pulmonary level have been described (Davies et al., 2011; Fontan & Baudet, 1971; Gewillig, 2005; Kreutzer et al., 1973). The idea of using a valve in the circuit has been abandoned with recognition that it was both unnecessary and potentially deleterious (Davies et al., 2011; Gewillig, 2005)

Over the years also the location of the connection has varied to some extent with constructions having been made with a posterior atrio-pulmonary connection, an anterior atrio-pulmonary connection or inclusion of a hypoplastic right ventricle when this was present. Often in these constructions long term follow up demonstrated dilation of the atrium that was included in the connection from systemic venous return to pulmonary artery. These are the patients who may end up with a failing Fontan involving a dilated right atrium possibly with atrial arrhythmias and atrial fibrillation and with thrombo-embolic events. For this reason, physicians caring for adult Fontan patients must have the operation notes and be familiar with the variety of circuits and their respective shortcomings.

In order to address this problem, more recently a total cavopulmonary connection is constructed with either an intra-atrial lateral tunnel or completely extra-cardiac prosthetic conduit (Gewillig, 2005; Hosein et al,. 2007; de Leval et al., 1988). Systemic venous blood from the superior vena cava drains directly into the pulmonary arteries. In the intra-atrial lateral tunnel modification, the inferior vena caval blood is routed via an intra-atrial conduit to the caudal side of the pulmonary artery. While a small amount of atrium remains in the circuit to provide growth potential, this atrial tissue is minimized to theoretically reduce the risk of atrial dilatation and arrhythmia. In the extra-cardiac conduit modification, a graft is interposed between the transsected inferior vena cava and the caudal side of the pulmonary artery (Marceletti et al., 1990). The concept for introduction of the extra-cardiac conduit modification was the need to avoid potential pulmonary and systemic venous obstruction in patients with small atrial chambers or malpositioned pulmonary or systemic veins. However, its ease of construction has led many surgeons to adopt it routinely.

As a rigid interposition graft, it shares many of the favourable energetics with the lateral tunnel procedure. However, studies using computational flow dynamics analyses have shown equivalent performance of both the lateral tunnel and extra cardiac conduit Fontan procedures (Bove et al., 2003). In addition, the assumption was made that the extra-cardiac conduit modification would be associated with less long-term postoperative arrhythmias; however, to this date no definitive benefit has been proven. Potential drawbacks of the extra-cardiac conduit Fontan modification include the lack of growth potential and the risk of thrombosis of the prosthetic conduit. Despite these concerns, midterm analyses have revealed essentially equivalent outcomes (Kumar et al., 2003).

Usually both modifications are performed as a staged procedure, comprising of neonatal palliation, partial cavopulmonary connection in the first year of life, and completion of total cavo-pulmonary connection in early childhood.

3.4 The failing Fontan

Although a Fontan circulation with the nowadays abandoned atrio-pulmonary or atrio-ventricular connection may have been initially successful, many patients develop complications during long-term follow up in adulthood. These may include systemic ventricular dysfunction, systemic atrio-ventricular valve dysfunction, subaortic obstruction, protein-losing enteropathy, elevated pulmonary vascular resistance, pulmonary arterio-venous malformations and thrombotic circuit events (Davies et al., 2011). In addition this concerns progressive right atrial dilatation and consequently atrial arrhythmias as well, resulting in a loss of atrial transport function and a further decrease of cardiac output in these patients.

Arrhythmias in these patients with a Fontan circulation are regarded to be the result of combination of atrial dilation, extensive atrial suture lines and cardiac dysfunction ion (Peters & Somerville, 1992). Percutaneous treatment of these arrhythmias is often limited by inability to access the appropriate cardiac chamber and has had only variable success (Walsh, 2007).

In an attempt to offer a further treatment to patients facing these problems, the total cavopulmonary connection, either with a lateral intra-atrial tunnel or with an extra-cardiac conduit, is also being applied as a conversion for the failing atrio-pulmonary or atrio-ventricular connection including a surgical maze procedure to treat the atrial arrhythmias (Mavroudis et al., 1998).

4. A history of maze surgery for atrial fibrillation

Maze surgery for atrial arrhythmias is characterised by a stepwise development in pioneering during the early years. Some of the present surgical procedures are being used based on limited experience and technical feasibility rather than true science (Ad 2007).

4.1 Left atrial isolation

In 1980, a left atrial isolation procedure was described, with confinement of atrial fibrillation to the left atrium (Ad, 2007). The right atrium and both of the ventricles continued to be in a synchronized sinus rhythm. This procedure was relatively effective in restoring regular ventricular rhythm without the need for a permanent pacemaker. This procedure also restored normal cardiac hemodynamics in patients with normal left ventricular function. The normalized right-sided cardiac output apparently was passed to the left atrium functioning as a conduit to the left ventricle. Unfortunately, the risk for systemic thrombo-embolism was unaffected because the left atrium stayed in fibrillation. Further steps in maze surgery for atrial fibrillation ideally needed to realise not only abolishing atrial fibrillation, but also re-establishing sinus rhythm, maintaining atrio-ventricular synchrony, restoring normal atrial transport function, and eliminating the risk of thrombo-embolic events.

4.2 Cox-maze procedure

The concept of the Cox-maze procedure resulted from animal studies by Cox et al. (Boineau et al., 1980; Cox et al., 1991a; Smith et al., 1985). The animal experiments suggested that a mechanism for atrial fibrillation could be found in large macro- re-entrant circuits around the orifice of the left atrial appendage and the ostia of the four pulmonary veins (Smith et al., 1985). Based on these findings, the atrial transsection procedure was introduced, consisting of an incision dorsally in the atria from the annulus of the tricuspid valve to the annulus of the mitral valve. By combining computerized mapping data in humans and data recorded in animal models, a better picture of the mechanisms of both atrial flutter and fibrillation evolved (Canavan et al., 1988; Cox et al., 1991a; Smith et al., 1985). It was documented that both in atrial flutter and fibrillation, three components could be identified: macro re-entrant circuit(s), passive atrial conduction in the atrium not involved in the macro re-entrant circuit(s), and atrioventricular conduction. The electrophysiological characteristics of these three components define a spectrum of atrial arrhythmias, from simple atrial flutter to complex atrial fibrillation. A surgical procedure capable of interrupting all macro re-entrant circuits that might potentially develop in the atria was developed. The procedure was designed to allow the sinus node to resume activity following surgery and to propagate the sinus impulse through both atria, and was first applied clinically in 1987 (Canavan et al., 1988; Cox et al., 1991a, Cox, 2011). This Cox-maze I procedure was associated with the late incidence of the inability to generate an appropriate sinus tachycardia in response to exercise, and with left atrial dysfunction. In order to deal with these drawbacks, the procedure was modified in steps to the Cox-maze III procedure (Cox, 1991; Cox et al., 1991b; Cox et al., 1995a; Cox et al., 1995b).

4.3 Cox-maze III

The Cox-maze III procedure was associated with a higher incidence of sinus rhythm, with improved long-term sinus node function, with fewer pacemaker implantations, and with improved long-term atrial transport function. In addition, the Cox-maze III procedure was technically somewhat less demanding than earlier procedures (Arcidi et al., 2000; Kosekai, 2000; McCarthy et al.,2000; Schaff et al., 2000). The Cox-maze III procedure proved to be effective in treating atrial fibrillation (Arcidi et al., 2000; Cox et al., 1996; Kosekai, 2000; McCarthy et al.,2000; Schaff et al., 2000).

Despite its success, the procedure has not been widely adopted, in part owing to its remaining complexity and technical difficulty. There was also a relatively high incidence of morbidity associated with the procedure, such as re-exploration for bleeding and a 10% incidence of pacemaker implantation. Because of the technical complexity of the original cut-and-sew Cox-maze procedure, it required a formal median sternotomy and cardiopulmonary bypass (Cox, 1991; Cox et al., 1996). As a result, only a few surgeons started to perform the procedure and gained sufficient experience, and many were waiting for less-invasive or simpler approaches to treat this extremely common arrhythmia.

4.4 Maze modifications

Over the years, a better understanding regarding atrial fibrillation pathophysiology evolved. In 1998, Haissaguerre and associates published a key work describing the pattern of the arrhythmogenic-foci-originating atrial fibrillation (Haissaguerre et al., 1998). In patients with paroxysmal atrial fibrillation, the pulmonary veins were found to be an important source of triggers initiating paroxysmal atrial fibrillation, which would probably respond to treatment with radiofrequency ablation. Based on these findings, a new strategy for non-pharmacological treatment was developed involving pulmonary vein isolation. However, some patients exhibit a much more complex pattern of initiation and maintenance of the arrhythmia, and the solution in certain cases is not as simple as pulmonary vein isolation only (Nademanee et al, 2004; Schmitt et al., 2002).

In the late 1990s, the first few cases of cryomaze procedure were performed. These were mainly application of cryoablation lines. The objective of the cryoablation was to replace the surgical incisions with transmural ablation lines to create conduction block. In 1999, the first non-cut-and-sew full Cox-maze procedure was performed using cryothermal energy as the only ablation modality. It was later that year that the Cox-maze III procedure was modified to what was later referred as the Cox-Maze IV. In this procedure, the pulmonary veins were isolated bilaterally and a connecting lesion was applied rather than performing the original box lesion. This modification was based on the findings of Haissaguerre and associates (Haissaguerre et al., 1998). The cryosurgical Cox-Maze procedure was also performed as a minimally invasive procedure through a right anterior thoracotomy (Cox &Ad, 2000). Most of the subsequent surgical modifications to the original Cox-Maze procedure were based on new surgical ablation devices, utilizing various ablative technologies. The new devices facilitated new surgical procedures to treat atrial fibrillation using different ablation protocols. Currently, it is a common approach to replace the surgical incisions with linear lines of ablation. Various ablation devices have been developed using different energy sources to perform the ablation, including radiofrequency (unipolar and bipolar) (Khargi et al., 2001; Gillinov et al., 2005), microwave (Kabbani et al., 2005), laser (Garrido et al., 2004), cryo-ablation Mack et al., 2009), and high-frequency ultrasound (Ninet et al., 2005). The concept behind these new technologies was to replace the surgical incisions with lines of transmural ablation creating conduction blocks. By using the ablation devices properly, the goal of the maze procedure to block re-entrant circuits can be maintained. However, various publications revealed that the various lesions applied on the heart under different conditions may result in non-transmural lesions (Damiano, 2003; Viola et al., 2002). Theoretically, the cut-and-sew Cox-maze procedure can be replaced by a more simple technique that is much less demanding technically and may be performed using less invasive tools.

4.5 Current surgical strategies

At present, a number of surgical approaches and procedures are described and being practised. Different options regarding surgical procedures are available (Ad, 2007). While the Cox-maze procedures were the product of a stepwise process, some of the present surgical procedures have only been based on limited experience and technical feasibility rather than true science (Ad, 2007). Some of the issues still under debate are, whether or not the maze procedure can be confined to the left atrium or to pulmonary vein isolation or that bi-atrial procedures are indicated, whether or not cardiopulmonary bypass is to be applied and which route of exposure facilitates an optimal result.

Although it was previously thought that atrial fibrillation was maintained by multiple macro-reentrant circuits, there is evidence that focal triggers can be responsible for the initiation of paroxysmal atrial fibrillation as well (Hocini et al., 2000; Nademannee et al., 2004). Therefore, preoperative electrophysiological diagnostic studies into areas of early activation, may allow surgeons to identify the particular triggers of atrial fibrillation in individual patients. Unfortunately, the analysis of multiple atrial electrocardiograms over long periods of time has been difficult. Thus, it usually is not possible to locate the precise focal point of origin responsible for the initiation or maintenance of AF in the majority of patients.

Nevertheless, modern atrial fibrillation surgery should include different surgical approaches to match the procedure to a given patient. Currently, surgery through a median sternotomy is being offered to patients with atrial fibrillation who are candidates for a concomitant cardiac surgical procedure. It is also be applied in patients who are candidates for an isolated maze procedure and who are at high risk for a minimally invasive approach. Generally, these patients should undergo a full biatrial maze lesion set. There is no place for the cut-and-sew technique anymore unless surgical ablation devices are not available. Any device that satisfies the operator in creating reliable transmural lesions can be used. Surgeons should be familiar with the limitations of each device.

In an effort to reduce cardiopulmonary bypass and cross clamp time, parts of the operation can be performed off bypass and before or after cross-clamping of the aorta. Right-sided lesions can be performed in every case before the patient is connected to cardiopulmonary bypass. One way of doing this is based on applying three purse-strings to the right atrial wall through which the ablation device can be introduced.

With left-sided lesions, there are two possible methods. The first is using the classical box lesion around all four pulmonary veins, as described in the original Cox-maze procedure. An endocardial approach for this lesion is usually performed in redo cases in which dissection of the epicardial adhesions around the pulmonary vein may be difficult. The other option is to encircle the right and left pulmonary veins from the epicardial side. This can be done off-bypass in some cases and with the support of cardiopulmonary bypass but without cross-clamping in others. Following isolation of the pulmonary veins and the necessary steps, the left atrium is opened and a connecting lesion and a mitral valve isthmus lesion to include the coronary sinus are created.

A minimally maze procedure through right anterior mini-thoracotomy can be performed for an isolated maze procedure or be combined with other procedures through the same approach [Garrido et al., 2004; Saltman et al., 2003]. The minimally invasive approach can also be considered in redo surgery, especially when a repeat median sternotomy may carry an increased risk. The procedure involves groin cannulation to connect the patients to cardiopulmonary bypass. The right sided lesions can be performed on a beating heart with or without cardiopulmonary support. Following cross-clamping, a vertical left atriotomy is performed, and the left sided lesions are made, creating a box lesion around all the pulmonary veins and a connecting lesion to the left atrial appendage and to the mitral valve isthmus with special attention to the coronary sinus. In the original technique, the left atrial appendage is resected, but increasingly the left atrial appendage orifice is oversewn from the endocardial side. Mitral valve procedures should be performed only after completion of the Cox-Maze procedure to ensure perfect left atrial isthmus ablation. In case of tricuspid valve surgery and repair of an atrial septal defect, double venous cannulation is required and the right atrium is opened, so the purse-string approach cannot be applied. When performed properly, the results obtained from the minimally invasive procedure are good (Ad, 2007).

Surgery to achieve pulmonary vein isolation only with or without left atrial appendage is now being performed and can be done as a totally endoscopic procedure using different ablation devices (Kabbani et al 2005; Saltman et al. 2003). Bilateral limited thoracotomies or mini sternotomy can also be used to control and isolate the pulmonary veins (Kawaguchi et al., 1996; Ninet et al., 2005). The major advantage of this approach is that it can be performed without the use of cardiopulmonary bypass, and in most instances, pulmonary vein isolation and left atrial appendage disarticulation can be offered. The experience gathered with this approach is fairly limited, and the follow-up in most reports is fairly short in a highly selected group of patients. It is clear that pulmonary vein isolation is not as successful in patients with more complex atrial fibrillation, such as permanent atrial fibrillation and enlarged left atrium, as in patients with paroxysmal atrial fibrillation (Hocini et al., 2000).

4.6 Prospects

Maze procedures are not guided by electrophysiological mapping and thus theoretically include some unnecessary lesions for some patients. Recent data has suggested that in some patients, there is a potential to cure their arrhythmia by performing procedures that are confined to the left atrium or include only isolation of the pulmonary veins (Nadamanee et al., 2004; Wolf et al., 2005). However, the success rate for these limited procedures is in general less than optimal (Barnett & Ad, 2006). Epicardial mapping systems may be developed that support the understanding of the pathophysiology of the arrhythmia and can be used to guide the surgeon to choose the appropriate procedure. Map-guided surgery has a great deal of potential; however, mapping patients in atrial fibrillation is complex, and the current intra-operative mapping devices would have to be minimized to allow minimally invasive surgery (Nitta et al., 2003).

5. Maze application in conversion-Fontan

When localised anatomic problems are associated with deteriorisation of a patient with a Fontan circulation, treatment (either surgical or interventional) should be considered. Recently, the total cavo-pulmonary connection, either with a lateral intra-atrial tunnel or with an extra-cardiac conduit, is also being applied as a conversion for the failing atrio-pulmonary connection or atrio-ventricular connection (Mavroudis et al., 1998). The combination of revision of the intracardiac form of Fontan to either a lateral tunnel or an extra-cardiac conduit, with an atrial reduction procedure, an appropriately modified maze procedure (see Figures 1 and 2) and the possibility of dual chamber pacing has been successful in a number of patients. It should be clear that following Fontan conversion morbidity is considerable and that mortality (up to 10%) is not insignificant, but those results continue to improve (Mavroudis et al., 2007). It should also be clear that an important number of Fontan failure patients are not amenable to revision or conversion.

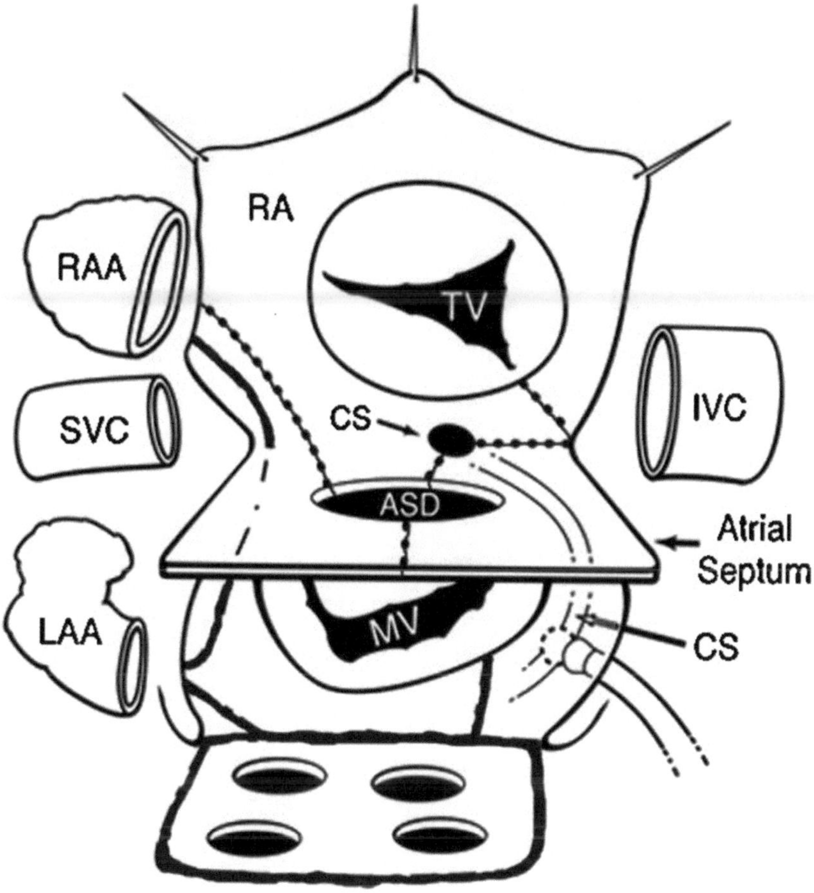

On the right side, the right atrial appendage (RAA) is amputated and the inferior caval vein (IVC) and superior caval vein (SVC) are transsected in connection with the right atriotomy. On the left side, the left atrial appendage (LAA) is amputated. With cryoablation, the right-sided lines from atrial septal defect (ASD) to the RAA, to the coronary sinus (CS) and through the crista terminalis to the posterior cut edge of the atrial wall and from the IVC to the CS and to the tricuspid valve annulus (TV) are made. The left-sided cryoablation lines consisted of lines from the pulmonary venous encircling to the LAA, to the mitral valve annulus (MV) and the CS cryoablation. In addition, a line from the base of the RAA to the base of the LAA across the domes of the right and left atria for the left atrial maze procedure was cryo-ablated.

Fig. 1. Diagram with atrial view from the right side of a modified right-sided maze procedure for right atrial re-entry tachycardia (continuous dotted lines) and a left atrial maze procedure for atrial fibrillation and left atrial re-entry tachycardia (continuous lines) (Adapted from Mavroudis et al., 2008).

At conversion, the atrial arrhythmias are in addition being treated by excision of a greater part of the dilated right atrial free wall and by intra-operative additional ablation of potential circuits of atrial arrhythmias. Intra-operative ablation consists of a right-sided maze operation for atrial flutter or the Cox-III maze operation for atrial fibrillation (Backer et al., 2006).

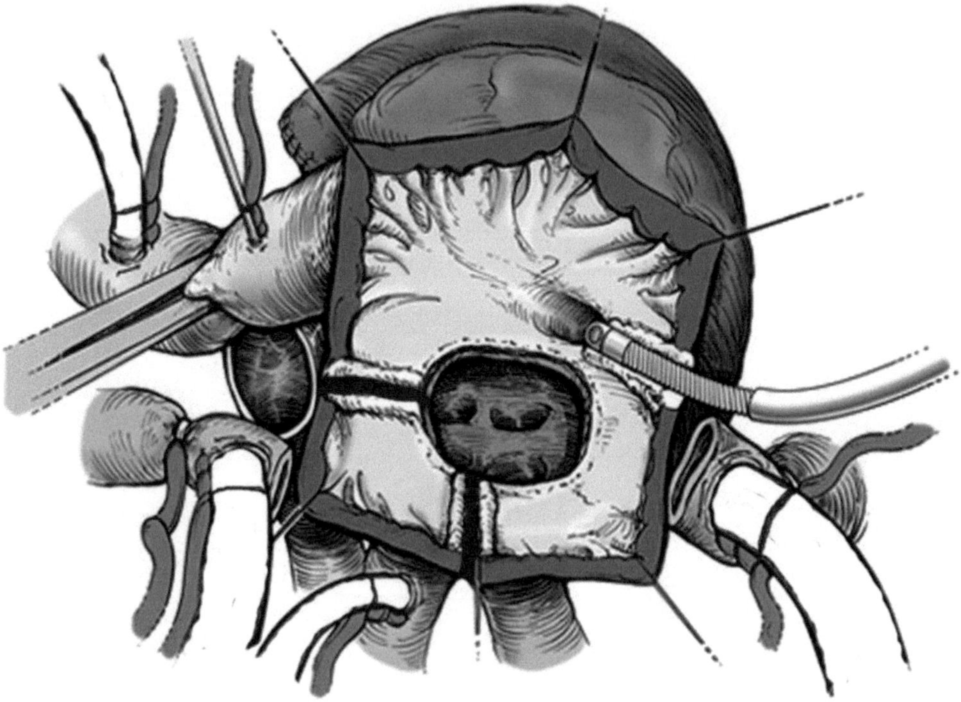

The inferior and superior venae cavae have been transected, the atrial wall excision has been performed, and the atrial septal patch has been removed. The right atrial appendage (when still present) is amputated. If the sino-atrial node is nonfunctional, no specific measures are taken for preservation of this structure. Cryoablation lesions are placed in three areas to complete the modified right-sided maze procedure. Cryoablation lesions are made to connect the superior portion of the atrial septal ridge with the incised area of the right atrial appendage and to connect the posterior portion of the atrial septal ridge with the posterior cut edge of the atrial wall, which extends through the crista terminalis. For the isthmus ablation, the lines are dependent on the anatomic substrate. In patients with tricuspid atresia, as noted here, the cryoablation lesion is placed to connect the postero-inferior portion of the coronary sinus orifice with the transected inferior vena cava.

In other anomalies, the isthmus block is completed by an additional line to connect the tricuspid valve annulus or common atrioventricular valve annulus with the transected inferior vena cava orifice.

Fig. 2. Atrial view from the right side of a patient who had an atrio-pulmonary Fontan procedure after aortic cross-clamping and cardioplegic arrest (Adapted from Mavroudis et al., 2008).

In addition, some authors propagate completion of surgery with an epicardial pacemaker system for further management of arrhythmias (Backer et al., 2006). The rationale is that transvenous access to the heart is not possible anymore and that frequently conversion concerns a more than once repeated sternotomy.

After conversion to a total cavo-pulmonary connection, most patients improve in New York Heart Association class (Backer et al., 2006; Bogers et al., 2008). This improvement may, however, take up to a year after surgery. Without anti-arrhythmic surgery, the recurrence rate of atrial arrhythmias is reported to be up to 76% (Backer et al., 2006). Among patients with a form of intracardiac Fontan and atrial dysrhythmias, conversion to an extra-cardiac conduit with a modified atrial maze procedure results in approximately 80% freedom from recurrence at 5 years of follow up (Deal et al., 2007). Moreover, recovery of atrial transport function, which is essential in the Fontan circulation, can be accomplished (Bogers et al., 2008)

6. Factors affecting the results of surgical maze procedures for atrial fibrillation

Taken into account that the different surgical strategies are usually the product of evolving techniques, the results from different series are in general not easy to accumulate or to compare, but results are fairly rewarding, not only with regard to restoring sinus rhythm, but also with regard to freedom of stroke and freedom of cardiovascular-related death on midterm follow up (Ad et al., 2000; Ballaux et al., 2006; Bando et al ., 2002, 2003; Cox et al., 1995a; Damiano et al., 2003; Fujita et al.,2010, Gaynor et al., 2007; Gillinov et al., 2007; Kim et al., 2007; Mokadam et al., 2004; Prasad et al., 2003; Rahman et al., 2010). In addition, differences in the reported success rate in restoring sinus rhythm are a continuing debate among cardiac surgeons and cardiologists on the outcome of maze procedures, because surgeons more often treat patients with chronic atrial fibrillation, while cardiologists choose more often to treat patients with paroxysmal atrial fibrillation.

The long-term success of maze procedures is limited in patients with well established predictors for failure. Arrhythmia duration prior to the procedure was found to be a predictor of failure. This may be related to a more significant adverse atrial tissue remodelling, resulting in extensive fibrosis and disparity of the action potential as well as enlargement of the left atrium. Increased size of the left or single atrium is also a powerful predictor for late failure, particularly in an atrium greater than 6 cm in diameter [Gaynor et al., 2005; Gillinov et al., 2006; Kawaguchi et al., 1996]. Increased age at the time of the procedure is another predictor for late failure, although not reported as such in all series (Damiano et al., 2003; Rahman et al., 2010). Other clinical variables that have been mentioned as having a negative impact on late success, such as structural heart disease, rheumatic heart disease, and the type of the atrial fibrillation, have not been consistently found by all centres to be significant (Ad, 2007). For these factors, the influence on outcome after maze surgery in conversion-Fontan is unknown.

Many problems encountered when the Cox-maze procedure was first developed are now being repeated in patients undergoing these less complex procedures. Therefore, in general a better classification of candidates for the procedure may enhance our understanding of the pathophysiology of atrial fibrillation and improve results of the modified procedures. This holds as well for congenital heart disease in general as well as for univentricular hearts after a Fontan palliation.

Before applying a maze procedure, a few variables should be discussed and investigated for their possible impact on the results of the surgical treatment in a certain patient. Important issues in this regard are: the type of atrial fibrillation, the duration in time of atrial fibrillation, the size of the left and right atria or single atrium, the presence of additional heart diseases (by definition in univentricular hearts), the procedure intended for curing atrial fibrillation, the treatment of atrial fibrillation in a combined procedure in which cardiopulmonary bypass is used (by definition in conversion-Fontan), the presence of clots in the left or single atrial appendage or a patent foramen ovale, limiting in general the ability to perform a procedure without cardio-pulmonary bypass.

Probably only a limited percentage of patients with lone atrial fibrillation will ever become candidates for the classical open-heart maze procedures (Ad, 2007). However, a number of device-based ablation procedures are being performed, which are less complex and technically less demanding in those patients. Therefore, the discussion concerning the complexity of the maze procedure should be shifted towards application with decision trees regarding specific maze procedures for specific clinical questions (such as the conversion-Fontan), e.g. type of maze procedure, timing of the maze procedure, type of equipment and energy source. The continuing effort to relieve the invasive downside of surgical maze procedures is warranted but with caution and without compromising the success rate (Ad, 2007). Surgery for atrial fibrillation should involve a true decision-making process, just as with any other surgical procedure. Therefore, combining all these variables and understanding the importance of each one of them may lead to a higher success rate, also in surgery for congenital heart disease.

7. Conclusion

Atrial fibrillation may result in significant symptoms in patients with a structurally normal heart, and in patients with a univentricular circulation atrial fibrillation can be deleterious. Nowadays symptomatic atrial fibrillation can be treated with catheter-based ablation, surgical ablation or hybrid approaches. On top of this maze experience, surgical ablation for atrial arrhythmias at conversion of atrio-pulmonary or ventriculo-pulmonary Fontan to a total cavopulmonary connection is feasible with recovery of both sinus rhythm as well as atrial transport function.

8. References

Ad N (2007) The Cox-maze procedure: history, results and predictors for failure. J Interv Card Electrophysiol 20:65–71

Ad N, Cox JL, Palazzo T., Kim YD, Syderhoud JP, Degroot KW, et al. (2000) Stroke prevention as an indication for the Maze procedure in the treatment of atrial fibrillation. Seminars Thorac Cardiovasc Surg 12:56–62

American College of Cardiology, American Heart Association, European Society of Cardiology (2002) Pocket Guidelines for the Management of Patients with Atrial Fibrillation

Arcidi JM Jr, Doty DB, Millar RC (2000) The Maze procedure: the LDS Hospital experience. Seminars Thorac Cardiovasc Surg 12:38–43

Backer CL, Deal BJ, Mavroudis C, Franklin WH, Stewart RD (2006) Conversion of the failedFontan circulation. Cardiol Young 16(suppl 1):85-91

Ballaux PKEW, Geuzebroek GSC, van Hemel NM, Kelder JC, Dossche KME, Ernst JMPG, et. al. (2006) Freedom from atrial arrhythmias after classic maze III surgery: A 10-year experience. J Thorac Cardiovasc Surg 132:1433–1440

Bando K, Kobayashi J, Hirata M, et al. (2003) Early and late stroke after mitral valve replacement with a mechanical prosthesis: Risk factor analysis of a 24-year experience. J Thorac Cardiovasc Surg 126:358-364

Bando K, Kobayashi J, Sasako Y, Tagusari O, Niwaya K, Kitamura S (2002) Effect of maze procedure in patients with atrial fibrillation undergoing valve replacement. J Heart Valve Dis 11:719–724

Barnett SD, Ad N (2006) Surgical ablation as treatment for the elimination of atrial fibrillation: A meta-analysis. J Thorac Cardiovasc Surg 131:1029–1035

Bogers AJJC, Kik C, de Jong PL, Meijboom FJ (2008). Recovery of atrial transport function after a maze procedure for atrial fibrillation in conversion of a failing Fontan circulation. Neth Heart J 16:170-172

Boineau JP, Schuessler RB, Mooney C, et al. (1980) Natural and evoked atrial flutter due to circus movement in dogs. Am J Cardiol 45,1167–1181

Bove EL, de Leval MR, Migliavacca F, Guadagni G, Dubini S (2003) Computational fluiddynamics in the evaluation of hemodynamic performance of cavopulmonary connections after the Norwood procedure for hypoplastic left heart syndrome, J Thorac Cardiovasc Surg 126:1040–1047.

Canavan TE, Schuessler RB, Cain ME, et al. (1998) Computerized global electrophysiological mapping of the atrium in a patient with multiple supraventricular arrhythmias. Ann Thorac Surg 46,223–231

Chugh SS, Blackshear JL, Shen WK, et al (2001). Epidemiology and natural history of atrial fibrillation: Clinical implications. J Am Coll Cardiol 37:371-378

Cox JL (1991) The surgical treatment of atrial fibrillation. IV. Surgical technique. J Thorac Cardiovasc Surg 101,584–592

Cox JL (2003) Atrial fibrillation I: A new classification system. J Thorac Cardiovasc Surg 126:1686-1692

Cox JL (2011) The first maze procedure. J Thorac Cardiovasc Surg 141:1093-1097

Cox JL, Ad N (2000) New surgical and catheter-based modifications of the Maze procedure. Seminars Thorac Cardiovasc Surg 12:68–73

Cox JL, Boineau J P, Schuessler RB, et al. (1995) Modifications of the Maze procedure for atrial flutter and atrial fibrillation. I. Rationale and surgical results. J Thorac Cardiovasc Surg 110:473–483

Cox JL, Canavan TE, Schuessler RB, et al. (1991a)The surgical treatment of atrial fibrillation. II. Intraoperative electrophysiologic mapping and description of the electrophysiologic basis of atrial flutter and atrial fibrillation. J Thorac Cardiovasc Surg 101, 406–426

Cox JL, Jaquiss RD, Schuessler RB, et al. (1995) Modifications of the Maze procedure for atrial flutter and atrial fibrillation. II. Surgical technique of the Maze III procedure. J Thorac Cardiovasc Surg 110,485–495

Cox JL, Schuessler RB, D'Agostino HJ J et al. (1991) The surgical treatment of atrial fibrillation: III Development of a definite surgical procedure. J Thorac Cardiovasc Surg 101, 569–583

Cox JL, Schuessler RB, Lappas DG, et al. (1996) An 8.5 year clinical experience with surgery for atrial fibrillation. Ann Surg 224,267–275

Damiano RJ Jr (2003) Alternative energy sources for atrial ablation: judging the newtechnology. Ann Thorac Surg 75:329–330

Damiano RJ Jr, Gaynor S., Bailey M, Prasad S, Cox J., Boineau J., et al. (2003) The long-term outcome of patients with coronary disease and atrial fibrillation undergoing the Cox maze procedure. J Thorac Cardiovasc Surg 126:2016–2021

Davies RR, Chen JM, Mosca R (2011) The Fontan procedure: evolution in technique; attendant imperfections and transplantation for "failure". Seminars Thorac Cardiovascular Surg 14:55-66

de Leval MR, Kilner P, Gewillig M, Bull C (1988) Total cavopulmonary connection: a logical alternative to atriopulmonary connection for Fontan operations. Experimental studies and early clinical experience. J Thorac Cardiovasc Surg 96:682-695

Deal BJ, Mavroudis C, Backer CL (2007) Arrhythmia management in the Fontan patient. Pediatr Cardiol 28:448–456.

Fontan F, Baudet E (1971) Surgical repair of tricuspid atresia. Thorax 26:240-248 Freedom RM, Li J, Yoo S.J (2003). Late complications following the Fontan operation. In: *Diagnosis and management of adult congenital heart disease*, Gatzoulis MA, Webb GD, Daubeney PEF (Eds.), pp. 85-92, Edinburgh, Churchill Livingstone, Edinburgh Fujita T, Kobayashi J, Toda K, Nakajima H, Iba Y, Shimahara Y, Yagihara T (2010) Long-term outcome of combined valve repair and maze procedure for nonrheumatic mitral regurgitation. J Thorac Cardiovasc Surg 140:1332-1337

Garrido MJ, Williams M, Argenziano M (2004) Minimally invasive surgery for atrial fibrillation: toward a totally endoscopic, beating heart approach. J Cardiac Surg 19:216–220

Gaynor SL, Schuessler RB, Bailey MS, Ishii Y, Boineau JP, Gleva MJ, et al. (2005) Surgical treatment of atrial fibrillation: predictors of late recurrence. J Thorac Cardiovasc Surg 129:104–111

Gewillig M (2005) The Fontan circulation. Heart 91:839–846

Gillinov AM, Bhavani S, Blackstone EH, Rajeswaran J, Svensson LG, Navia JL, et al. (2006) Atrial fibrillation: impact of patient factors and lesion set. Ann Thorac Surg 82:502–513

Gillinov AM, McCarthy PM, Blackstone EH, Rajeswaran J, Pettersson G, Sabik JF, et al. (2005) Surgical ablation of atrial fibrillation with bipolar radiofrequency as the primary modality. J Thorac Cardiovasc Surg 129:1322–1329

Haissaguerre M, Jais P, Shah DC, Takahashi A, Hocini M, Quiniou G, et al. (1998) Spontaneous initiation of atrial fibrillation by ectopic beats originating in the pulmonary veins. New Eng J Med 339:659–666

Hocini M, Haissaguerre M, Shah D, et al. (2000) Multiple sources initiating atrial fibrillation from a single pulmonary vein identified by a circumferential catheter. Pacing Clin Electrophysiol 23:1828-31

Hosein RB, Clarke AJ, McGuirk SP, griselli M, Stumper O, de Giovanni JV, barron DJ, BrawnWJ (2007) Factors influencing early and late outcome following the Fontan procedure in the current era: The 'two commandments'?, Eur J Cardiothorac Surg 31:344–352.

Kabbani SS, Murad G, Jamil H, Sabbagh A, Hamzeh K (2005) Ablation of atrial fibrillationusing microwave energy–early experience. Asian Cardiovasc Thorac Ann 13:247–250

Kawaguchi AT, Kosakai Y, Isobe F, Sasako Y, Eishi K, Nakano K, et al. (1996) Factors affecting rhythm after the maze procedure for atrial fibrillation. Circulation 94(9 Suppl):II139–II14

Khargi K, Deneke T, Haardt H, Lemke B, Grewe P, Muller KM, et al. (2001) Saline-irrigated, cooled-tip radiofrequency ablation is an effective technique to perform the maze procedure. Ann Thorac Surg 72:S1090–S1095

Kim KC, Cho KR, Kim YJ, Sohn DW, Kim KB (2007) Long-term results of the Cox-Maze III procedure for persistent atrial fibrillation associated with rheumatic mitral valve disease: 10-year experience. Eur J Cardio-Thorac Surg 31:261–266

Kosakai, Y (2000) Treatment of atrial fibrillation using the Maze procedure: the Japanese experience. Seminars Thorac Cardiovasc Surg 12:44–52

Kreutzer G, Galindez E, Bono H, de Palma C, Laura JP (1973) An operation for the correction of tricuspid atresia, J Thorac Cardiovasc Surg 66: 613–621

Kumar SP, Rubinstein CS, Simsic JM, Taylor AB, Saul JP, Bradley SM (2003) Lateral tunnel versus extracardiac conduit Fontan procedure: a concurrent comparison. Ann Thorac Surg 76:1389–1396

Mack CA, Milla F, Ko W, Girardi LN, Lee LY, Tortolani A, et al. (2009) Surgical treatment of atrial fibrillation using argon-based cryoablation during concomitant cardiac procedures. Circulation 112(9 Suppl):I1–I6

Marcelletti C, Corno A, Giannico S, Marini B (1990) Inferior vena cava-pulmonary artery extracardiac conduit: a new form of right heart bypass. J Thorac Cardiovasc Surg 100:228–232

Mavroudis C, Backer CL, Deal BJ, Johnsrude CL (1998) Fontan conversion to cavopulmonary connection and arrhytmhia circuit cryoablation. J Thorac Cardiovasc Surg 115:547-556

Mavroudis C, Deal BJ, Backer CL, Stewart RD, Franklin WH, Tsao S, Ward K. DeFreitas RA (2007) J Maxwell Chamberlain Memorial Paper for congenital heart surgery. 111 Fontan conversions with arrhythmia surgery: surgical lessons and outcomes. Ann Thorac Surg 84:1457–1465.

Mavroudis C, Backer CL, Deal BJ (2008) Late reoperations for Fontan patients: state of theart invited review. Eur J Cardiothorac Surg 34:1034-40

McCarthy PM, Gillinov AM, Castle L, Chung M, Cosgrove D III (2000) The Cox-Maze procedure: the Cleveland Clinic experience. Seminars Thorac Cardiovasc Surg 12:25–29

Mokadam NA, McCarthy PM, Gillinov AM, et al. (2004) A prospective multicenter trial of bipolar radiofrequency ablation for atrial fibrillation: Early results. Ann Thorac Surg 78:1665-1670

Nademanee K, McKenzie J, Kosar E, et al. (2004) A new approach for catheter ablation of atrial fibrillation: mapping of the electrophysiologic substrate. J Am Coll Cardiol 2004;43:2044–2053

Ninet J, Roques X, Seitelberger R, Deville C, Pomar JL, Robin J, et al. (2005) Surgical ablation of atrial fibrillation with off-pump, epicardial, high-intensity focused ultrasound: Results of a multicenter trial. J Thorac Cardiovasc Surg 130:803-809

Nitta T, Ohmori H, Sakamoto S, Miyag, Y, Kanno S, Shimizu K (2003) Map-guided surgeryfor atrial fibrillation. J Thorac Cardiovasc Surg 129:291–299

Peters NS, Somerville J (1992) Arrhythmias after the Fontan procedure. Br Heart J 68:199–204

Prasad SM, Maniar HS, Camillo CJ, Schuessler RB, Boineau JP, Sundt TM III, et al. (2003) The Cox maze III procedure for atrial fibrillation: long-term efficacy in patientsundergoing lone versus concomitant procedures. J Thorac Cardiovasc Surg 126:1822–1828

Rahman NM, Chard RB, Thomas SP (2010) Outcomes for surgical treatment of atrial fibrillation using cryoablation during concomitant procedures. Ann Thorac Surg 90:1523-8

Saltman AE, Rosenthal LS, Francalancia NA, Lahey S (2003) A completely endoscopic approach to microwave ablation for atrial fibrillation. Heart Surg Forum 6:E38– E41

Schaff HV, Dearani JA, Daly RC, Orszulak TA, Danielson GK (2000). Cox-Maze procedure for atrial fibrillation: Mayo Clinic experience. Seminars Thorac Cardiovasc Surg 2000;12:30–37

Schmitt C, Ndrepepa G, Weber S, Schmieder S, Weyerbrock S, Schneider M, et al. (2002)Biatrial multisite mapping of atrial premature complexes triggering onset of atrial fibrillation. Am J Cardiol 89:1381–1387

Smith PK., Holman WL, Cox JL (1985) Surgical treatment of supraventricular tachyarrhythmias. Surgical Clinics North America 65,553–570

Steinberg JS: Atrial fibrillation: an emerging epidemic? Heart 2004; 90:239-240

van Gelder IC, Hagens VE, Bosker HA, et al. (2002) A comparison of rate control and rhythm control in patients with recurrent persistent atrial fibrillation. N Engl J Med 347:1834-1840

Viola N, Williams M, Oz MC (2002) The technology in use for the surgical ablation of atrial fibrillation. Seminars Thorac Cardiovasc Surg 14:198–205

Walsh EP (2007) Interventional electrophysiology in patients with congenital heart disease. Circulation 115:3224–3234

Wolf RK, Schneeberger EW, Osterday R, Miller D, Merrill W, Flege JB Jr, et al. (2005) Video-assisted bilateral pulmonary vein isolation and left atrial appendage exclusion for atrial fibrillation. J Thorac Cardiovasc Surg 130:797–802

3

Definition, Diagnosis and Treatment of Tachycardia

Anand Deshmukh
The Cardiac Center of Creighton University, Omaha, Nebraska
USA

1. Introduction

1.1 Anatomy of the human cardiac conduction system

1.1.1 Sinoatrial node

Sinoatrial node (SAN) serves as the natural pacemaker of the heart. It is a spindle shaped structure that is located at the junction of the superior vena cava and right atrium.

The electrical excitation during sinus heart rhythm originates from the SAN and spreads to the other regions of the heart. It receives arterial supply from either the right coronary artery (60 % of the time) or the left circumflex coronary artery (40-45% of the time). It is innervated with postganglionic adrenergic and cholinergic nerve terminals. The discharge rate of SAN is modulated by stimulation of beta adrenergic and muscarinic (cholinergic) receptors. Stimulation of beta-1 and beta-2 receptors results in positive chronotropic response where as stimulation of muscarinic M2 receptors results in negative chronotropic response.

1.1.2 Atrioventricular node

Atrioventricular node (AVN) is located right above the insertion of the septal leaflet of the tricuspid valve beneath the right atrial endocardium. It receives arterial supply from the AV nodal branch of the right coronary artery (85%-90% of the time) or left circumflex coronary artery (15 % of the time). Action potential from the SAN travels through the atrial myocardium to the AVN. The AVN serves to delay the atrial impulse transmission to the ventricles and thus coordinates atrial and ventricular contractions.

1.2 Bundle of His and bundle branches

Bundle of His is the continuation of the penetrating portion of the atrioventricular bundle on the ventricular side. It divides into the right and left bundle branches. It is supplied by the left anterior descending and posterior descending arteries. Thus it is relatively protected from ischemic damage.

The bundle branches begin at the superior margin of the muscular interventricular septum and divide into the left bundle branch, which may further divide into the anterosuperior branch and central branch and the right bundle branch, which traverses along the right side of the interventricular septum.

1.3 Purkinje fibers

These fibers form an interweaving network on the endocardial surface of the myocardium and are connected to the ends of the bundle branches. They conduct the cardiac impulse simultaneously to both the ventricles.

1.4 Normal sinus rhythm

Normal sinus rhythm refers to generation of impulse from the SAN at a rate of 60-100 beats/min in an adult (Fig 1). In adults, rates below 60 beats/min are referred to as bradycardia and rates above 100 beats/min are referred to as tachycardia. The normal sequence of electrical activation originates from the SAN and spreads through the atria to the AVN and His Purkinje system and finally to the ventricular myocardium.

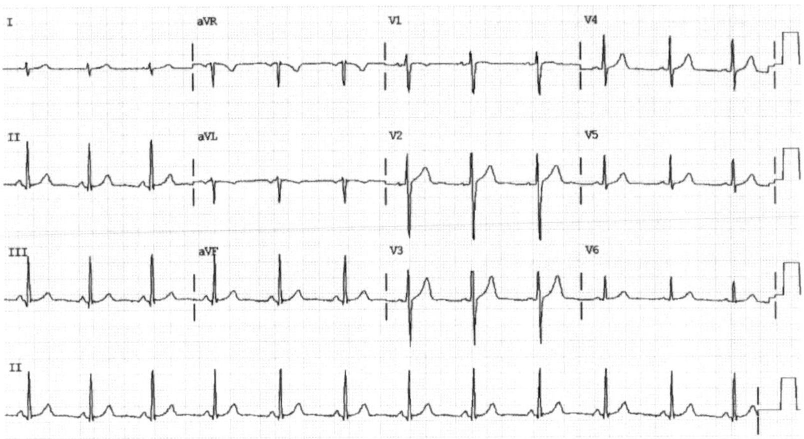

Fig. 1. Normal sinus rhythm

2.Tachycardia

Tachycardias are characterized on the basis of origin; those that originate above the ventricle are referred to as supraventricular tachycardias (SVTs) and those that originate from the ventricle or purkinje fibers are characterized as ventricular tachycardias. The distinction between the two types of tachycardias is critical at the beginning due to difference in their prognosis. Ventricular tachycardias overall have grave prognosis and usually result from significant heart disease. On the other hand, SVTs are usually nonlethal and have a more benign prognosis.

2.1 Narrow and wide complex tachycardia

Based on the duration of QRS complex on electrocardiogram (ECG), tachycardias can be divided into narrow and wide QRS complex tachycardias. Narrow QRS complex tachycardias have a QRS complex duration of less than 120 ms and wide QRS complex tachycardias have a QRS complex duration of more than 120 ms. Wide complex tachycardias are due to ventricular origin of the tachycardia. Ventricular origin of the tachycardia results in slow conduction of electrical impulses across the ventricular myocardium due to longer conduction velocity of the ventricular myocardium unlike narrow complex tachycardia which are conducted over the normal conduction system which has faster conduction velocity resulting in narrow QRS complex on the surface electrocardiogram. Wide complex tachycardia however can be supraventricular in origin if there is pre-existing bundle branch block in either of bundles or if there is activation of the ventricles over the accessory bypass tract and subsequent spread of electrical activation through the ventricular myocardium resulting in a wider QRS complex.

2.2 Sinus tachycardia

Sinus tachycardia as the name suggests originates from the SAN and has a rate of more than 100 beats/min (Fig 2).

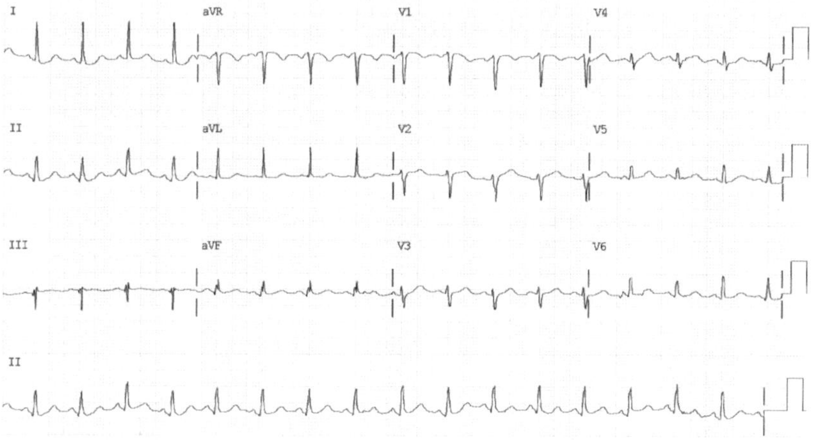

Fig. 2. Sinus tachycardia

It has a gradual onset and termination. It is characterized by presence of sinus P waves prior to each QRS complex on ECG. It is usually caused by increase in adrenergic discharge or decrease in parasympathetic discharge.

It is common during infancy and childhood. The maximum heart rate achieved is higher in young individuals and decreases with age. In adults, it occurs in response to various physiologic or pathological stresses such as exercise, fever, anxiety, thyrotoxicosis, anemia and shock. It may result from consumption of drugs such as atropine, amphetamines, caffeine and alcohol. Sinus tachycardia is often benign by itself and is usually a manifestation of underlying causes as mentioned above. Thus treatment of sinus tachycardia requires treatment of the underlying cause.

2.3 Inappropriate Sinus Tachycardia (IST)

Is a syndrome that can occur due to increased automaticity of the SAN or an automatic atrial focus present near the SAN. It may occur due to an imbalance in the vagal and sympathetic control of the SAN. Treatment of IST involves treatment with beta-blockers or calcium channel blockers that decrease the SAN automaticity. Radiofrequency ablation of the SAN may be indicated in severe drug-refractory cases of inappropriate sinus tachycardia.

2.4 Postural Orthostatic Tachycardia Syndrome (POTS)

Refers to orthostatic decrease in blood pressure and sinus tachycardia in the absence of drugs or hypovolemia (1).

3. Atrial Fibrillation

Atrial fibrillation (AF) is a type of supraventricular arrhythmia characterized by presence of low amplitude fibrillatory waves on the ECG (Fig 3). The fibrillatory waves exhibit variable amplitude and shape and are placed irregularly. They are generated at a rate of 300-600 beats/min. The resulting ventricular rhythm is irregularly irregular. However, the ventricular rhythm may be regular in AF in the patients with third degree atrioventricular block with an escape pacemaker or artificial pacemaker.

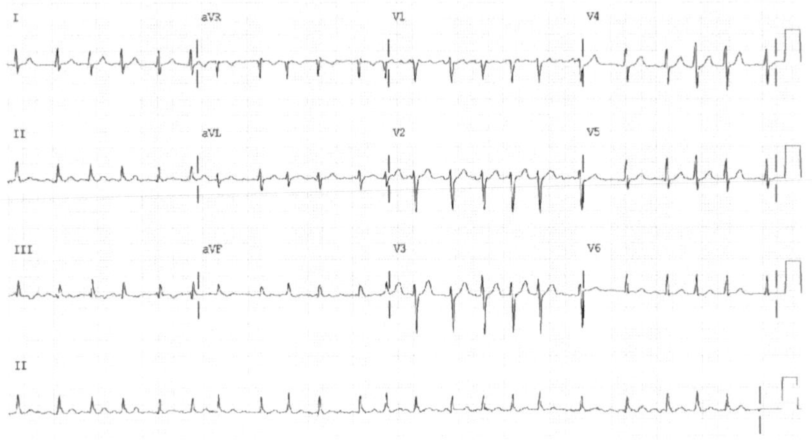

Fig. 3. Atrial fibrillation

3.1 Classification

AF is considered to be *paroxysmal* if it terminates spontaneously within 7 days. If it continues for more than 7 days, it is considered to be *persistent*. *Permanent* AF persists for more than a year and is resistant to cardioversion. *Lone* AF is a term used to describe the occurrence of AF in patients younger than 60 years of age that do not have hypertension or evidence of any structural heart disease.

3.2 Epidemiology

AF is the most common cardiac arrhythmia encountered in clinical practice. It is also the most common cause of hospitalization among all the arrhythmias. Advanced age, obesity, hypertension, congestive heart failure, mitral and aortic valve disease are independent risk factors for development of AF.

3.3 Causes of AF

Hypertension and hypertensive heart disease is by far the most common cause of AF. Other causes include ischemic heart disease, mitral valve disease, hypertrophic cardiomyopathy, dilated cardiomyopathy, pulmonary hypertension, and obesity with resultant obstructive sleep apnea. AF may be caused by reversible temporary causes such as excessive alcohol intake *(holiday heart syndrome)*, myocardial infarction, pulmonary embolism, thoracic surgery, pericarditis and myocarditis. Hyperthyroidism is one of the correctable causes of AF.

3.4 Clinical features

AF may be symptomatic or asymptomatic. The most common symptoms of AF are palpitation, shortness of breath, tiredness and lightheadedness. It is often asymptomatic in elderly patients and those with persistent AF. Patients with AF may experience syncope at the conversion of AF to normal sinus rhythm from long sinus pause. Cerebrovascular accident (CVA) may be the initial manifestation of AF in patients with asymptomatic AF due to predisposition to thrombus formation in the atria, predominantly in the left atrial appendage due to chaotic and asynchronous atrial activity. It may also manifest as congestive heart failure due to tachycardia induced cardiomyopathy.

3.5 Physical examination

On physical examination, patients with AF often have irregularly irregular pulse. Patients often have pulse deficit, which is discordance between peripheral pulse and apical impulse. It results from short diastolic filling period for the ventricles during rapid AF resulting in low stroke volume and absence of peripheral pulse. There is variability in the intensity of the first heart sound on auscultation due to variable diastolic filling of the ventricles.

3.6 Diagnostic evaluation

History should be directed to assess the nature of AF (paroxysmal or persistent), nature of triggers, correctable causes such as excessive alcohol or caffeine intake, severity, frequency and duration of episodes of AF.

Twenty-four hour Holter monitoring may be helpful in patients with frequent episodes of AF whereas an event monitor would be helpful in patients with sporadic symptoms for detection of the episodes of AF.

Laboratory evaluation should include thyroid function tests to evaluate the thyroid function as a cause of AF. An echocardiogram is helpful to determine the left atrial size, left ventricular function and valvular heart disease. A stress test may be helpful for evaluation of ischemic heart disease as a cause of AF.

3.7 Thromboembolic complications

As described above, AF predisposes to thromboembolic complications such as CVA. However, the risk of these complications is not the same in all the individuals with AF. Thus it is imperative to stratify the risk of developing these complications. The risk for CVA is highest in patients with prior history of ischemic CVA and mitral stenosis whereas it is lower in patients with lone AF. Gage et al developed a simple clinical scheme to stratify the patients on the basis of major risk factors. It is known by the acronym *CHADS-2* that includes *C*ongestive heart failure, *H*ypertension, *A*ge ≥ 75 years , *D*iabetes mellitus and previous *S*troke. Each of the first four risk factors is assigned 1 point and prior ischemic stroke or transient ischemic attack is assigned 2 points (2). There is a direct relationship between the annual risk of stroke and CHADS-2 score (Table 1).

Score	Annual risk (%)
0	1.9
1	2.8
2	4.0
3	5.9
4	8.5
5	12.5
6	18.2

CHADS-2 score is calculated by adding 1 point for each of recent congestive heart failure, hypertension, age 75 years and older, diabetes mellitus and 2 points for history of stroke or transient ischemic attack.

Table 1. Annual stroke risk according to CHADS-2 score (2).

The risk of thromboembolic complications is similar in patients with paroxysmal and persistent AF (3).

3.8 Prevention of thromboembolic complications

As discussed above, the risk of stroke increases with increase in the CHADS-2 score in patients with AF. The annual risk of stroke in patients with CHADS-2 score of 0 is approximately 1.9 %. In these patients, aspirin therapy alone is adequate due to the lower annual risk of stroke. Warfarin therapy is superior to aspirin in prevention of stroke (61 % vs. 18 %), however the risk of hemorrhagic complications is also higher and falls in the same range of 1-2 % annually (4, 5). Thus, considering the risk benefit ratio, aspirin therapy alone would be adequate in these patients.

In patients with CHADS -2 score of 1, the annual risk of stroke is 2.8 %. The decision to use aspirin alone or warfarin therapy should be individualized and patient preference may be taken into consideration. The dose of aspirin used for prevention of stroke ranges from 81-325 mg daily.

In patients with CHADS-2 score >1, aspirin therapy alone is inadequate to decrease the risk of stroke. These patients should receive warfarin for prevention of stroke. The target international normalized ratio (INR) should be 2.0-3.0 during warfarin therapy. The risk of major bleeding with warfarin is between 1-2 % annually as described above and it increases with INR >3.0 (6). Advanced age should not be a deterrent to starting warfarin therapy (7).

US-Federal Drug Administration (FDA) F recently approved direct thrombin inhibitors such as dabigatran for prevention of stroke in patients with non-valvular AF. It offers the advantage of fixed dosing and lack of the requirement for INR testing during therapy. Dabigatran given at a dose of 110 mg twice daily was associated with similar rates of stroke and systemic embolism as with warfarin and lower rates of major bleeding. When it was administered at a dose of 150 mg twice daily, it was associated with lower rates of stroke and systemic embolism but similar rates of major hemorrhage (8).

4. Acute management of AF

In patients who present with an episode of AF and rapid ventricular response, control of ventricular rate should be the priority. It can be achieved with intravenous diltiazem or beta-blockers such as esmolol. However, if the patient is hemodynamically unstable, emergent transthoracic electric direct current (DC) cardioversion is appropriate.

The decision to restore sinus rhythm after control of ventricular rate should be individualized based on nature of AF (paroxysmal or persistent), duration of AF, presence of symptoms, age, prior episodes and antiarrhythmic and anticoagulation therapy.

The decision making for restoration of sinus rhythm in patients with AF has two components: one is early vs. late cardioversion and second is electrical cardioversion vs. pharmacologic cardioversion.

Early cardioversion is attempted in patients with AF lasting less than 48 hours and those who have been on therapeutic anticoagulation of 3-4 weeks prior to cardioversion. Late cardioversion is attempted in patients with left atrial appendage thrombus on transesophageal echocardiography (TEE), if the duration of AF is > 48 hours or if the duration is unclear and those with suspected correctable cause of AF. When the duration of AF is > 48 hours or unclear, the other option to avoid delayed cardioversion is TEE for surveillance of left atrial thrombus followed by cardioversion if there is no evidence of thrombus.

Cardioversion can be done using either electrical or pharmacologic means. Pharmacologic cardioversion can be performed by intravenous administration of ibutilide (success rate 60-70 %), amiodarone (success rate 40-50%) or procainamide (success rate 30 %). After infusion of ibutilide, patients should be monitored for polymorphic ventricular tachycardia that can occur as an adverse effect. In patients without structural heart disease, oral agents such as propafenone (300-600mg) or flecainide (100-200mg) can be administered for cardioversion. The success rate of transthoracic electrical cardioversion is very high (95 %). In some cases, electrical cardioversion may be required after administration of antiarrhythmics for maintenance of sinus rhythm.

4.1 Long-term management of AF

As far as long-term management of AF is considered, several studies have compared rate control (controlling ventricular rate) strategy vs. rhythm control (restoration of sinus rhythm) strategy. The largest of these trials (AFFIRM) failed to show any benefit of rhythm control strategy over rate control strategy. Rhythm control strategy in this study was associated with higher rates of hospitalization and adverse drug effects of antiarrhythmic therapy that were used for restoration of sinus rhythm (9). However, the decision to pursue rate control or rhythm control strategy is a complex one and should be individualized after taking several factors into account including, age, comorbidities, duration of AF, left atrial dimensions, presence of symptoms, response to prior cardioversions. In patients > 65 years of age with asymptomatic or minimally symptomatic AF, it would be reasonable to pursue rate control strategy whereas symptomatic AF in younger and older age patients should be offered the option of rhythm control.

As far as antithrombotic therapy is considered, all patients with either paroxysmal or persistent AF should receive antithrombotic therapy with either aspirin or warfarin based on their risk stratification irrespective of their symptom status as described above.

4.2 Pharmacologic rate control

The goal for heart rate control in AF is to maintain heart rate less than 80 beats/min at rest and less than 110 beats /min during activity. Oral agents available for heart rate control in AF include digitalis, beta-blockers, calcium channel blockers and amiodarone. The first line agents for rate control are beta-blockers such as metoprolol and calcium channel blockers such as diltiazem and verapamil. Digitalis is useful to control heart rates due to its vagotonic effects but may not be adequate as a single agent for rate control during exertion. It is useful in patients with systolic heart failure due to its effects on prevention of heart failure hospitalization. Although amiodarone is not routinely used for rate control, it is useful in patients with contraindications for calcium channel blockers (such as systolic heart failure) and beta-blockers (such as reactive airway disease).

4.3 Pharmacologic rhythm control

A pharmacologic rhythm control strategy consists of either chronic prophylactic therapy with antiarrhythmic drugs or single pill in the pocket approach at each symptomatic recurrence of AF by typically using class IC (flecainide, propafenone) drugs depending on the frequency and severity of symptoms. Amiodarone is by far the most effective agent for rhythm control (maintenance of sinus rhythm) among all the antiarrhythmic agents. Its adverse effects including pulmonary and liver toxicity and effects on thyroids limit its use.

Ventricular arrhythmias are common from all the antiarrhythmic agents and they are poorly tolerated due to their adverse effects. Use of antiarrhythmic therapy for rhythm control should be individualized based on comorbidities such as hypertension, left ventricular hypertrophy, congestive heart failure and ischemic heart disease.

4.4 Catheter ablation of AF

Catheter ablation of AF should be offered to patients but requires appropriate selection of patients. Patients with lone paroxysmal AF and minimal structural heart disease are the ideal candidates for this procedure. It may be appropriate to consider this approach as first line therapy in patients younger than 35 years of age with symptomatic AF and SAN dysfunction that complicates antiarrhythmic drug therapy. Patients with persistent and symptomatic AF and minimal structural heart disease who have failed at least one antiarrhythmic drug therapy may be offered catheter ablation.

Isolation of pulmonary veins alone is often sufficient in patients with paroxysmal AF. However, in patients with persistent AF, a variety of ablation strategies have been used. The success rate for AF ablation is higher for paroxysmal AF (70-80%) than persistent AF (50 %). The risk of major complication after AF ablation is approximately 5-6 % and most common complications include cardiac tamponade, pulmonary vein stenosis and stroke. Atrioesophageal fistula is a rare but lethal complication of this procedure.

4.5 Other nonpharmacologic approaches to AF management

AV nodal ablation and insertion of pacemaker may be considered in patients with persistent AF and inadequate ventricular rate control with medications or intolerance to medications, and those with failed attempt at catheter ablation of AF.

Maze procedure is a surgical procedure developed by Cox that involves multiple incisions involving the right and left atria but requires open thoracotomy and cardiopulmonary bypass (10). It may be considered concomitantly in patients who are undergoing coronary bypass graft surgery or valvular repair or replacement.

5. Atrial tachycardia

Atrial tachycardias are broadly classified into focal and macroreentrant types based on management. Focal atrial tachycardias originate from activation of one particular focus in the atria where as macroreentrant tachycardias use a relatively large reentrant circuit using conduction barriers for creation of the circuit.

5.1 Atrial flutter

Atrial flutter is the most common type of macroreentrant atrial tachycardia. The reentrant circuit of atrial flutter is constrained anteriorly by the tricuspid annulus and posteriorly by the crista terminalis and eustachian ridge. A typical atrial flutter circulates in a counterclockwise fashion around the tricuspid annulus and atypical flutter circulates in a clockwise fashion

Atrial rate during atrial flutter varies between 200-300 beats/min. Ventricular response to atrial flutter is determined by factors such as conduction through the AVN and concomitant antiarrhythmic drug therapy. On ECG, atrial flutter manifests as recurring, regular, saw tooth flutter waves (Fig 4).

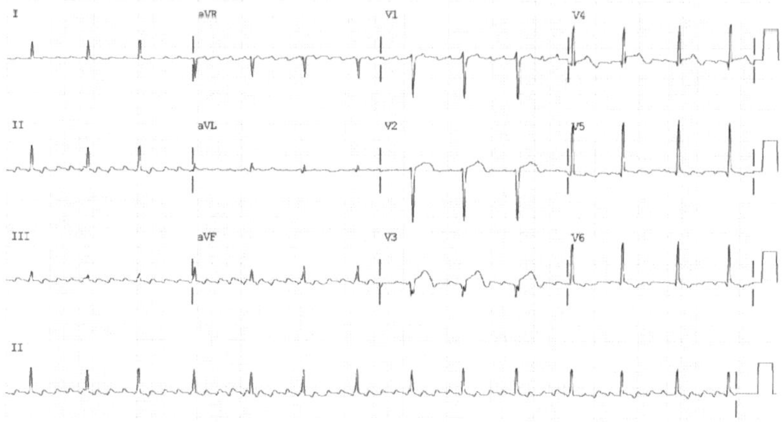

Fig. 4. Typical atrial flutter

5.2 Clinical features

Atrial flutter occurs as a result of valvular heart disease such as mitral and tricuspid stenosis, pulmonary embolism, prior AF ablations, atrial septal defects that result in atrial dilation, thyrotoxicosis, alcoholism and following surgeries for congenital heart disease. Patients in atrial flutter often describe symptoms such as palpitations, diaphoresis, lightheadedness and dizziness.

On physical examination, patients have constant intensity of the first heart sound if the ventricular response is constant and rapid jugular venous pulsations. Carotid sinus massage often slows down the ventricular response but does not terminate it.

5.3 Management

Atrial flutter is much more difficult to rate control than AF. Thus, transthoracic synchronous DC cardioversion may be offered as an initial treatment to patients with atrial flutter. Pharmacologic agents such as procainamide and ibutilide are often successful in conversion of atrial flutter to sinus rhythm, however ibutilide is associated with *Torsades de pointes (Tdp)* arrhythmia. If atrial flutter persists despite cardioversion, class IA and IC agents or low dose amiodarone may be helpful for prevention of recurrences. However, patients should be on AV nodal blocking agent during this therapy to prevent faster ventricular response after slowing of atrial flutter rate that may allow more frequent AV nodal conduction.

The success rate for ablation of cavo-tricuspid isthmus dependent atrial flutter is 90-100%, thus it may be offered as an alternative to drug therapy as an initial therapy in patients with these types of atrial flutter.

As far as acute management of atrial flutter is considered, ventricular rate control can be attempted with intravenous diltiazem and verapamil or beta-blockers such as esmolol and metoprolol. Digoxin may be added if the combination of beta-blockers and calcium channel blockers is inadequate for ventricular rate control. Intravenous amiodarone has been found to be successful in rate control of atrial flutter.

The recommendations for antithrombotic therapy in patients with atrial flutter are the same as AF.

6. Focal atrial tachycardia

Focal atrial tachycardias originate from a single atrial focus and generally exhibit atrial rates between 150-200 beats/min. They typically occur in short bursts, however, may be incessant. On ECG, focal atrial tachycardia is differentiated from sinus tachycardia by P wave morphologies that are characteristically different in contour compared to sinus P wave morphology and from atrial flutter by presence of isoelectric interval in all the ECG leads. Right atrial tachycardias produce positive or biphasic P waves in lead V1 where as left atrial tachycardias produce negative P waves.

Focal atrial tachycardia occurs commonly in patients with structural heart disease, cor pulmonale, digitalis toxicity and electrolyte abnormalities. Stimulants such as caffeine can precipitate focal atrial tachycardia.

On examination, patients have variable intensity of the first heart sound due to variable conduction through the AVN with resultant variable R-R interval, and increased number of *a* waves on the jugular venous pulse. Carotid sinus massage or intravenous adenosine results in increased vagal activity and decrease in ventricular response but rarely terminates it.

Focal atrial tachycardia in patients on digitalis can be due to toxicity. Digitalis should be discontinued in these patients and electrolyte abnormalities such as hypokalemia should be corrected. Administration of digitalis antibodies should be considered in patients with rapid ventricular response after correction of electrolyte abnormalities. In patients who are not taking digitalis, beta-blockers, calcium channel blockers or digitalis may be considered for control of ventricular response. Persistent atrial tachycardia may require administration of class IA, IC or III agents. Patients intolerant of antiarrhythmic therapy or non compliant with antiarrhythmic therapy can be offered catheter ablation for elimination of the tachycardia based on the location of the focus and local expertise in ablation.

7. Multifocal (chaotic) atrial tachycardia

Multifocal atrial tachycardia is characterized by presence of variable P wave morphologies and PR intervals due to origin of this tachycardia from multiple foci (Fig 5). At least 3 different types of P wave contours are necessary for the diagnosis.

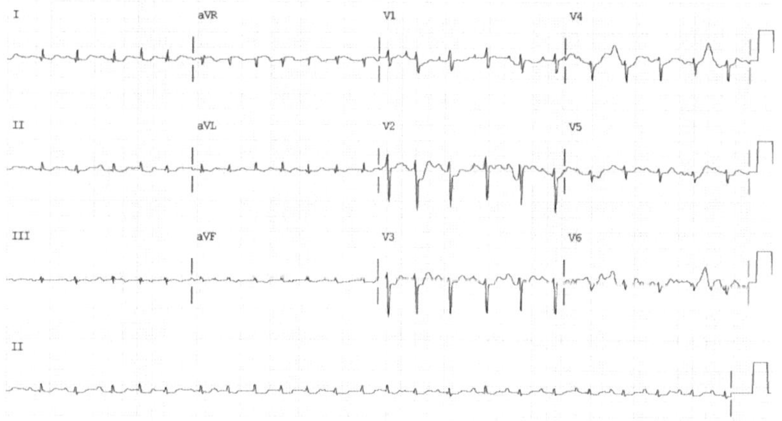

Fig. 5. Multifocal atrial tachycardia

It occurs in elderly patients with chronic obstructive pulmonary disease and congestive heart failure. It may be rarely caused by digitalis or theophylline administration.

Management of this tachycardia should be directed at treatment of underlying disease. Calcium channel blockers such as verapamil and diltiazem or amiodarone are helpful in management. Potassium and magnesium should be replaced. Beta-blockers are avoided in patients with reactive airway disease.

8. AV nodal reentrant tachycardia

AV nodal reentrant tachycardia (AVNRT) is a reentrant form of SVT involving AV junction. On surface ECG, it is characterized by presence of regular R-R intervals, narrow QRS complexes (in absence of previous conduction defects), sudden onset and termination and ventricular rates between 150-250 beats/min (Fig 6).

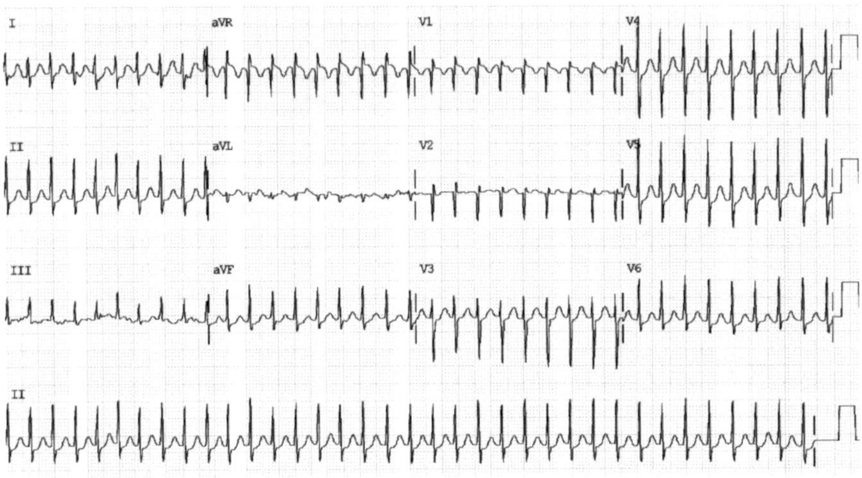

Fig. 6. AV nodal reentrant tachycardia

Conduction of the electrical impulses from the atria to the AVN occurs over slow and fast pathways. A premature atrial complex (PAC) or rarely a premature ventricular complex (PVC) often initiates this tachycardia. PAC conducts to the ventricle over the slow pathway during the refractory period of the fast pathway resulting in prolonged PR interval before the initiation of the tachycardia. After conduction over the slow pathway it returns and conducts over the fast pathway, which is no longer refractory and thus initiating the circus movement. This is the mechanism of a typical AVNRT. Atypical form of AVNRT is characterized by anterograde conduction to the ventricles over the fast pathway and retrograde conduction to the atrial over the slow pathway. Thus atrial activation is slightly before, during or slightly after the activation of QRS complex. If atrial activation occurs after the QRS complex, it manifests on the surface ECG as pseudo-r′ in lead V1 and pseudo-S waves in leads II, III and aVF.

Typical form of AVNRT is characterized by short ventriculoatrial conduction (VA) interval due to near simultaneous activation of atria and ventricles where as atypical form of AVNRT is characterized by longer VA interval due to activation of ventricles over the fast pathway and retrograde activation of atria over the slow pathway. Typical AVNRT is a short R-P type of SVT due to faster retrograde conduction to the atria over the fast pathway whereas atypical AVNRT is a long R-P type SVT due to longer retrograde conduction to the atria over the slow pathway.

8.1 Clinical features

AVNRT usually occurs in patients with no structural heart disease. It manifests with symptoms such as palpitations, lightheadedness, anxiety, syncope, diaphoresis, angina and worsening of presence of new heart failure symptoms. It occurs in third or fourth decade of life. It is more prevalent in women than in men.

8.2 Management of acute attack

Patients with infrequent episodes of AVNRT that are well tolerated can be simply reassured. Vagal maneuvers such as carotid sinus massage, gagging, and Valsalva maneuver may sometimes be helpful in termination of the episode. Adenosine administered in doses of 6-12 mg is the initial drug of choice in patients with suspected AVNRT. However, it should be kept in mind that adenosine is contraindicated in patients with asthma. Calcium channel blockers such as diltiazem or verapamil administered intravenously may also be helpful in termination of the acute attack. Digitalis is rarely used in acute attack due to its slower onset of action. However, it may increase the success rate of vagal maneuvers. Beta-blockers are rarely used due to their inferior efficacy as compared to calcium channel blockers in termination of acute episode. DC synchronized cardioversion may be required in patients with hemodynamic instability due to AVNRT.

8.3 Prevention of recurrences

Long term medical therapy or radiofrequency ablation for prevention of recurrences is recommended in patients with frequent and severe episodes of AVNRT. Long acting calcium channel blockers, long acting beta-blockers or digitalis may be helpful in prevention of recurrence.

Radiofrequency ablation can be offered as an initial therapy in patients who are symptomatic from frequent and severe episodes. It should also be offered in patients who are intolerant or reluctant to pharmacologic therapy for prevention of recurrences. It has a very high success rate (95 %) and very low complication rate.

9. AV reciprocating (reentrant) tachycardia

AV reciprocating tachycardia (AVRT) occurs due to reentry over accessory pathways that connect the atrium or AVN to the ventricle outside the normal AVN and His- Purkinje system. These pathways can conduct impulses either anterogradely from the atria to the ventricles or retrogradely from the ventricles to the atria. When the conduction occurs anterogradely over the accessory pathway (manifest conduction), it results in pre-excited QRS complex where as if the accessory pathway conducts only retrogradely (concealed conduction), it does not produce ventricular preexcitation. Preexcited QRS complex with tachycardia is referred to as Wolf Parkinson White (WPW) syndrome.

9.1 Reentry over a concealed pathway (Orthodromic AVRT)

Orthodromic AVRT results from anterograde conduction from the atria to the ventricles over the normal AV nodal conduction system and retrograde conduction from the ventricles to the atria over the accessory pathway. Thus there is no ventricular preexcitation during the tachycardia and the accessory pathway is considered to be concealed.

On ECG, this results in retrograde P waves that occur in the ST segment or T wave portion of the ECG. The contour of P waves is different from sinus P waves due to eccentric activation of the atria in most cases.

Diagnosis is usually done during an electrophysiology study (EPS), where a PVC activates the atria prior to activation of the His bundle. Also if the PVC activates the atria when His bundle is supposed to be refractory, presence of accessory pathway is almost certain. The VA interval remains constant over a wide range of coupling intervals of the PVC as most of the accessory pathways exhibit all or none conduction unlike conduction over the AVN which shows decremental property at higher rates. The VA interval is < 50% of R-R interval.

9.2 Clinical features

Tachycardia rates in these patients tend to be faster than AVNRT and are around 200 beats/min. Patients can present with palpitations, anxiety, presyncope or syncope. On physical examination, they have regular pulse and constant intensity first heart sound due to constant R-R interval.

9.3 Management

As the tachycardia circuit involves the AVN and the fact that conduction over the accessory pathway occurs only retrogradely, the acute management of orthodromic AVRT is similar to AVNRT. Vagal maneuvers, adenosine, calcium channel blockers or digitalis that produce transient AV block may result in termination of this tachycardia. Chronic prophylactic therapy involves administration of antiarrhythmic drugs that prolong the conduction over the accessory pathway such as class I and class III drugs or radiofrequency ablation. Radiofrequency ablation of the accessory pathway has high success rates, low complication rate and should be considered for symptomatic patients early in their management or those with intolerance to antiarrhythmic therapy.

10. Preexcitation syndrome

Preexcitation syndrome results from activation of the ventricle in part or entirely from atrial impulses that are conducted over the accessory pathway that conducts anterogradely. Three features of WPW syndrome are -

1. PR interval less than 120 ms
2. Presence of slow up or down sloping QRS complex in some leads, often called as *delta* waves
3. Secondary ST-T wave changes that are generally directed in direction opposite to the major delta or QRS vector.

Accessory pathways can be *atriohisian* that connect the atria to the His bundle, *atriofascicular* that connect atria to one of the fascicles, *nodofascicular* that connect the AVN to the fascicles, or *fasciculoventricular* that connect the fascicles to the ventricle. *Mahaim fibers* are atriofascicular or nodofascicular fibers that exhibit progressive increase in the AV interval in response to atrial overdrive pacing unlike the usual atrioventricular accessory pathway.

Location of the accessory pathways can be predicted by careful analysis of the ECG. Accessory pathways that conduct to the right ventricle produce negative delta waves and QRS in lead V1 whereas those conducting to the left ventricle produce positive delta wave and QRS in lead V1. Posteroseptal pathways produce negative delta waves or QRS complex in leads II, III and aVF. Left free wall pathways produce negative or isoelectric delta wave in lateral leads.

Right free wall pathways produce left axis deviation where as if the accessory pathway is located in the right ventricle, presence of inferior axis indicates anteroseptal pathway.

Accessory pathways have a longer refractory period during long cycle lengths. Thus a PAC can result in conduction over the normal AVN and His bundle complex as the accessory pathway is refractory but when the impulse arrives to the ventricles, it has recovered excitability and can conduct retrogradely resulting in reciprocating orthodromic AVRT. If the conduction occurs anterogradely over the accessory pathways and retrogradely over the AVN-His bundle, it is referred to as antidromic AVRT.

10.1 Permanent form of AV junctional reciprocating tachycardia (PJRT)

Rfrom very slowly conducting posteroseptal accessory pathway. It is maintained by anterograde conduction over the AVN and retrograde conduction over the accessory pathway.

10.2 Clinical features

Incidence of preexcitation syndrome is approximately 1.5/1000 among healthy adults. Left free wall accessory pathway is the most common type of accessory pathway. Patients with Ebstein anomaly often have right-sided accessory pathways. The prevalence is higher in men and decreases with age. The frequency of tachycardia however increases with age with reciprocating tachycardia being the most common (80 %) of patients followed by AF (15-30 %). The incidence of sudden death is very rare (<0.1 %). Patients who have ventricular fibrillation (VF) have ventricular cycle lengths in the range of 240 ms or less. Presence of only intermittent preexcitation during sinus rhythm, abrupt loss of conduction during administration of procainamide are suggestive of longer refractory period of accessory pathway.

10.3 Management of preexcitation syndrome and tachycardia

Patients who have preexcitation on ECG with no history of palpitations or tachycardia may be managed conservatively without any further electrophysiologic evaluation. However, patients with preexcitation on the ECG and history of palpitations or documented tachycardia need further treatment. Therapeutic options include pharmacologic management and radiofrequency ablation.

While considering pharmacologic management of preexcited tachycardia and patients with accessory pathway (concealed or manifest), it is important to understand the effects of various drugs on these pathways. Class IA drugs increase the refractoriness of accessory pathways. Calcium channel blockers, adenosine, and digitalis act on AVN where as class IC agents (flecainide, propafenone) and class III agents such as amiodarone and sotalol increase the refractoriness of both AVN and accessory pathway.

10.4 Management of acute episode

Management of orthodromic AVRT (using the concealed accessory pathway) has been discussed above.

Patients with preexcited tachycardias suspected by presence of anomalous QRS complexes, or know prior history of preexcitation from previous ECGs, require drugs that prolong the refractoriness of the accessory pathway (such as procainamide) often coupled with drugs that prolong the refractoriness of AVN to break the reentry circuit. However, patients that are hemodynamically unstable require electrical DC cardioversion.

10.5 Prevention of recurrence

Radiofrequency ablation of the accessory pathway has become the treatment of choice in patients with accessory pathway for prevention of recurrence due to its high success rate and low complication rate. However, if transvenous catheter ablation is unsuccessful epicardial ablation or surgical interruption of the accessory pathway may be necessary.

Drug therapy is an alternative approach to ablation however the effect of drugs on accessory pathways is unpredictable. Class IC agents, amiodarone and sotalol or combination of class IC agent and beta blocker may be effective as they prolong refractoriness in the accessory pathway as well as AVN. Further testing (such as exercise, isoproterenol infusion) is essential to be certain that ventricular response is controlled in patients with AF that are started on these agents.

11. Ventricular tachycardia

Ventricular tachycardia (VT) is defined as 3 or more consecutive premature ventricular complexes. It is considered to be nonsustained if it lasts less than 30 seconds and sustained if it last more than 30 seconds or requires termination due to hemodynamic collapse.

VT originates distal to His bundle in the ventricular muscle, specialized conduction system or combination of both tissues. It can occur in patients with no structural heart disease, as a part of inherited syndromes or in patients with structural heart disease.

On ECG, it is characterized by wide QRS complexes that are mostly regular, with rates varying between 70-250 beats/min and ST-T vector directed opposite to the QRS vector (Fig 7).

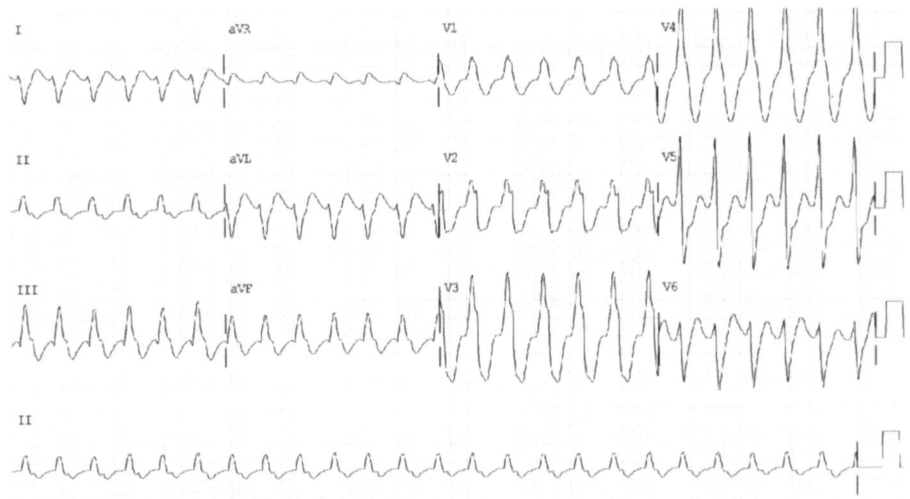

Fig. 7. Ventricular tachycardia

11.1 Wide QRS complex tachycardia and differentiation of VT from SVT with aberrant conduction

Differential diagnosis of wide QRS complex tachycardia includes VT, SVT with aberrant conduction due to rate dependent bundle branch block, SVT with preexisting bundle branch block, SVT /AF with anterograde conduction over the accessory pathway, or antidromic AVRT. VT is however the most common cause of tachycardia with wide QRS complex.

The features that favor the diagnosis of VT include –

1. Presence of underlying structural heart disease, or myocardial infarction
2. Duration of QRS complex greater than 140 ms
3. Presence of fusion beats (QRS complexes originating from co-activation of ventricles by ventricular and supraventricular rhythm on ECG)
4. Presence of capture beats (ventricular activation from supraventricular beats with contour different from rest of the complexes)
5. Presence of conduction disturbances on the baseline ECG and QRS complexes different in configuration compared to baseline ECG
6. AV dissociation i.e. no relation between ventricular and supraventricular rhythm; it is highly specific but not very sensitive
7. Positive or negative concordance in precordial leads (all QRS complexes in precordial leads are either negative or positive)
8. In the presence of right bundle branch block pattern, the initial pattern of activation is different from activation by sinus initiated QRS complexes, larger amplitude of R wave compared to R' and rS or QS pattern in lead V6
9. In the presence of left bundle branch block, R wave in V1 is longer than 30 ms and duration of start of R wave to nadir of S wave in V1 is longer than 60 ms and qR or qS pattern in lead V6
10. Extreme left axis deviation ("northwest axis") on the ECG

Electrophysiologic characteristics of VT include negative HV interval and dissociated His bundle deflections from ventricular activation.

11.2 Clinical features

VT can occur as nonsustained or sustained episode. Nonsustained VT is usually well tolerated, however patients may complain of palpitations and presyncopal symptoms. Sustained VT can be hemodynamically stable or it may present has unstable runs finally degenerating into ventricular fibrillation.

Ischemic heart disease is by far the most common cause of VT followed by cardiomyopathy. Patients with sustained monomorphic VT have myocardial substrate different from patients with ventricular fibrillation and often have reduced left ventricular ejection fraction, slowed intraventricular conduction and previous myocardial infarction.

Reduced left ventricular function, inducibility of sustained VT during electrophysiologic study, T wave alternans are some of the strong predictors of poor outcome in patients with VT (11).

Prognosis of patients with idiopathic VT, in absence of structural heart disease is good.

11.3 Acute management of sustained ventricular tachycardia

Sustained VT in hemodynamically stable patients can be terminated pharmacologically with administration of one of the antiarrhythmics such as amiodarone, lidocaine, procainamide or sotalol. Amiodarone administered by intravenous infusion is often effective. If the arrhythmia is non responsive to medical therapy or if patient is hemodynamically unstable, electrical DC cardioversion can be used. Ventricular pacing using transvenous catheter inserted into the right ventricle at rates faster than VT can terminate VT however runs the risks of degenerating VT into ventricular flutter or fibrillation.

After stabilization of the patient, one should look for reversible conditions such as ischemia, electrolyte abnormalities, and drugs as a cause of VT.

11.4 Therapy for prevention of recurrences

Symptomatic nonsustained VT in patients with normal left ventricular function can be treated with beta-blockers. Patients refractory to beta-blockers can be treated with class IC agents, sotalol or amiodarone.

Asymptomatic nonsustained VT in a patient with no evidence of structural heart disease does not require treatment.

11.5 Primary prevention

Patients with nonsustained VT and structural heart disease with a left ventricular ejection fraction of <0.35 to 0.40 should undergo EPS and implantable cardioverter defibrillator (ICD) implantation if they have inducible VT (12,13).

Patients with nonsustained VT, prior myocardial infarction and left ventricular ejection fraction of <0.30 do not require EPS and can directly undergo ICD placement (14)

Patients with ischemic and non-ischemic cardiomyopathy, left ventricular ejection fraction of <0.35 and NYHA class II or III heart failure should undergo ICD implantation due to 7 % absolute decrease in mortality (15). Amiodarone is the next best therapy in patients with heart failure, non-ischemic cardiomyopathy ejection fraction of <0.40, and frequent PVCs (16).

11.6 Secondary prevention

Survivors of sudden cardiac arrest or patients with sustained VT resulting in hemodynamic compromise and poor left ventricular function should be offered ICD implantation (17, 18). Patients who refuse ICD implantation, treatment with amiodarone is the next best therapy (19).

Optimal therapy for patients with sustained VT and normal left ventricular function is unknown however empiric amiodarone appears to be safe.

Radiofrequency ablation is effective in patients with idiopathic VT; however it is less effective in patients with structural heart disease and depressed LV function. It may be effective as an adjunctive therapy in patients with recurrent ICD shocks due to VT that is not responsive to combination of antiarrhythmic therapy.

12. Ventricular arrhythmia in arrhythmogenic right ventricular cardiomyopathy

Arrhythmogentic right ventricular cardiomyopathy (ARVC) is familial and progressive cardiomyopathy of the right ventricle. VT in ARVC is caused by reentry. It has left bundle branch contour due and often resembles right ventricular outflow tract tachycardia. Patients may be asymptomatic or may manifest signs and symptoms of right heart failure. ECG during sinus rhythm shows right bundle branch block pattern and T wave inversions in leads V1 through V3. Epsilon wave (which is a terminal notch in the QRS) can be present in these leads. ICDs are preferable for the treatment of this condition due to progressive nature of the disease.

13. Inherited arrhythmia syndromes

13.1 Catecholaminergic polymorphic ventricular tachycardia

Catecholaminergic polymorphic ventricular tachycardia (CPVT) is an inherited VT that occurs in children and adolescents without any structural heart disease or surface electrocardiographic abnormalities. It is stress induced and patients present with syncope or aborted sudden death. VT is bidirectional in nature and may eventually degenerate into polymorphic VT with exercise. The treatment of choice is beta-blockers and ICD. Patients should be instructed to avoid vigorous exercise.

13.2 Brugada syndrome

It is an inherited form of idiopathic ventricular fibrillation that occurs commonly in young healthy Southeast Asians. These patients have no structural heart disease. On ECG, they have ST segment elevation in the precordial leads at rest. Mutations in the sodium channel genes (SCN5A) and calcium channel have been identified in several families. Phase 2 reentry due to heterogenous loss of action potential dome is thought to be responsible for ventricular arrhythmias. There is no pharmacologic treatment available and ICD implantation is the only treatment that is effective for prevention of sudden death.

13.3 Torsades de pointes

Tdp refers to a VT characterized by presence of QRS complexes with varying amplitude that twist around the isoelectric baseline (Fig 8). The rate usually varies from 200-250 beats/min. It occurs in patients with prolonged ventricular repolarization manifesting as prolonged QT interval.

VT that is similar to *Tdp* but occurs in patients without QT prolongation is called polymorphic ventricular tachycardia.

Tdp can occur in two settings. Late PVCs may discharge during termination of long T wave that precipitates the episode of VT or short coupled variant occurring due to close-coupled PVC. *Tdp* is thought to occur from early afterdepolarizations.

The common predisposing factors for *Tdp* include severe bradycardia, hypokalemia, use of class IA or III antiarrhythmic drugs, QT interval prolonging drugs or congenital long QT syndrome.

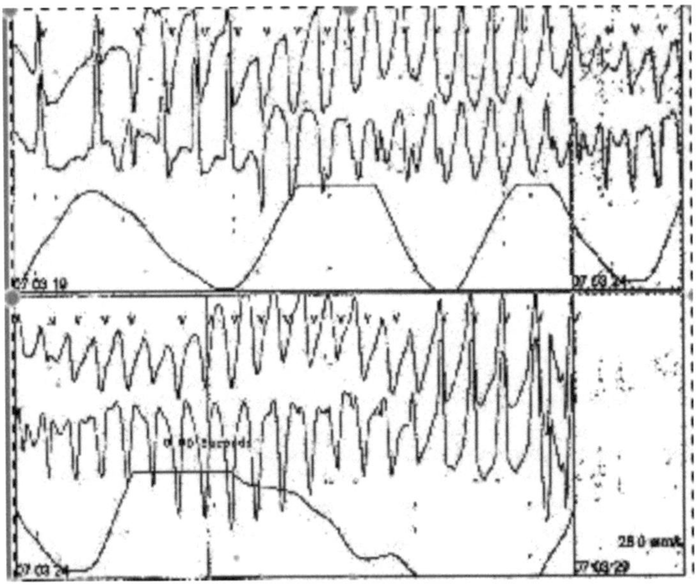

Fig. 8. Torsades de pointes

In patients with *Tdp*, the reversible cause should be corrected such as discontinuing Class IA or III antiarrhythmic, or QT prolonging drug. In patients with acquired long QT syndrome, intravenous magnesium should be given. This is followed by temporary atrial or ventricular pacing. Isoproterenol infusion can be tried prior to starting pacing.

Polymorphic VT however can be treated with standard antiarrhythmic drugs.

13.4 Long Q-T syndrome

Corrected long QT interval (QTc) is less than 460 ms for men and 470 ms for women. Patients with long QT syndrome have prolonged QT interval and the risk for life threatening arrhythmias increases with length of QTc.

Long QT syndrome can be congenital or acquired. Congenital long QT syndrome is usually due to inherited channelopathies. Acquired form of long QT syndrome as described above is caused by electrolyte abnormalities such as hypokalemia, drugs such as class IA and III antiarrhythmics, tricyclic antidepressants, phenothiazines, central nervous system lesions, and severe bradyarrhythmias.

Patients with long QT syndrome may present with syncope, however sudden death may the initial manifestation in pediatric patients. High risk factors for sudden death in patients with long QT syndrome include family history of sudden death and prior history of syncopal episodes.

In patients with idiopathic long QT syndrome, stress testing, electrocardiographic monitoring during various stimuli such as auditory stimuli, psychological stress, sudden exposure to cold valsalva maneuver can all be helpful to determine the risk of life threatening arrhythmias. ECG should be obtained for all family members in the presence of symptoms in the proband.

Tdp often develops during bradycardia in patients with acquired forms of long QT syndrome.

Idiopathic long QT syndrome patients, who are asymptomatic, have no family history of sudden cardiac death, and QTc shorter than 500ms need no therapy, however beta-blockers are generally recommended.

Patients with above risk factors but no syncopal episodes or aborted sudden death should be treated with beta-blockers.

Patients with syncope and aborted sudden death require ICD implantation. These patients should also be treated with beta-blockers.

Patients who continue to have symptoms despite maximal therapy can be treated with left sided cervicothoracic sympathetic ganglionectomy.

For treatment of *Tdp* from acquired long QT syndrome, refer to the discussion above.

13.5 Short QT syndrome

QT interval less than 350 ms at heart rates less then 100 beats/min is generally accepted as short QT interval. Short QT interval syndrome is an inherited disorder due to gain of function mutations in the genes that are responsible for long QT syndrome. It is associated with increased risk of ventricular fibrillation and sudden death. Patients are also predisposed to development of AF. In patients with short QT interval, high-risk features include history of syncope, family history of sudden death, palpitations, or AF. Reversible causes of short QT interval such as hyeprcalcemia, hyperthermia, and digitalis need to be excluded before making the diagnosis. ICDs are the treatment of choice in symptomatic patients with short QT syndrome. Antiarrhythmic agents such as quinidine have been found to be effective (20).

14. Idiopathic ventricular tachycardia and ventricular fibrillation

Idiopathic VT is a monomorphic VT occurring in patients with no structural heart disease. There are three distinct forms - outflow tract VT, annular VT, and fascicular VT. Prognosis for these patients is good and they are often amenable to ablation.

Idiopathic ventricular fibrillation occurs in less than 10 % cases of out of hospital cardiac arrest. Association with early repolarization has been suggested in some studies (21). Recurrences can occur and ICD implantation is the treatment of choice. It can occur due to short-coupled PVCs in which case ablation of PVC might be helpful to prevent recurrences.

14.1 Bidirectional ventricular tachycardia

It is characterized by QRS complexes with right bundle branch block pattern with alternating polarity and regular rhythm. It occurs in patients with digitalis toxicity and CPVT. In patients with digitalis excess, digoxin-binding antibodies should be given in addition to antiarrhythmic therapy such as lidocaine or phenytoin.

15. Bundle branch reentrant ventricular tachycardia

It is reentrant tachycardia due to a circuit established over the bundle branches or fascicles. It results in monomorphic sustained VT and is usually seen in patients with structural heart disease. Therapy is similar to other types of VT. Pace termination is effective in acute setting and radiofrequency ablation is effective in elimination of VT.

15.1 Ventricular flutter and ventricular fibrillation

Ventricular flutter is characterized by regular large oscillations occurring at a rate of 150 -300 beats/min where as ventricular fibrillation is characterized by irregular undulations of varying amplitude and contour (Fig 9).

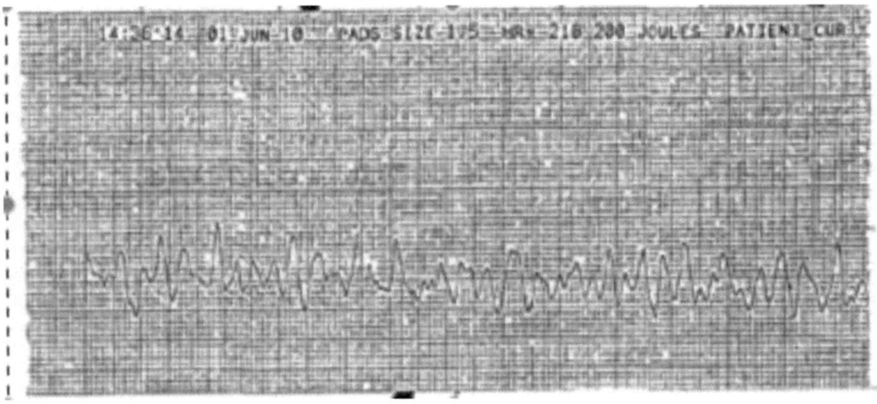

Fig. 9. Ventricular fibrillation

15.2 Clinical features

VT often precedes ventricular fibrillation; however it is not a rule. It is most commonly caused by coronary artery disease. Other causes include hypoxia, and antiarrhythmic drug therapy. It may occur during pace termination of VT that may degenerate into ventricular fibrillation.

Patients with ventricular fibrillation present with fainting episode, syncope, loss of consciousness, apnea and if the corrective measures are not taken, the event is fatal within 3-5 minutes.

15.3 Prognosis

Poor prognostic factors in resuscitated patients from ventricular fibrillation include decreased left ventricular ejection fraction, regional wall motion abnormalities, congestive heart failure, presence myocardial infarction in absence of an acute event and patients with anterior myocardial infarction complicated by ventricular fibrillation. Overall, prognosis of resuscitated patients from ventricular fibrillation patients is better than those presenting with asystole.

15.4 Management

There are three components to management of patients with sudden cardiac arrest from ventricular fibrillation - immediate resuscitation, search for etiology of the event and prevention of recurrence.

First of all, immediate resuscitative measures should be undertaken in patients with sudden cardiac arrest as per the advanced life support guidelines. The key to better outcome and survival in patients with ventricular fibrillation is early defibrillation. Nonsynchronized direct current shock (defibrillation) using 200 to 400 Joules is usually adequate. The shock energy required is low if defibrillation is done early.

After patients are stabilized, further evaluation should be directed towards the etiology of the event and correcting it if possible (such as correction of ischemia, or electrolyte abnormalities).

Pharmacologic approaches to prevent recurrences include intravenous administration of antiarrhythmic agents such as amiodarone, lidocaine or procainamide. Amiodarone tends to be the most effective of all. Pharmacologic approaches for prevention of recurrences should be used until the etiology of the event is identified. Patients with continued risk of VT or VF should be offered ICD placement if the etiology of the event is irreversible.

16. References

[1] Brady PA, Low PA, Shen WK. Inappropriate sinus tachycardia, postural orthostatic tachycardia syndrome, and overlapping syndromes. Pacing Clin Electrophysiol 2005; 28:1112 - 1121

[2] Gage BF, Waterman AD, Shannon W, et al. Validation of clinical classification schemes for predicting stroke: results from the National Registry of Atrial Fibrillation. JAMA 2001; 285:2864-70

[3] Nieuwlaat R, Dinh T, Olsson SB, et al. Should we abandon the common practice of withholding oral anticoagulation in paroxysmal atrial fibrillation? Eur Heart J 2008 29:915-22

[4] Lip GY, Edwards SJ. Stroke prevention with aspirin, warfarin and ximelagatran in patients with non-valvular atrial fibrillation: A systematic review and meta-analysis. Thromb Res 2006; 118:321 - 33

[5] van Walraven C, Hart RG, Wells GA et al. A clinical prediction rule to identify patients with atrial fibrillation and a low risk for stroke while taking aspirin. Arch Intern Med 2003; 163:936-43

[6] Oden A, Fahlen M, Hart RG. Optimal INR for prevention of stroke and death in atrial fibrillation: A critical appraisal. Thromb Res 2006; 117:493-9

[7] Mant J, Hobbs FD, Fletcher K, et al. Warfarin versus aspirin for stroke prevention in an elderly community population with atrial fibrillation (the Birmingham Atrial Fibrillation Treatment of the Aged, BAFTA): A randomized controlled trial. Lancet 2007; 370; 493-503

[8] Connolly SJ, Ezekowitz MD, Yusuf S, et al. Dabigatran versus warfarin in patients with atrial fibrillation. N Engl J Med 2009; 361:1139-51

[9] Wyse DG, Waldo AL, DiMarco JP, et al. A comparison of rate control and rhythm control in patients with atrial fibrillation. N Engl J Med 2002; 347:1825-33

[10] Cox JL, Boineau JP, Schuessler RB, et al. Electrophysiologic basis, surgical development, and clinical results of the maze procedure for atrial flutter and atrial fibrillation. Adv Card Surg 1995; 6:1-67

[11] Chow T, Kerelakes DJ, Bartone C, et al. Prognostic utility of microvolt T-wave alternans in risk stratification of patients with ischemic cardiomyopathy. J Am Coll Cardiol 2006; 47: 1820-7

[12] Buxton AE, Lee KL, DiCarlo L, et al. Electrophysiologic testing to identify patients with coronary artery disease who are at risk for sudden death. Multicenter Unsustained Tachycardia Trial Investigators. N Engl J Med 2000; 342(26): 1937-45

[13] Moss AJ, Hall WJ, Cannom DS, et al. Improved survival with an implanted defibrillator in patients with coronary disease at high risk for ventricular arrhythmia. Multicenter Automatic Defibrillator Implantation Trial Investigators. N Engl J Med 1996; 335(26): 1933-40.

[14] Moss AJ, Zareba W, Hall WJ, et al. Prophylactic implantation of a defibrillator in patients with myocardial infarction and reduced ejection fraction. N Engl J Med 2002; 346(12): 877-83

[15] Bardy GH, Lee KL, Mark DB, et al. Amiodarone or an implantable cardioverter-defibrillator for congestive heart failure. N Engl J Med. 2005; 352(3): 225-37

[16] Singh SN, Fletcher RD, Fisher SG, et al. Amiodarone in patients with congestive heart failure and asymptomatic ventricular arrhythmia. N Engl J Med 1995; 333(2): 77-82

[17] The Antiarrhythmics versus Implantable Defibrillators (AVID) Investigators. A comparison of antiarrhythmic-drug therapy with implantable defibrillators in patients resuscitated from near-fatal ventricular arrhythmias. N Engl J Med1997; 337(22): 1576-8

[18] Connolly SJ, Gent M, Roberts RS, et al. Canadian implantable defibrillator study (CIDS): a randomized trial of the implantable cardioverter defibrillator against amiodarone. Circulation2000; 101(11): 1297-302

[19] The CASCADE Investigators. Randomized antiarrhythmic drug therapy in survivors of cardiac arrest (the CASCADE Study). Am J Cardiol. 1993; 72(3): 280-7

[20] Gaita F, Giustetto C, Bianchi F, et al. Short QT syndrome: pharmacological treatment. J Am Coll Cardiol. 2004; 43(8): 1494-9.

[21] Haissaguerre M, Derval N, Sacher F, et al. Sudden cardiac arrest associated with early repolarization. N Engl J Med. 2008; 358(19): 2016-23

4

Ryanodine Receptor Channelopathies: The New Kid in the Arrhythmia Neighborhood

María Fernández-Velasco[1], Ana María Gómez[2], Jean-Pierre Benitah[2] and Patricia Neco[2]

[1]*Instituto de Investigacion Hospital La Paz, IdiPAZ, Madrid*

[2]*Inserm, Univ. Paris-Sud 11, IFR141, Labex Lermit, Châtenay-Malabry,*

[1]*Spain*

[2]*France*

1. Introduction

Cardiac arrhythmia is a major mortality cause in both acquired and inherited cardiomyopathy, accounting for more than 750.000 deaths per year (~ 0.1% of total recorded deaths) in Europe and the USA (Priori SG, 2002). The 2008 WHO rapport has foreseen that cardiovascular disease will be the world leading death cause in the near future, surpassing infectious diseases.

Some of these cardiac diseases are acquired as cardiac hypertrophy, which develops as an adaptation of the heart to diseases that challenge the heart work chronically. Cardiac hypertrophy often degenerates in heart failure (HF), the final outcome of most cardiovascular diseases. Chronic HF prevalence is increasing in western countries, with only 25% of men and 38% of women surviving 5 years after the onset of clinical signs. Quality of life is hampered by the reduced pump function, which can also lead to death. However, half of deceases in HF patients are sudden due to cardiac arrhythmia. During cardiac pathology, altered activity of the cardiac, type 2, ryanodine receptor (RyR2) may generate arrhythmia and sudden death. This risk is high in HF where there is a profound remodeling of Ca^{2+} cycling, and alterations in transmembrane Ca^{2+} influx, Ca^{2+} release or/and sarcoplasmic reticulum (SR) Ca^{2+}-load underlie systolic dysfunction (Gómez *et al.*, 1997; Bénitah JP, 2002). Thus, when dealing with HF and poor cardiac outcomes, it is a need to better understand the mechanisms of cardiac arrhythmia in order to efficiently treat these patients. However, a large number of inherited arrhythmogenic syndromes that cause sudden death have been characterised. Some are associated with structural heart disease, such as familial hypertrophic cardiomyopathy and arrythmogenic right ventricular cardiomyopathy type 2 (ARVD2). Others do not produce structural heart disease and so are difficult to detect. Most of these cardiomyopathies are due to mutations in plasmalemmal cardiac ion channels, mainly the Na^{+} channel and several K^{+} channels (Lehnart *et al.*, 2007). These mutations promote arrhythmogenesis by altering the action potential (AP) duration, which therefore may enhance the propensity of arrhythmic activity via the development of early after depolarizations (EADs). However, the recent finding of mutations in the Ca^{2+} release channel (RyR2) associated with catecholaminergic polymorphic ventricular tachycardia

(CPVT) and ARVD2 has opened a new view of arrhythmogenesis, evidencing that alterations in intracellular Ca^{2+} cycling can generate arrhythmia (Priori SG, 2001). CPVT is a familial arrhythmogenic disorder characterised by syncopal events and Sudden Cardiac Death occurring in children and young adults during physical stress or emotion in the absence of structural heart disease. In addition to the severe phenotype, CPVT exhibits a cumulative mortality of 30 - 50% by 35 years. To date, more than 145 RyR2 mutations have been identified as causative of CPVT in affected individuals, which appear clustered in 3 "hot spots". Some of these mutations have been investigated in several *in vitro* systems (lipid bilayers, HEK293 cells, HL1-cardiomyocytes), suggesting that CPVT-linked RyR2 mutations produced an increase of the RyR2 activity, termed as RyR2 Ca^{2+} leakage, under beta-adrenergic stimulation (Lehnart *et al.*, 2004). This abnormal SR Ca^{2+} release during diastole would activate the Na^{+}-Ca^{2+} exchanger (NCX) to extrude Ca^{2+} out of the cell. Since NCX is electrogenic, a net inward current is generated for each Ca^{2+} ion extruded, which could develop delayed after depolarizations (DADs) and evoke triggered activity if they reach threshold. This abnormality may promote arrhythmogenesis in CPVT patients, where the increased RyR2 activity may generate DADs through the activation of NCX (Nakajima *et al.*, 1997). This mechanism is interestingly very similar to the one that has been suggested in HF, where chronic hyperadrenergic state generates an inadequate diastolic Ca^{2+} release (Ca^{2+} leak) and SR Ca^{2+} depletion, leading to a decreased myocardial contractility. Recently, Priori's laboratory has developed a knock-in mouse model carrying a highly penetrant R4496C mutation in the RyR2 (equivalent to the human R4497C mutation), identified in an Italian family with CPVT. Previous reports have shown that these mice developed bidirectional and polymorphic ventricular tachycardia under the injection of isoproterenol (β-adrenergic agonist) and caffeine (Cerrone *et al.*, 2005). Interestingly, the presence of DADs was detected after high pacing rates and under the application of isoproterenol, in isolated ventricular myocytes (Liu *et al.*, 2006). Our laboratory has also performed experiments using this mouse model and, in addition to other findings, we observed abnormal cytosolic Ca^{2+} release and spontaneous triggering activity, in ventricular myocytes paced at high rates or treated with isoproterenol (Fernandez-Velasco M, et al 2009). In this chapter, we will review the latest knowledge on the role of intracellular Ca^{2+} on cardiac arrhythmia in acquired and inherited diseases, paying special attention to the molecular and cellular mechanisms of the disease.

2. Involvement of RyR in cardiac arrhythmias

The cardiac RyR is the major Ca^{2+} release channel in the ventricle and it is central in activating contraction by the mechanism of Ca^{2+} -induced Ca^{2+} release during the excitation-contraction process. It is located in the membrane of the SR, mainly in the junctional SR, facing the L-type Ca^{2+} channels located in the membrane invaginations termed trasverse tubules. During cardiac excitation-contraction coupling (ECC), the membrane depolarization during the AP activates Ca^{2+} influx via sarcolemmal L-type Ca^{2+} channels, providing enough Ca^{2+} to activate the RyR (Fabiato, 1983; Bers, 2002). By this mechanism, the initial Ca^{2+} signal is greatly amplified, then providing enough Ca^{2+} for contraction. Relaxation occurs when calcium is removed from cytosol, mainly by NCX and SR Ca^{2+}-ATPase (SERCA). The sarcolemmal Ca^{2+} ATPase, different from SERCA, can also extrude some Ca^{2+}. However, its contribution appears to be minor (about 3% of total Ca^{2+} removal) and its physiological significance has yet to be determined. For equilibrium to occur, the amount of Ca^{2+} extruded through the NCX should be equivalent to the amount of Ca^{2+} entering the cell through DHPRs, and the amount of Ca^{2+}

transported by SERCA should be equivalent to Ca^{2+} released by the SR. For each Ca^{2+} extruded, the NCX enters 3 Na^{+}, generating thus an inward current. In cases of Ca^{2+} overload, spontaneous SR Ca^{2+} release through RyRs produces Ca^{2+} waves, activating transient inward currents (Iti), (Berlin *et al.*, 1989) which if they reach threshold may trigger an action potential (triggered activity). The NCX is centrally involved in this current (Venetucci *et al.*, 2007). Triggered activity-derived arrhythmias are produced by after depolarizations that can occur early during the repolarization phase of the action potential (early after depolarization, EAD) or late, after completion of the repolarization phase (delayed after depolarization, DAD) (Figure 1). When either type of after depolarization is large enough to reach the threshold potential for activation of a regenerative inward current, a new AP is generated, which is named as triggered activity.

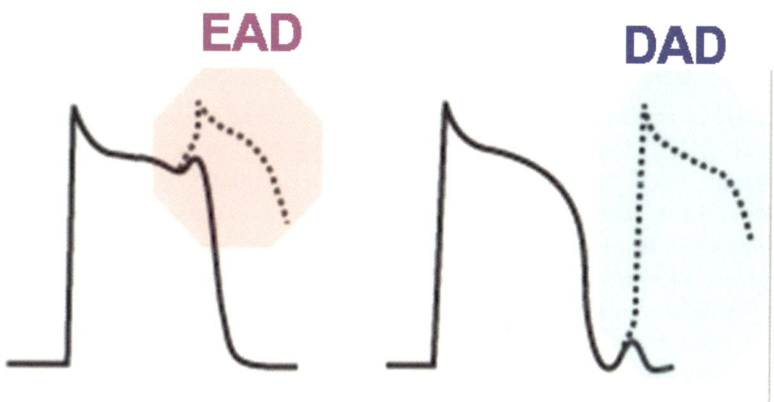

Fig. 1. Example of an early after depolarization (EAD) and delayed after depolarization (DAD) leading to triggered activity.

3. Involvement of RyR in cardiac arrhythmias in the hypertrophied and failing heart

Half of the deaths in heart failure patients are due to sudden death and cardiac hypertrophy has also an elevated risk of sudden death, which may arise as a consequence of ventricular arrhythmia. The ventricular cardiomyocytes of these hearts are prolonged, which favors the occurrence of early EADs. EADs are believed to be dependent on the L-type Ca^{2+} channel. DADs are common of Ca^{2+} overloaded cells, which is uncommon in heart failure. However, the RyR activity is altered, which may favor DADs. Several modifications that happen in the RyR of the failing hearts have been shown to promote diastolic Ca^{2+} leak and be arrhythmogenic. These modulations include phosphorylation (PKA and/or CaMKII), oxidation, decreased nitrosylation, lost of its accessory protein FKBP12.6 (calstabin 2) and unzipping. However, the RyR leakiness would not be enough to provoke arrhythmia, because it should be compensated by the reduction in SR Ca^{2+} load (Venetucci *et al.*, 2008). Hyperphosphorylation of RyR by PKA was found in humans at end stage heart failure and different models of heart failure (Marx *et al.*, 2000; Reiken *et al.*, 2003) and related to sudden death (Marks, 2001), although controversed (Jiang *et al.*, 2002). RyR phosphorylation increases activity of RyR, making RyR leaky and thus favoring arrhythmia. The RyR is also hyperphosphorylated at the CaMKII site (Ai *et al.*, 2005) during heart failure, which may be involved in the propensity to arrhythmias. In this sense, CaMKII blockade repressed the spontaneous Ca^{2+} waves in heart failure cardiomyocytes (Curran *et al.*).

RyR phosphorylation in heart failure has been suggested to unbind the RyR from its regulatory protein, the FKBP12.6 (Marx *et al.*, 2000). While the direct correlation with phosphorylation is a matter of debate (Maier *et al.*, 2003; Blayney *et al.*, 2010), the cardiac expression of FKBP12.6 is reduced in heart failure, causing diastolic Ca^{2+} leak that may result in higher propensity of DADs and consequent triggered arrhythmias (Shou *et al.*, 1998; Yano *et al.*, 2000; Reiken *et al.*, 2001; Xin *et al.*, 2002; Wehrens *et al.*, 2004; Ai *et al.*, 2005; Wehrens *et al.*, 2005; Yano *et al.*, 2005; Huang *et al.*, 2006; Yano *et al.*, 2006; Gomez *et al.*, 2009). Supporting the role of FKBP12.6 in arrhythmia, stabilizing FKBP12.6 binding to RyR by FKBP12.6 overexpression prevents triggered arrhythmias in normal hearts, probably by reducing diastolic SR Ca^{2+} leakage (Gellen *et al.*, 2008). Conversely, FKBP12.6 knockouts exhibited exercise induced ventricular arrhythmia (Wehrens *et al.*, 2003).

Other alterations during heart failure may affect RyR function. In this sense, RyR oxidation in a canine model of sudden death are involved in arrythmogenic $[Ca^{2+}]_i$ transients alternans (Belevych *et al.*, 2009). Moreover, the increase in xantine oxidase activity also reduces the level of S-nytrosilation. The RyR hyponitrosylation has also been involved in the Ca^{2+} leak from SR in experimental heart failure (Gonzalez *et al.*, 2010). This alteration might contribute to the arrhythmogenesis in heart failure. In this sense, it has been shown that NOS1-/- mice show RyR hyponitrosylation with consequent SR Ca^{2+} leak and an arrhythmic phenotype, without altering the FKBP12.6 stoichiometry (Gonzalez *et al.*, 2007). Consistent with these findings, NOS1 overexpression protected the mice in a model of heart failure by preserving Ca^{2+} cycling (Loyer *et al.*, 2008). However, others have found that RyR is hypernitrosilated in a model of muscular dystrophy, where arrhythmias are frequent, suggesting that hypernytrosilated RyR is leaky. It should be noted that in this model the binding to FKBP12.6 was also decreased (Fauconnier *et al.*, 2010), which may account for the RyR leakiness.

The N and central domains of the RyR interact with each other in a process called "zipping", which stabilizes the channel in its closed state (Ikemoto & Yamamoto, 2002). In heart failure, the RyR is unzipped favoring its phosphorylation and unbinding to FKBP12.6 (Oda *et al.*, 2005).

Besides these direct alterations of the RyR, this channel may be "sensitized" in some conditions by an increase in the local $[Ca^{2+}]$ around it, from either side of the SR membrane. In this sense, the increase in the IP3R expression in the junctional SR during heart failure might, under certain circumstances, locally increase the $[Ca^{2+}]_i$ in the neighboring RyRs and facilitate Ca^{2+} waves propagation (Harzheim *et al.*, 2009). Increasing the $[Ca^{2+}]_i$ in the luminal side, as by an increase in SERCA activity, might also sensitize the RyR and participate in Ca^{2+} waves formation (Keller *et al.*, 2007) although SERCA activity is thought to be depressed in heart failure.

4. Involvement of RyR in inherited cardiac arrhythmias

4.1 Catecholaminergic polymorphic ventricular tachycardia

CPVT is a rare arrhythmogenic disease characterized by exercise or stress induced ventricular tachyarrhythmia, syncope, or sudden death that appear in individuals with structural normal hearts (Leenhardt *et al.*, 1995; Coumel, 1997; Priori *et al.*, 2002). Because the electrocardiogram (ECG) of CPVT patients is unremarkable under basal conditions, the diagnosis is established in symptoms and the detection of stress-induced arrhythmias during exercise test or Holter recording. Although some CPVT patients develop polymorphic ventricular tachycardia (VT), the bidirectional VT is considered the diagnostic marker of CPVT (Priori *et al.*, 2002). Interestingly, bidirectional VT occurs during digitalis intoxication, where the Na^+/K^+ ATPase pump is inhibited, increasing the intracellular Na^+ concentration that in turn, by NCX induces an intracellular Ca^{2+} overload, triggering arrhythmogenic DADs (Rosen & Danilo, 1980). Thus, it was reasonable to postulate that bidirectional VT in CPVT patients can be due to changes in the intracellular calcium handling. Indeed, several reports have associated CPVT with mutations in genes encoding key-proteins involved in the control of intracellular calcium handling, such as RyR2 and calsequestrin (CASQ2), causative of CPVT1 and CPVT2, respectively (Lahat *et al.*, 2001a; Priori *et al.*, 2002).

4.2 RyR2 mutations in CPVT

The gene encoding RyR2 (chromosome 1q42.1–43) consists of 105 exons, which encodes 4967 amino acids (~560 kDa) and it is one of the largest and most intricate in the human genome. The RyR2 is a homotetramer with hydrophobic segments of the four identical subunits forming a central Ca^{2+} pore (Wagenknecht, 1989). Currently more than 145 RyR2 mutations have been reported as causative of CPVT, and they continue growing since the first mutations was reported a decade ago (Priori SG, 2001) - an updated database is shown in the 'Gene connection for the heart' website (http://www.fsm.it/cardmoc/). Some of these RyR2 mutations have been identified in patient groups screened for Long QT syndrome (Tester DJ, 2005), and ARVD2 (Tiso *et al.*, 2001). CPVT-related arrhythmias are by far reproduced during an exercise stress test, by isoproterenol infusion, or by other forms of adrenergic stimulation (Sumitomo *et al.*, 2003; Vyas *et al.*, 2006). A genetic screening of RyR2 is necessary to verify the disease in patients suspicious of CPVT1, although this strategy is time consuming and expensive. However, screening for RyR2 mutations could be simplified due to the circumstance that CPVT mutations used to cluster in certain exons, and a tiered scan of these exons can be used to lower the cost (Medeiros-Domingo A, 2009). RyR2 mutations linked to CPVT are clustered into 3 discrete protein regions or "hot spots": N-terminus (32%), central domain (30%) and C-terminus (38%) (Yano *et al.*, 2006; George CH, 2007). Similar mutation clustering is observed in the *RYR1* gene, which encodes the skeletal muscle RyR1 and is linked to malignant hyperthermia and central core disease (Dirksen, 2002). The N-terminus (also called domain I: amino acids 77-466) is a domain particularly susceptible to conformational change. It contains the cytoplasmic loop, which it is postulated that interacts with the central domain (zipping) stabilizing RyR2 activity during diastole (Yamamoto T, 2000). The central domain (domain II: amino acids 2246-2534) contains an FKBP12.6 binding domain (1636–1937) and it is supposed to interact with the N-terminus domain (zipping-unzipping). The C-terminus domain (domain III: amino acids 3778-4201 and domain IV: amino acids 4497 to 4959) contains the transmembrane regions of the Ca^{2+} channel and an hydrophobic region which it is postulated to transduce cytoplasmic events to regulate the Ca^{2+} pore forming domain (George CH., 2006). Only a small number of mutations are located in regions of RyR2 outside these portions. By contrast to other channelopathies, most of the RyR2 mutations described in CPVT are single nucleotide replacements ("point mutations") leading to an amino acid substitution.

4.3 Functional alterations of CPVT related mutations in the RyR

Although the phenotypic manifestation of CPVT is usually the stress-induced development of bidirectional or polymorphic ventricular tachycardia, patient symptoms are heterogeneous, presenting in some cases high variability among affected subjects within the same family (d'Amati & King, 2005). However in other cases, patients with point mutations located in the same RyR2 cluster present similar CPVT symptoms, probably because they affect RyR2 function in a common way. To improve the current knowledge of RyR2 complexity and to provide an adequate treatment to CPVT patients, it is necessary to study the molecular mechanisms of all sudden cardiac death (SCD)-linked mutations screened. A number of studies on them have been undertaken. Most of them have been analyzed in heterologous systems, but some transgenic mice have been constructed, allowing the exploration of the cardiac function.

CPVT-linked mutations have been expressed in various heterologous systems (lipid bilayer, HEK293 cells, HL1-cardiomyocytes). Specifically, HEK293 cells (human embryonic kidney cell line) have been widely used as an expression system. This cell line presents some weak points such as it lacks ECC proteins and the contractile machinery that characterizes heart cells. However, it presents several advantages: 1) it is easy to transfect using conventional methods and, 2) as it does not express native RyR, they cannot interfere with expressed constructs.

Some human N-terminus mutations (R176Q/T2504M and L433P), central domain mutations (S2246L and R2474S), and C-terminus mutations (N4104K, Q4201R, R4496C, I4867M and N4895D) have been explored using HEK293 cells. These RyR2 mutations showed an increased frequency of spontaneous Ca^{2+} oscillations and a reduced Ca^{2+} store content, thus displaying gain-of-function (Jiang *et al.*, 2004; Jiang D, 2005). In addition, most mutated RyR2 incorporated into lipid bilayers displayed an increased sensitivity to luminal Ca^{2+}, although the two N-terminus mutants were 10-fold less sensitive than the others (Jiang D, 2005). However, some RyR2 mutants displayed an increased sensitivity to cytosolic Ca^{2+} and caffeine. This is the case for S2246L, N4104K and R4497C mutations expressed in HEK293 cells or HL-1 cells, where it was also shown a gain-of-function RyR2 activity, while there was no change in SR Ca^{2+} load (George CH., 2006). In some cases, differences in RyR2 mutants' response to agonists are closely dependent on the mutational locus. This may be the case of a report from Thomas and coworkers, who have observed marked differences in caffeine-dependent Ca^{2+} release in N-terminal and central domain ARVD2-linked RyR2 mutations (L433P, N2386I and R176Q/T2504M) (Thomas *et al.*, 2004; George CH & .2005). Interestingly, one of these 3 mutations (L433P) was not associated with gain-of-function, but rather with loss-of-function (George CH & . 2005).

It is of note that the characterization of RyR2 mutations according to the mutational locus may be of large interest because this permits to design a model which integrates domain-specific arrhythmogenic mechanisms. The result model could extrapolate how new mutations may affect RyR2 function, allowing for a common therapy that restores channel activity. Table 1 shows a classification of SCD-linked mutations characterized so far.

Location in RyR2	Mutation	Disease	Characterization	System	RyR2 defect
N-Terminal	R176Q	ARVD / SUO	Enhanced SOICR increased sensitivity to luminal Ca^{2+} (Jiang D, 2005); R176Q/T2504M increase caffeine-dependent sensibility to cytosolic Ca2+ (Thomas, 2005); myocytes elicited oscillatory Ca^{2+} signals under β-adrenergic stimulation. (Kannankeril *et al.*, 2006)	HEK293 Lipid bilayers Knock-in mice	Gain-of-function
N-Terminal	E189D	CPVT	Increases the propensity of SOICR and enhance caffeine sensitivity. (Jiang D, 2010)	HEK293	Gain-of-function
N-Terminal	G230C	CPVT	Increased sensibility to cytosolic Ca^{2+}, decreased FKBP-12.6 binding (Meli, 2011)	HEK293 Lipid bilayers	Gain-of-function
N-Terminal	L433P	ARVD	Enhanced SOICR, increased sensitivity to luminal Ca^{2+} (Jiang D, 2005)	HEK293 Lipid bilayers	Gain-of-function
			Decrease caffeine-dependent, sensibility to cytosolic Ca^{2+} (Thomas, 2005), desensitized response to caffeine (Thomas *et al.*, 2004)	HEK293	Loss-of-function
Cytoplasmic loop	G1885E	ARVC	Enhanced SOICR, reduced RyR2 activity in G1885E/G1886S double mutant. (Koop, 2008)	HEK293	Gain-of-function
Cytoplasmic loop	G1886S	ARVC	Enhanced SOICR, reduced RyR2 activity in G1885E/G1886S double mutant. (Koop, 2008)	HEK293	Gain-of-function
Cytoplasmic loop	S2246L	CPVT/IVF	PKA-dependent increased RyR2 activity (Wehrens *et al.*, 2003); PKA and caffeine-dependent increased RyR2 activity (George *et al.*, 2003);abnormal domain interaction (George CH., 2006);enhanced SOICR, increased sensitivity to luminal Ca2+ (Jiang *et al.*, 2004)	HEK293 Lipid bilayers CHO HL-1	Gain-of-function
Cytoplasmic loop	R2267H	CPVT	PKA-dependent increased sensitivity to cytosolic Ca^{2+} (Tester, 2007)	HEK293 Lipid bilayers	Gain-of-function
FKBP binding dom.	P2328S	CPVT	Decreased FKBP-12.6 binding, PKA-dependent increased RyR2 activity (Lehnart *et al.*, 2004)	HEK293 Lipid bilayers	Gain-of-function
FKBP binding dom.	N2386I	ARVD	Increase caffeine-dependent, sensibility to low cytosolic Ca2+ (Thomas, 2005)	HEK293	Gain-of-function

Location in RyR2	Mutation	Disease	Characterization	System	RyR2 defect
FKBP binding dom	R2474S	CPVT	Enhanced SOICR, increased sensitivity to luminal Ca^{2+} (Jiang D, 2004); (Wehrens *et al.*, 2003); abnormal zipping-unzipping interaction, increase caffeine-dependent, sensibility to cytosolic Ca^{2+} (Yang, 2006); increased frequency of spontaneous Ca^{2+} transients and increased sensitivity to luminal Ca^{2+} mediated by defective interdomain interaction. (Uchinoumi *et al.*, 1998)	HEK293 Lipid bilayers Permeabilized myocytes from rats Knock-in mice	Gain-of-function
FKBP binding dom.	T2504M	ARVD	R176Q/T2504M increase caffeine-dependent sensibility to cytosolic Ca^{2+} (Thomas, 2005); R176Q/T2504M enhance SOICR and increase sensitivity to luminal Ca^{2+} (Jiang D, 2005)	HEK293 Lipid bilayers	Gain-of-function
TM Domain	N4104K	CPVT	PKA and caffeine-dependent increased RyR2 activity (George *et al.*, 2003); abnormal I domain interaction (George CH., 2006); enhanced SOICR (Jiang D, 2005); increased sensitivity to luminal Ca2+ (Jiang D, 2004)	HEK293 Lipid bilayers CHO HL-1	Gain-of-function
TM Domain	Q4201R	CPVT	Ehanced SOICR, increased sensitivity to luminal Ca^{2+} (Jiang D, 2005); decreased FKBP-12.6 binding, PKA-dependent increased RyR2 activity (Lehnart *et al.*, 2004)	HEK293 Lipid bilayers	Gain-of-function
TM Domain	R4497C	CPVT	PKA-dependent increased RyR2 activity (Wehrens *et al.*, 2003); PKA and caffeine-dependent increased RyR2 activity (George *et al.*, 2003); abnormal I domain interaction (Uchinoumi *et al.*, 1998); enhanced SOICR (Jiang D, 2005); increased sensitivity to luminal Ca2+ (Jiang *et al.*, 2004); increased sensitivity to low cytosolic Ca^{2+}, caffeine-dependent increased RyR2 (Jiang *et al.*, 2002); Increased sensitivity to cytosolic Ca^{2+} , triggering activity in ventricular myocytes in presence of high pacing rate and isoproterenol. (Fernandez-Velasco *et al.*, 2009)	HEK-293 Lipid bilayer CHO HL-1 Knock-in ce	Gain-of-function

Location in RyR2	Mutation	Disease	Characterization	System	RyR2 defect
TM Domain	V4653F	CPVT	Decreased FKBP-12.6 binding, PKA-dependent increased RyR2 activity (Lehnart *et al.*, 2004); Increased sensitivity to cytosolic Ca^{2+} (Tester, 2007)	HEK293 Lipid bilayers	gain-of-function
TM Domain	A4860G	IVF	Reduced sensitivity to luminal Ca^{2+}, reduced SOICR activity (Jiang D, 2007)	HEK293 Lipid bilayers	Loss-of-function
C-term	I4867M	CPVT	Enhanced SOICR, increased sensitivity to luminal Ca^{2+} (Jiang D, 2005)	HEK293 Lipid bilayers	Gain-of-function
C-term	N4895D	CPVT	Enhanced SOICR, increased sensitivity to luminal Ca^{2+} (Jiang D, 2004)	HEK293 Lipid bilayers	Gain-of-function

Table 1. RyR2 mutations linked to SCD disease characterized so far. Amino acid mutations are listed in order according to the mutational locus. CPVT=Catecholaminergic Polymorphic Ventricular Tachycardia; ARVD=Arrhythmogenic Right Ventricular Dysplasia; IVF = Idiopathic Ventricular Fibrillation induced by emotion or exercise. TM = Transmembrane domain; SUO = syncope of unknown origin;; SOICR = Store-operated induced- Ca2+ release; HEK293 = Human embrionic kidney cell line; CHO = Chinese hamster ovary cell line; HL-1 = cardiac myocyte cell line.

Because animal's models can contribute to the better understanding of the molecular mechanisms involved in the arrhythmogenic disease, transgenic mice models that harbor some of the most important RyR2 mutations observed in CPVT patients were developed (Uchinoumi *et al.*, ; Cerrone *et al.*, 2005; Kannankeril *et al.*, 2006).

These animals mimic several of the abnormal electrical events observed in CPVT subjects. Indeed, delayed after depolarization (DADs) and triggered activity have been detected in knock-in models of CPVT (Liu *et al.*, 2006). It has been proven by different authors that cardiac myocytes isolated from CPVT models show abnormal diastolic Ca^{2+} release (Ca^{2+} leak) as Ca^{2+} sparks and/or Ca^{2+} waves, which may conduce to arrhythmia by DADs (Uchinoumi *et al.*, ; Kannankeril *et al.*, 2006; Fernandez-Velasco *et al.*, 2009).

One mice model that harbor RyR2 (R2474S) mutation leading to CPVT upon exercise and β-adrenergic stimulation was developed by Lehnart et al., (Lehnart *et al.*, 2008). Cardiomyocytes isolated from R2474S mice exhibited abnormal calcium diastolic leak, calcium waves, APs and inward currents upon isoproterenol treatment. Tonic-clonic seizures were identified in these mice, consistent with the neurological dysfunction including epilepic seizures detected in CPVT patients (Leenhardt *et al.*, 1995; Postma *et al.*, 2005; Lehnart *et al.*, 2008).

Another mechanism by which mutation can alter the calcium handling in CPVT is the disruption of protein-protein interaction. In this context, Wehrens et al., established a direct link between FKBP12.6 and CPVT process (Wehrens *et al.*, 2004). FKBP12.6 (calstabin 2) is an accessory subunit that maintains the RyR2 closed, avoiding calcium leak during diastole. Wehrens et al., proposed that CPVT mutations induce the dissociation of FKBP12.6 from RyR2 upon β-adrenergic stimulation. Therefore, this effect induces a deregulation of the

RyR2 gating, increasing the calcium diastolic release and promoting cardiac arrhythmias by delayed after depolarizations (Marx SO, 2000). Indeed, these authors showed that the presence of different CPVT mutations decreases the affinity of FKBP12.6 binding to RyR, leading to calcium leak (Marx SO, 2000; Wehrens *et al.*, 2003; Lehnart *et al.*, 2008)}. However, these findings have not been confirmed by others groups (Tiso *et al.*, 2002; George *et al.*, 2003; Liu *et al.*, 2006; Xiao *et al.*, 2007; Guo *et al.*, 2010).

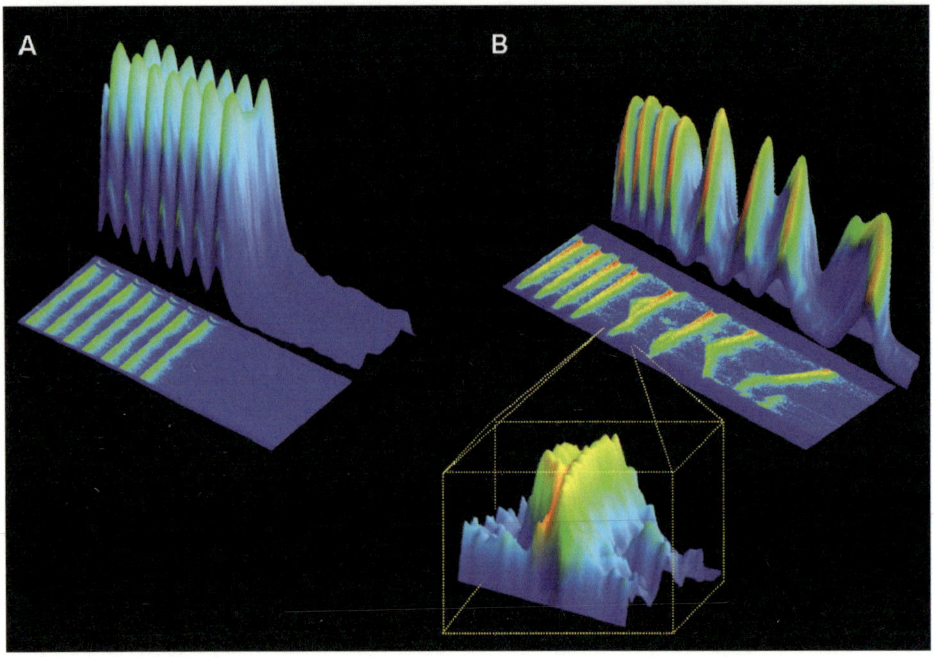

Fig. 2. Triggered activity observed in RyR2R4496C myocytes. 3D line-scan images of ventricular myocytes isolated from (A) a wild type mouse and (B) RyR^{R4496C} mouse during electrical stimulation (4Hz). RyR^{R4496C} cell shows Ca^{2+}-waves that induce consistent with DADs. Finally Matsusaki's group has described altered interdomain RyR2 interactions in CPVT (Ikemoto & Yamamoto, 2000; Tateishi *et al.*, 2009). They proposed that under physiological conditions, N and central terminal domains of RyR2 interact, maintaining the channel closed. CPVT-linked mutations in the N or central domain, causing a disruption of the interaction (domain unzipping), rendering the channel more sensitive to changes in luminal or cytosolic calcium. So, it is reasonable to hypothesize that mutations in these regions of RyR2 could affect the physiological conformational states, resulting in channel dysfunction, as occurs in CPVT (Lobo & Van Petegem, 2009; Tung *et al.*, 2010).

On the other hand, our group using a *knock-in* mice model that express R4496C mutation in the cardiac RyR2 (the equivalent mutation found in CPVT patients, R4497C) demonstrated an enhanced of Ca^{2+} sensitivity of the mutant RyR2 (Fernandez-Velasco *et al.*, 2009). This mice model mimics extraordinarily the clinical manifestations of patients presenting the RyR2R4497C mutation, including the bidirectional VT. RyR2R4496C cardiomyocytes exposed to adrenaline and caffeine developed DADs, suggesting that triggered arrhythmias are elicited by adrenergic activation (Nakajima *et al.*, 1997; Liu *et al.*, 2006). We demonstrated that untreated RyR2R4496C myocytes have increased spontaneous Ca^{2+} release in diastole during electrical pacing, due to the enhanced Ca^{2+} sensitivity of mutant RyR2; this abnormality is further augmented by exposure to isoproterenol and increasing pacing rates (Figure 2).

4.4 Mutations in calsequestrin 2 linked to CPVT

As previously mentioned, alterations in the control of Ca^{2+} release by changes in luminal calcium can induce serious disruptions in the Ca^{2+} cycling. This is what happens in the recessive form of CPVT associated with mutations in calsequestrin (CASQ2) (Eldar *et al.*, 2003). CASQ2 is a polymer with a low-affinity and high capacity of calcium binding located in the luminal side of SR (Beard *et al.*, 2004; Gyorke & Terentyev, 2008). Although it is documented that CASQ2 interacts with RyR2 via triadin and junctin, and acts as luminal calcium sensor by inhibiting RyR2 function at low luminal calcium concentration (Gyorke *et al.*, 2004; Terentyev *et al.*, 2007), the exact mechanism by which this protein exerts their function is not completely understood.

To date, 12 CASQ2-mutations and 3 non synonymous polymorphisms have been detected in CPVT subjects (http://www.fsm.it/cardmoc/). Although some of these mutations affect the protein synthesis, reducing significantly the CASQ2 expression in the heart, others induce a defective protein expression and alter the ability of SR calcium buffering (Postma *et al.*, 2002; Terentyev *et al.*, 2003; di Barletta *et al.*, 2006; Knollmann *et al.*, 2006; Terentyev *et al.*, 2006). Related to this, different authors have shown in murine cardiomyocytes and in heterologous systems, that mutants of CASQ2 including CASQ2 (L167H), CASQ2 (G112+5X), CASQ2 (R33Q), CASQ2-/- and CASQ2 (D307H) induce a deregulation of SR Ca^{2+} release, leading to arrhythmogenic DADs (Lahat *et al.*, 2001a; Lahat *et al.*, 2001b; Terentyev *et al.*, 2003; di Barletta *et al.*, 2006; Knollmann *et al.*, 2006; Terentyev *et al.*, 2006; Dirksen *et al.*, 2007). These observations are consistent with the ECG pattern observed in CPVT patients (Napolitano & Priori, 2007).

Missense and nonsense CASQ2 mutations have been reported. Regarding missense mutations, CASQ2 (D307H), CASQ2 (R33Q) and CASQ2 (L67H) have been found in CPVT subjects (Terentyev *et al.*, 2006; Kim *et al.*, 2007; Qin *et al.*, 2008; Terentyev *et al.*, 2008). These mutations alter the CASQ2 interaction with RyR2, compromising its ability to store Ca^{2+} in the SR. So far, it has been reported that there are four nonsense mutations that cause the protein to be reduced or deleted (di Barletta *et al.*, 2006). In vivo, CASQ2-/- mice exhibit CPVT with a bidirectional QRS pattern, the classic ECG feature observed in their human disease (Knollmann *et al.*, 2006).

Cellular arrhythmias were detected in cardiomyocytes expressing CASQ2 mutants under β-adrenergic stimulation (Terentyev *et al.*, 2003; di Barletta *et al.*, 2006; Dirksen *et al.*, 2007). These results are consistent with the arrhythmogenic storm elicited by the emotional or physical stress in CPVT patients.

Because there is a correlation between the spontaneous Ca^{2+} release and the DADs, the question is why the spontaneous calcium release occurs. Different approaches address that mutations in CASQ2 compromise the two principal functions described for this protein: as a SR Ca^{2+} storage site and as modulator of RyR2 activity (Kubalova *et al.*, 2005; Terentyev *et al.*, 2006; Terentyev *et al.*, 2008; Knollmann, 2009). Both mechanisms elicited an abnormal control of RyR2 by luminal Ca^{2+} required to effective termination of SR Ca^{2+} release, promoting the spontaneous Ca^{2+} release during diastole. Studies using transgenic CPVT mice models with CASQ2 mutations confirm that the underlying mechanism of ventricular arrhythmias are DADs caused by spontaneous Ca^{2+} release under adrenergic stress (Mohamed *et al.*, 2007). However, it is important to note that compensatory changes observed in the CASQ2 transgenic mice can alter the junctin and/or triadin function and may affect the manifestation of CPVT under chronic procedures. (Knollmann *et al.*, 2006; Song *et al.*, 2007).

5. Supraventricular arrhythmias in CPVT

CPVT patients often develop supraventricular arrhythmias as resting bradycardia and His-Purkinje block (Sumitomo *et al.*, 2003; Cerrone M, 2007; Sumitomo *et al.*, 2007; Kazemian P, 2011; Sy RW, 2011). Supraventricular arrhythmias (SVAs) are an important issue to underline during following-up patients with CPVT. Although the risk for SCD in CPVT patients is expected to be associated with ventricular arrhythmias, supraventricular abnormalities as sinus node dysfunction, atrioventricular block and supraventricular tachyarrhythmias result in significant increase of morbidity. Moreover, the frequent association of supraventricular arrhythmias in CPVT patients, which has been reported to precede or coexist with ventricular tachycardia, suggests that SVAs may be an important risk factor for SCD in this patient population (Sumitomo *et al.*, 2007; Sy RW, 2011). These SVAs in single point mutations of RyR2 are usually bradycardia, atrial tachycardia, atrial fibrillation and atrioventricular reentry (Sumitomo *et al.*, 2003; Sumitomo *et al.*, 2007; Kazemian P, 2011; Sy RW, 2011). Additionally, Bhuiyan and coworkers found CPVT patients from 2 unlinked families with a deletion of 35 peptides in RyR2 exon-3, who presented also SVAs (sinus bradycardia, sinus block or arrest, atrioventricular block, atrial fibrillation and atrial standstill). Interestingly, these patients also presented left ventricular dysfunction and dilatation, which are rare in CPVT patients.

Additionally, prevention of SVAs is also important in CPVT disease due to potential complications with implantable cardioverter- defibrillators (ICD) therapy. In CPVT, beta-blockers are recommended, together with exercise restraint. Despite beta-blocker therapy, ICD are implanted in patients with previous cardiac arrest, or with recurrent syncope or documented ventricular tachycardia. However, SVAs are not benign arrhythmias in patients with CPVT; they potentially can trigger fast ventricular tachycardias and inappropriate ICD discharges that may lead to fatal ventricular arrhythmias (Pizzale *et al.*, 2008). In the study by Sy and co-workers (Sy RW, 2011), one patient died of refractory ventricular tachycardia/ventricular fibrillation caused by inappropriate ICD shocks of rapidly conducting atrial fibrillation.

The cellular mechanism of sinus bradycardia in CPVT is still unexplored. One possibility is that the function of one or several ion channels that participate in the Ca^{2+} clock mechanism is altered (i.e. NCX, L-type Ca^{2+} channel, etc.) and this abnormality may correspond to a Ca^{2+} and voltage clock uncoupling. It has been reported that the CPVT-linked mutation R4496C presents an increased "SR Ca^{2+} leak" in ventricular myocytes isolated from a transgenic mice (Fernandez-Velasco *et al.*, 2009). A combined genetic and functional approach would be highly required to explore the involvement of RyR mutations on bradycardia and sino-atrial node dysfunction in CPVT disease.

6. Purkinje conduction system

The His-Purkinje system is responsible of the propagation for the action potential to the ventricles. The electrical properties of Purkinje cells are different from those of nodal cells, because they displayed low pacemaker activity and even slower conduction rate. However, Purkinje cells exhibit long action potential duration (APD) and therefore they are prone to EAD and DAD formation (Makarand Deo, 2010). This long APD provides sufficient time for L-type calcium channel reactivation, leading to EAD or DAD formation, which can lead to ectopic beats. Although EADs formation in Purkinje fibers has been quite explored (Fedida D, 2006), little is known concerning the development of DADs in these cardiac conducting fibers (GR., 1980; Gough WB, 1989). It has been recently described that DADs are associated to the development of CPVT disease (Liu *et al.*, 2006; Fernandez-Velasco *et al.*, 2009), but the mechanism of how DADs induce bidirectional VT is unknown. To fulfill this question, Cerrone and co-workers performed whole-heart optical mapping in heart isolated from knock-in mice carrying the R4496C mutation, and they found that bidirectional VT was caused by two foci in the distal His-Purkinje system, one in the right ventricle and the other in the left ventricle, activating the ventricles alternatively (Cerrone M, 2007). Polymorphic VT was initially multifocal but eventually became reentrant and degenerated into ventricular fibrillation. Moreover, chemical ablation of the right ventricular His-Purkinje system with Lugol solution converted bidirectional VT to monomorphic VT in mice. The same group further demonstrated in an additional report that Purkinje cells are more sensitive to the R4496C RyR2 mutation than ventricular myocytes, which strongly supports the idea that Purkinje cells are responsible of the arrhythmia in CPVT (Herron TJ, 2010). The latter result was further explored by other work, which has also tested that Flecainide reduce spontaneous Ca^{2+} release in Purkinje cells (Kang G, 2010).

6.1 Treatment of CPVT

Although β-adrenergic blockers is the most common treatment chosen for CPVT patients, they are incompletely effective with up to 30% of subjects requiring implantable cardioverter-defibrilators (ICDs) (Priori *et al.*, 2002). In severe cases of CPVT, the nondihydropyridine Ca^{2+} channels blockers may also be effective (Swan *et al.*, 2005; Rosso *et al.*, 2007).

Dantrolene, a drug used to prevent malignant hyperthermia in patients with mutations in RyR1 who have been exposed to volatile anaesthetics, has been proposed to have therapeutic potential in heart disease by causing "rezipping" of the amino and central domains of RyR2 (Kobayashi *et al.*, 2009; Kobayashi *et al.*, 2010).

More recently, a protective effect of flecainide was proposed for CPVT treatment, thus this drug is able to block Ca^{2+} leak from RyR2 in CASQ2 deficient mice (Watanabe *et al.*, 2009).

Finally, the use of drugs (JTV519) with selective action on FKBP 12.6 is still remaining in discrepancy, because diverging data to this respect were obtained.

7. Arrhythmogenic right ventricular dysplasia

Arrhythmogenic right ventricular dysplasia (ARVD) is a genetic form of cardiomyopathy that by contrast to CPVT, primarily affects the right ventricle (RV) and is characterized by the abnormal replacement of myocytes by adipose and fibrous tissue (Basso *et al.*, 2009). The estimated prevalence of ARVD in general population ranges from 1 in 2000 to 1 in 5000 (Corrado *et al.*, 1997) and is more frequent in men than in women, being a major cause of sudden death in the young and in athletes.

ARVD was initially believed to be a developmental defect of the RV myocardium, leading to the original designation of dysplasia (Basso *et al.*, 1996). The diagnostic of ARVD patients including MRI, echocardiography, electrocardiography and right ventricle biopsy (McKenna *et al.*, 1994). ARVD is characterized by functional abnormalities of the right ventricle, with abnormal depolarization/repolarization, leading to syncope, ventricular arrhythmias and sudden death (Rossi *et al.*, 1982). Interestingly, in a high percent of patients left ventricular dysfunction was found (Corrado *et al.*, 1997).The most typical clinical presentation of ARVD is symptomatic ventricular arrhythmias of right ventricular origin, usually triggered by effort.

ARVD can be inherited as an autosomal dominant disease with reduced penetrance and variable expression, although autosomal recessive forms also have been detected (Rampazzo *et al.*, 2002). Mutations in genes encoding for different molecules have been linked to ARVD. To this regard, mutations in adhesion proteins (plakoglobin, desmoplakin, plakophilin-2 and desmoglein-2), in cytokines (Transforming grow factor beta 3), in transmembrane protein 43 and in RyR2 have been detected in ARVD subjects (Tiso *et al.*, 2001; Rampazzo *et al.*, 2002; Gerull *et al.*, 2004; Beffagna *et al.*, 2005; Pilichou *et al.*, 2006; Merner *et al.*, 2008).

Regarding RyR2 mutations, ARVD patients with mutations in RyR2 tend to have mild ARVD symptoms and are classified as ARVD2. The R176Q mutation has been associated with the ARVD disease and also carries out a second mutation of T2504M (Tiso *et al.*, 2001). Both mutations induced the increased RyR activity in vitro (Thomas *et al.*, 2004).

The mice model that harbors R176Q mutation allowed for the better understanding of this arrhythmogenic disease. Hearts from R176Q heterozygous mice were structurally normal, but under β-adrenergic stimulation, myocytes elicited oscillatory Ca^{2+} signals, leading to mice VT (Kannankeril *et al.*, 2006).

7.1 Treatment of ARVD

There is not a curative treatment, instead, the aim is to detect patients with high risk and prevent complications.

The four therapeutic options are pharmacological agents (first choice), catheter ablation (if the patient is refractory to drug treatment or the disease is localized), implantable cardioverter-defibrillators (in refractory subject at risk for sudden death) and surgery as the last option (ventriculotomy and disconnection of the RV free wall) or cardiac transplantation (if severe terminal heart failure) (McKenna *et al.*, 1994).

As we mentioned, the first option for ARVD patients is the pharmacological treatment, including ACEI, anticoagulants, antiarrhythmic agents as sotalol, verapamil, beta-blockers, amiodarone and flecainide.

In conclusion, genetic analysis is essential in both CPVT and ARVD patients, because if a pathogenic mutation is identified, a pre-symptomatic diagnosis of the disease among family members might be provided and also the development of the disease can be monitored to assess the risk of transmitting them offspring.

8. References

Ai X, Curran JW, Shannon TR, Bers DM & Pogwizd SM. (2005). Ca^{2+}/calmodulin-dependent protein kinase modulates cardiac ryanodine receptor phosphorylation and sarcoplasmic reticulum Ca^{2+} leak in heart failure. *Circ Res* 97, 1314-1322.

Basso C, Corrado D, Marcus FI, Nava A & Thiene G. (2009). Arrhythmogenic right ventricular cardiomyopathy. *Lancet* 373, 1289-1300.

Basso C, Thiene G, Corrado D, Angelini A, Nava A & Valente M. (1996). Arrhythmogenic right ventricular cardiomyopathy. Dysplasia, dystrophy, or myocarditis? *Circulation* 94, 983-991.

Beard NA, Laver DR & Dulhunty AF. (2004). Calsequestrin and the calcium release channel of skeletal and cardiac muscle. *Prog Biophys Mol Biol* 85, 33-69.

Beffagna G, Occhi G, Nava A, Vitiello L, Ditadi A, Basso C, Bauce B, Carraro G, Thiene G, Towbin JA, Danieli GA & Rampazzo A. (2005). Regulatory mutations in transforming growth factor-beta3 gene cause arrhythmogenic right ventricular cardiomyopathy type 1. *Cardiovasc Res* 65, 366-373.

Belevych AE, Terentyev D, Viatchenko-Karpinski S, Terentyeva R, Sridhar A, Nishijima Y, Wilson LD, Cardounel AJ, Laurita KR, Carnes CA, Billman GE & Gyorke S. (2009). Redox modification of ryanodine receptors underlies calcium alternans in a canine model of sudden cardiac death. *Cardiovasc Res* 84, 387-395.

Benitah JP KB, Vassort G, Richard S, Gómez AM. (2002). Altered communication between L-type calcium channels and ryanodine receptors in heart failure. *Front Biosci* 7, e263-275.

Berlin JR, Cannell MB & Lederer WJ. (1989). Cellular origins of the transient inward current in cardiac myocytes. Role of fluctuations and waves of elevated intracellular calcium. *Circ Res* 65, 115-126.

Bers DM. (2002). Cardiac excitation-contraction coupling. *Nature* 415, 198-205.

Blayney LM, Jones JL, Griffiths J & Lai FA. (2010). A mechanism of ryanodine receptor modulation byFKBP12/12.6, protein kinase A, and K201. *Cardiovasc Res* 85, 68-78.

Cerrone M, Colombi B, Santoro M, di Barletta MR, Scelsi M, Villani L, Napolitano C & Priori SG. (2005). Bidirectional ventricular tachycardia and fibrillation elicited in a knock-in mouse model carrier of a mutation in the cardiac ryanodine receptor. *Circ Res* 96, e77-82.

Cerrone M NS, Tolkacheva EG, Talkachou A, O'Connell R, Berenfeld O, Anumonwo J, Pandit SV, Vikstrom K, Napolitano C, Priori SG, Jalife J. (2007). Arrhythmogenic mechanisms in a mouse model of catecholaminergic polymorphic ventricular tachycardia. *Circ Res* 101, 1039-1048.

Corrado D, Basso C, Thiene G, McKenna WJ, Davies MJ, Fontaliran F, Nava A, Silvestri F, Blomstrom-Lundqvist C, Wlodarska EK, Fontaine G & Camerini F. (1997). Spectrum of clinicopathologic manifestations of arrhythmogenic right ventricular cardiomyopathy/dysplasia: a multicenter study. *J Am Coll Cardiol* 30, 1512-1520.

Coumel P. (1997). Polymorphous ventricular tachyarrhythmias in the absence of structural heart disease. *Pacing Clin Electrophysiol* 20, 2065-2067.

Curran J, Brown KH, Santiago DJ, Pogwizd S, Bers DM & Shannon TR. (2010). Spontaneous Ca waves in ventricular myocytes from failing hearts depend on Ca(2+)-calmodulin-dependent protein kinase II. *J Mol Cell Cardiol* 49, 25-32.

d'Amati G, Bagattin, A., Bauce, B., Rampazzo, A., Autore, C., Basso, C., & King K, Romeo, M.D., Gallo, P., Thiene, G. Danieli GA, Nava A. . (2005). Juvenile sudden death in a family with polymorphic ventricular arrhythmias caused by a novel RyR2 gene mutation: evidence of specific morphological substrates. *Hum Pathol* 36, 761–767.

di Barletta MR, Viatchenko-Karpinski S, Nori A, Memmi M, Terentyev D, Turcato F, Valle G, Rizzi N, Napolitano C, Gyorke S, Volpe P & Priori SG. (2006). Clinical phenotype and functional characterization of CASQ2 mutations associated with catecholaminergic polymorphic ventricular tachycardia. *Circulation* 114, 1012-1019.

Dirksen RT, & Avila, G. (2002). Altered ryanodine receptor function in central core disease: leaky or uncoupled Ca(2+) release channels? *Trends Cardiovasc Med* 12, 189–197.

Dirksen WP, Lacombe VA, Chi M, Kalyanasundaram A, Viatchenko-Karpinski S, Terentyev D, Zhou Z, Vedamoorthyrao S, Li N, Chiamvimonvat N, Carnes CA, Franzini-Armstrong C, Gyorke S & Periasamy M. (2007). A mutation in calsequestrin, CASQ2D307H, impairs Sarcoplasmic Reticulum Ca2+ handling and causes complex ventricular arrhythmias in mice. *Cardiovasc Res* 75, 69-78.

Eldar M, Pras E & Lahat H. (2003). A missense mutation in the CASQ2 gene is associated with autosomalrecessive catecholamine-induced polymorphic ventricular tachycardia. *Trends Cardiovasc Med* 13, 148-151.

Fabiato A. (1983). Calcium-induced release of calcium from the cardiac sarcoplasmic reticulum. *Am J Physiol* 245, C1-14.

Fauconnier J, Thireau J, Reiken S, Cassan C, Richard S, Matecki S, Marks AR & Lacampagne A. (2010). Leaky RyR2 trigger ventricular arrhythmias in Duchenne muscular dystrophy. *Proc Natl Acad Sci U S A* 107, 1559-1564.

Fedida D OP, Hesketh JC, Ezrin AM. (2006). The role of late I and antiarrhythmic drugs in EAD formation and termination in Purkinje fibers. *J Cardiovasc Electrophysiol* Suppl 1, S71-S78.

Fernandez-Velasco M, Rueda A, Rizzi N, Benitah JP, Colombi B, Napolitano C, Priori SG, Richard S & Gomez AM. (2009). Increased Ca2+ Sensitivity of the Ryanodine Receptor Mutant RyR2R4496C Underlies Catecholaminergic Polymorphic Ventricular Tachycardia. *Circ Res* 104, 201-209.

Gellen B, Fernandez-Velasco M, Briec F, Vinet L, LeQuang K, Rouet-Benzineb P, Benitah JP, Pezet M, Palais G, Pellegrin N, Zhang A, Perrier R, Escoubet B, Marniquet X, Richard S, Jaisser F, Gómez AM, Charpentier F & Mercadier JJ. (2008). Conditional FKBP12.6 overexpression in mouse cardiac myocytes prevents triggered ventricular tachycardia through specific alterations in excitation-contraction coupling. *Circulation* 117, 1778-1786.

George CH, Higgs GV & Lai FA. (2003). Ryanodine receptor mutations associated with stress-induced ventricular tachycardia mediate increased calcium release in stimulated cardiomyocytes. *Circ Res* 93, 531-540.

George CH JH, Thomas NL, Fry DL, Lai FA. (2007). Ryanodine receptors and ventricular arrhythmias: Emerging trends in mutations, mechanisms and therapies. *J Mol and Cell Cardiol* 42, 34-50.

George CH, Thomas NL, FA. L (2005) Ryanodine receptor dysfunction in arrhythmia and sudden cardiac death. Future Cardiol 1:531–541

George CH. JH, Walters N, Thomas NL, West RR, & Lai FA. (2006). Arrhythmogenic mutation-linked defects in ryanodine receptor autoregulation reveal a novel mechanism of Ca^{2+} release channel dysfunction. *Circ Res* 98, 88–97.

Gerull B, Heuser A, Wichter T, Paul M, Basson CT, McDermott DA, Lerman BB, Markowitz SM, Ellinor PT, MacRae CA, Peters S, Grossmann KS, Drenckhahn J, Michely B, Sasse-Klaassen S, Birchmeier W, Dietz R, Breithardt G, Schulze-Bahr E & Thierfelder L. (2004). Mutations in the desmosomal protein plakophilin-2 are common in arrhythmogenic right ventricular cardiomyopathy. *Nat Genet* 36, 1162-1164.

Gomez AM, Rueda A, Sainte-Marie Y, Pereira L, Zissimopoulos S, Zhu X, Schaub R, Perrier E, Perrier R, Latouche C, Richard S, Picot MC, Jaisser F, Lai FA, Valdivia HH & Benitah JP. (2009). Mineralocorticoid Modulation of Cardiac Ryanodine Receptor Activity Is Associated With Downregulation of FK506- Binding Proteins. *Circulation* 119, 2179-U2189.

Gómez AM, Valdivia HH, Cheng H, Lederer MR, Santana LF, Cannell MB, McCune SA, Altschuld RA & Lederer WJ. (1997). Defective excitation-contraction coupling in experimental cardiac hypertrophy and heart failure. *Science* 276, 800-806.

Gonzalez DR, Beigi F, Treuer AV & Hare JM. (2007). Deficient ryanodine receptor S-nitrosylation increases sarcoplasmic reticulum calcium leak and arrhythmogenesis in cardiomyocytes. *Proc Natl Acad Sci U S A* 104, 20612-20617.

Gonzalez DR, Treuer AV, Castellanos J, Dulce RA & Hare JM. (2010). Impaired S-nitrosylation of the ryanodine receptor caused by xanthine oxidase activity contributes to calcium leak in heart failure. *J Biol Chem* 285, 28938-28945.

Gough WB e-SN. (1989). Dependence of delayed afterdepolarizations on diastolic potentials in ischemic Purkinje fibers. *Am J Physiol* 257, H770-777.

GR. F. (1980). Effects of transmembrane potential on oscillatory afterpotentials induced by acetylstrophanthidin in canine ventricular tissues. *J Pharmacol Exp Ther* 215, 332-341.

Guo T, Cornea RL, Huke S, Camors E, Yang Y, Picht E, Fruen BR & Bers DM. (2010). Kinetics of FKBP12.6 binding to ryanodine receptors in permeabilized cardiac myocytes and effects on Ca sparks. *Circ Res* 106, 1743-1752.

Gyorke I, Hester N, Jones LR & Gyorke S. (2004). The role of calsequestrin, triadin, and junctin in conferring cardiac ryanodine receptor responsiveness to luminal calcium. *Biophys J* 86, 2121-2128.

Gyorke S & Terentyev D. (2008). Modulation of ryanodine receptor by luminal calcium and accessory proteins in health and cardiac disease. *Cardiovasc Res* 77, 245-255.

Harzheim D, Movassagh M, Foo RS, Ritter O, Tashfeen A, Conway SJ, Bootman MD & Roderick HL. (2009). Increased InsP3Rs in the junctional sarcoplasmic reticulum augment Ca^{2+} transients and arrhythmias associated with cardiac hypertrophy. *Proc Natl Acad Sci U S A* 106, 11406-11411.

Herron TJ MM, Anumonwo J, et al. (2010). Purkinje cell calcium dysregulation is the cellular mechanism that underlies catecholaminergic polymorphic ventricular tachycardia. *Heart Rhythm* 7, 1122–1128.

Huang F, Shan J, Reiken S, Wehrens XH & Marks AR. (2006). Analysis of calstabin2 (FKBP12.6)-ryanodine receptor interactions: rescue of heart failure by calstabin2 in mice. *Proc Natl Acad Sci U S A* 103, 3456-3461.

Ikemoto N & Yamamoto T. (2000). Postulated role of inter-domain interaction within the ryanodine receptor in Ca(2+) channel regulation. *Trends Cardiovasc Med* 10, 310-316.

Ikemoto N & Yamamoto T. (2002). Regulation of calcium release by interdomain interaction within ryanodine receptors. *Front Biosci* 7, d671-683.

Jiang D CW, Wang R, Zhang L, Chen SR. (2007). Loss of luminal Ca^{2+} activation in the cardiac ryanodine receptor is associated with ventricular fibrillation and sudden death. *Proc Natl Acad Sci U S A* 104, 18309-18314.

Jiang D JP, Davis DR, Gow R, Green MS, Birnie DH, Chen SR, Gollob MH. (2010). Characterization of a novel mutation in the cardiac ryanodine receptor that results in catecholaminergic polymorphic ventricular tachycardia. *Channels (Austin)* 4(4), 302-310.

Jiang D XB, Yang D, Wang R, Choi P, Zhang L, Cheng H, Chen SR. (2004). RyR2 mutations linked to ventricular tachycardia and sudden death reduce the threshold for store-overload-induced Ca^{2+} release (SOICR). *Proc Natl Acad Sci U S A* 101, 13062-13067.

Jiang D XB, Zhang L, Chen SR. (2005). Enhanced basal activity of a cardiac Ca^{2+} release channel (ryanodine receptor) mutant associated with ventricular tachycardia and sudden death. *Circ Res* 97, 1173-1181.

Jiang D, Xiao B, Yang D, Wang R, Choi P, Zhang L, Cheng H & Chen SR. (2004). RyR2 mutations linked to ventricular tachycardia and sudden death reduce the threshold for store-overload-induced Ca2+ release (SOICR). *Proc Natl Acad Sci U S A* 101, 13062-13067.

Jiang MT, Lokuta AJ, Farrell EF, Wolff MR, Haworth RA & Valdivia HH. (2002). Abnormal Ca^{2+} release, but normal ryanodine receptors, in canine and human heart failure. *Circ Res* 91, 1015-1022.

Kang G GS, Liu N, Liu FY, Zhang J, Priori SG, Fishman GI. (2010). Purkinje cells from RyR2 mutant mice are highly arrhythmogenic but responsive to targeted therapy. *Circ Res* 107, 512-519.

Kannankeril PJ, Mitchell BM, Goonasekera SA, Chelu MG, Zhang W, Sood S, Kearney DL, Danila CI, De Biasi M, Wehrens XH, Pautler RG, Roden DM, Taffet GE, Dirksen RT, Anderson ME & Hamilton SL. (2006). Mice with the R176Q cardiac ryanodine receptor mutation exhibit catecholamine-induced ventricular tachycardia and cardiomyopathy. *Proc Natl Acad Sci U S A* 103, 12179-12184.

Kazemian P GM, Pantano A, Oudit GY. (2011). A Novel Mutation in the RYR2 Gene Leading to Catecholaminergic Polymorphic Ventricular Tachycardia and Paroxysmal Atrial Fibrillation: Dose- Dependent Arrhythmia-Event Suppression by β-Blocker Therapy. *Can J Cardiol* In press.

Keller M, Kao JP, Egger M & Niggli E. (2007). Calcium waves driven by "sensitization" wave-fronts. *Cardiovasc Res* 74, 39-45.

Kim E, Youn B, Kemper L, Campbell C, Milting H, Varsanyi M & Kang C. (2007). Characterization of human cardiac calsequestrin and its deleterious mutants. *J Mol Biol* 373, 1047-1057.

Knollmann BC. (2009). New roles of calsequestrin and triadin in cardiac muscle. *J Physiol* 587, 3081-3087.

Knollmann BC, Chopra N, Hlaing T, Akin B, Yang T, Ettensohn K, Knollmann BE, Horton KD, Weissman NJ, Holinstat I, Zhang W, Roden DM, Jones LR, Franzini-Armstrong C & Pfeifer K. (2006). Casq2 deletion causes sarcoplasmic reticulum volume increase, premature Ca^{2+} release, and catecholaminergic polymorphic ventricular tachycardia. *J Clin Invest* 116, 2510-2520.

Kobayashi S, Yano M, Suetomi T, Ono M, Tateishi H, Mochizuki M, Xu X, Uchinoumi H, Okuda S, Yamamoto T, Koseki N, Kyushiki H, Ikemoto N & Matsuzaki M. (2009).

Dantrolene, a therapeutic agent for malignant hyperthermia, markedly improves the function of failing cardiomyocytes by stabilizing interdomain interactions within the ryanodine receptor. *J Am Coll Cardiol* 53, 1993-2005.

Kobayashi S, Yano M, Uchinoumi H, Suetomi T, Susa T, Ono M, Xu X, Tateishi H, Oda T, Okuda S, Doi M, Yamamoto T & Matsuzaki M. (2010). Dantrolene, a therapeutic agent for malignant hyperthermia, inhibits catecholaminergic polymorphic ventricular tachycardia in a RyR2(R2474S/+) knock-in mouse model. *Circ J* 74, 2579-2584.

Koop AG, Petra; Chen, S. R. Wayne; Thieleczek, Rolf; Varsanyi, Magdolna . . (2008). ARVC-Related Mutations in Divergent Region 3 Alter Functional Properties of the Cardiac Ryanodine Receptor. *Biophysical J* 94, 4668–4677.

Kubalova Z, Terentyev D, Viatchenko-Karpinski S, Nishijima Y, Gyorke I, Terentyeva R, da Cunha DN, Sridhar A, Feldman DS, Hamlin RL, Carnes CA & Gyorke S. (2005). Abnormal intrastore calcium signaling in chronic heart failure. *Proc Natl Acad Sci U S A* 102, 14104-14109.

Lahat H, Eldar M, Levy-Nissenbaum E, Bahan T, Friedman E, Khoury A, Lorber A, Kastner DL, Goldman B & Pras E. (2001a). Autosomal recessive catecholamine- or exercise-induced polymorphic ventricular tachycardia: clinical features and assignment of the disease gene to chromosome 1p13-21. *Circulation* 103, 2822-2827.

Lahat H, Pras E, Olender T, Avidan N, Ben-Asher E, Man O, Levy-Nissenbaum E, Khoury A, Lorber A, Goldman B, Lancet D & Eldar M. (2001b). A missense mutation in a highly conserved region of CASQ2 is associated with autosomal recessive catecholamine-induced polymorphic ventricular tachycardia in Bedouin families from Israel. *Am J Hum Genet* 69, 1378-1384.

Leenhardt A, Lucet V, Denjoy I, Grau F, Ngoc DD & Coumel P. (1995). Catecholaminergic polymorphic ventricular tachycardia in children. A 7-year follow-up of 21 patients. *Circulation* 91, 1512-1519.

Lehnart SE, Ackerman MJ, Benson DW, Jr., Brugada R, Clancy CE, Donahue JK, George AL, Jr., Grant AO, Groft SC, January CT, Lathrop DA, Lederer WJ, Makielski JC, Mohler PJ, Moss A, Nerbonne JM, Olson TM, Przywara DA, Towbin JA, Wang LH & Marks AR. (2007). Inherited arrhythmias: a National Heart, Lung, and Blood Institute and Office of Rare Diseases workshop consensus report about the diagnosis, phenotyping, molecular mechanisms, and therapeutic approaches for primary cardiomyopathies of gene mutations affecting ion channel function. *Circulation* 116, 2325-2345.

Lehnart SE, Mongillo M, Bellinger A, Lindegger N, Chen BX, Hsueh W, Reiken S, Wronska A, Drew LJ, Ward CW, Lederer WJ, Kass RS, Morley G & Marks AR. (2008). Leaky Ca^{2+} release channel/ryanodine receptor 2 causes seizures and sudden cardiac death in mice. *J Clin Invest* 118, 2230-2245.

Lehnart SE, Wehrens XH, Laitinen PJ, Reiken SR, Deng SX, Cheng Z, Landry DW, Kontula K, Swan H & Marks AR. (2004). Sudden death in familial polymorphic ventricular tachycardia associated with calcium release channel (ryanodine receptor) leak. *Circulation* 109, 3208-3214.

Liu N, Colombi B, Memmi M, Zissimopoulos S, Rizzi N, Negri S, Imbriani M, Napolitano C, Lai FA & Priori SG. (2006). Arrhythmogenesis in catecholaminergic polymorphic ventricular tachycardia: insights from a RyR2 R4496C knock-in mouse model. *Circ Res* 99, 292-298.

Lobo PA & Van Petegem F. (2009). Crystal structures of the N-terminal domains of cardiac and skeletal muscle ryanodine receptors: insights into disease mutations. *Structure* 17, 1505-1514.

Loyer X, Gomez AM, Milliez P, Fernandez-Velasco M, Vangheluwe P, Vinet L, Charue D, Vaudin E, Zhang W, Sainte-Marie Y, Robidel E, Marty I, Mayer B, Jaisser F, Mercadier JJ, Richard S, Shah AM, Benitah JP, Samuel JL & Heymes C. (2008). Cardiomyocyte overexpression of neuronal nitric oxide synthase delays transition toward heart failure in response to pressure overload by preserving calcium cycling. *Circulation* 117, 3187-3198.

Maier LS, Zhang T, Chen L, DeSantiago J, Brown JH & Bers DM. (2003). Transgenic CaMKIIdeltaC overexpression uniquely alters cardiac myocyte Ca^{2+} handling: reduced SR Ca^{2+} load and activated SR Ca^{2+} release. *Circ Res* 92, 904-911.

Makarand Deo PMB, Albert M. Kim and Edward J. Vigmond. (2010). Arrhythmogenesis by single ectopic beats originating in the Purkinje system. *Am J Physiol Heart Circ Physiol* 299, H1002-H1011.

Marks AR. (2001). Ryanodine receptors/calcium release channels in heart failure and sudden cardiac death. *J Mol Cell Cardiol* 33, 615-624.

Marx SO, Reiken S, Hisamatsu Y, Jayaraman T, Burkhoff D, Rosemblit N & Marks AR. (2000). PKA phosphorylation dissociates FKBP12.6 from the calcium release channel (ryanodine receptor): defective regulation in failing hearts. *Cell* 101, 365-376.

Marx SO RS, Hisamatsu Y, Jayaraman T, Burkhoff D, Rosemblit N, Marks AR. (2000). PKA phosphorylation dissociates FKBP12.6 from the calcium release channel (ryanodine receptor): defective regulation in failing hearts. *Cell* 101, 365-376.

McKenna WJ, Thiene G, Nava A, Fontaliran F, Blomstrom-Lundqvist C, Fontaine G & Camerini F. (1994). Diagnosis of arrhythmogenic right ventricular dysplasia/cardiomyopathy. Task Force of the Working Group Myocardial and Pericardial Disease of the European Society of Cardiology and of the Scientific Council on Cardiomyopathies of the International Society and Federation of Cardiology. *Br Heart J* 71, 215-218.

Medeiros-Domingo A BZ, Tester DJ, et al. . (2009). The RYR2-encoded ryanodine receptor/calcium release channel in patients diagnosed previously with either catecholaminergic polymorphic ventricular tachycardia or genotype negative, exercise-induced long QT syndrome: a comprehensive open reading frame mutational analysis. . *J Am Coll Cardiol* 54, 2065–2074.

Meli ACR, Marwan M.; Dura,Miroslav; Reiken, Steven; Wronska,Anetta; Wojciak, Julianne; Carroll, Joan; Scheinman, Melvin M.; Marks Andrew R. . (2011). A Novel Ryanodine Receptor Mutation Linked to Sudden Death Increases Sensitivity to Cytosolic Calcium. *Circ Res* published online Jun 9.

Merner ND, Hodgkinson KA, Haywood AF, Connors S, French VM, Drenckhahn JD, Kupprion C, Ramadanova K, Thierfelder L, McKenna W, Gallagher B, Morris-Larkin L, Bassett AS, Parfrey PS & Young TL. (2008). Arrhythmogenic right ventricular cardiomyopathy type 5 is a fully penetrant, lethal arrhythmic disorder caused by a missense mutation in the TMEM43 gene. *Am J Hum Genet* 82, 809-821.

Mohamed U, Napolitano C & Priori SG. (2007). Molecular and electrophysiological bases of catecholaminergic polymorphic ventricular tachycardia. *J Cardiovasc Electrophysiol* 18, 791-797.

Nakajima T, Kaneko Y, Taniguchi Y, Hayashi K, Takizawa T, Suzuki T & Nagai R. (1997). The mechanism of catecholaminergic polymorphic ventricular tachycardia may be triggered activity due to delayed afterdepolarization. *Eur Heart J* 18, 530-531.

Napolitano C & Priori SG. (2007). Diagnosis and treatment of catecholaminergic polymorphic ventricular tachycardia. *Heart Rhythm* 4, 675-678.

Oda T, Yano M, Yamamoto T, Tokuhisa T, Okuda S, Doi M, Ohkusa T, Ikeda Y, Kobayashi S, Ikemoto N & Matsuzaki M. (2005). Defective regulation of interdomain interactions within the ryanodine receptor plays a key role in the pathogenesis of heart failure. *Circulation* 111, 3400-3410.

Pilichou K, Nava A, Basso C, Beffagna G, Bauce B, Lorenzon A, Frigo G, Vettori A, Valente M, Towbin J, Thiene G, Danieli GA & Rampazzo A. (2006). Mutations in desmoglein-2 gene are associated with arrhythmogenic right ventricular cardiomyopathy. *Circulation* 113, 1171-1179.

Pizzale S, Gollob MH, Gow R & Birnie DH. (2008). Sudden death in a young man with catecholaminergic polymorphic ventricular tachycardia and paroxysmal atrial fibrillation. *J Cardiovasc Electrophysiol* 19, 1319-1321.

Postma AV, Denjoy I, Hoorntje TM, Lupoglazoff JM, Da Costa A, Sebillon P, Mannens MM, Wilde AA & Guicheney P. (2002). Absence of calsequestrin 2 causes severe forms of catecholaminergic polymorphic ventricular tachycardia. *Circ Res* 91, e21-26.

Postma AV, Denjoy I, Kamblock J, Alders M, Lupoglazoff JM, Vaksmann G, Dubosq-Bidot L, Sebillon P, Mannens MM, Guicheney P & Wilde AA. (2005). Catecholaminergic polymorphic ventricular tachycardia: RYR2 mutations, bradycardia, and follow up of the patients. *J Med Genet* 42, 863-870.

Priori SG AE, Blømstrom-Lundqvist C, Bossaert L, Breithardt G, Brugada P, Camm JA, Cappato R, Cobbe SM, Di MC, Maron BJ, McKenna WJ, Pedersen AK, Ravens U, Schwartz PJ, Trusz-Gluza M, Vardas P, Wellens HJ, Zipes DP. (2002). Task Force on Sudden Cardiac Death, European Society of Cardiology. *Europace* 4, 3-18.

Priori SG, Napolitano C, Memmi M, Colombi B, Drago F, Gasparini M, DeSimone L, Coltorti F, Bloise R, Keegan R, Cruz Filho FE, Vignati G, Benatar A & DeLogu A. (2002). Clinical and molecular characterization of patients with catecholaminergic polymorphic ventricular tachycardia. *Circulation* 106, 69-74.

Priori SG NC, Tiso N, Memmi M, Vignati G, Bloise R, Sorrentino V, Danieli GA. (2001). Mutations in the cardiac ryanodine receptor gene (hRyR2) underlie catecholaminergic polymorphic ventricular tachycardia. *Circulation* 103, 196-200.

Qin J, Valle G, Nani A, Nori A, Rizzi N, Priori SG, Volpe P & Fill M. (2008). Luminal Ca^{2+} regulation of single cardiac ryanodine receptors: insights provided by calsequestrin and its mutants. *J Gen Physiol* 131, 325-334.

Rampazzo A, Nava A, Malacrida S, Beffagna G, Bauce B, Rossi V, Zimbello R, Simionati B, Basso C, Thiene G, Towbin JA & Danieli GA. (2002). Mutation in human desmoplakin domain binding to plakoglobin causes a dominant form of arrhythmogenic right ventricular cardiomyopathy. *Am J Hum Genet* 71, 1200-1206.

Reiken S, Gaburjakova M, Gaburjakova J, He Kl KL, Prieto A, Becker E, Yi Gh GH, Wang J, Burkhoff D & Marks AR. (2001). beta-adrenergic receptor blockers restore cardiac calcium release channel (ryanodine receptor) structure and function in heart failure. *Circulation* 104, 2843-2848.

Reiken S, Gaburjakova M, Guatimosim S, Gómez AM, D'Armiento J, Burkhoff D, Wang J, Vassort G, Lederer WJ & Marks AR. (2003). Protein kinase A phosphorylation of the cardiac calcium release channel (ryanodine receptor) in normal and failing hearts. Role of phosphatases and response to isoproterenol. *J Biol Chem* 278, 444-453.

Rosen MR & Danilo P, Jr. (1980). Effects of tetrodotoxin, lidocaine, verapamil, and AHR-2666 on Ouabain-induced delayed afterdepolarizations in canine Purkinje fibers. *Circ Res* 46, 117-124.

Rossi P, Massumi A, Gillette P & Hall RJ. (1982). Arrhythmogenic right ventricular dysplasia: clinical features, diagnostic techniques, and current management. *Am Heart J* 103, 415-420.

Rosso R, Kalman JM, Rogowski O, Diamant S, Birger A, Biner S, Belhassen B & Viskin S. (2007). Calcium channel blockers and beta-blockers versus beta-blockers alone for preventing exercise-induced arrhythmias in catecholaminergic polymorphic ventricular tachycardia. *Heart Rhythm* 4, 1149-1154.

Shou W, Aghdasi B, Armstrong DL, Guo Q, Bao S, Charng MJ, Mathews LM, Schneider MD, Hamilton SL & Matzuk MM. (1998). Cardiac defects and altered ryanodine receptor function in mice lacking FKBP12. *Nature* 391, 489-492.

Song L, Alcalai R, Arad M, Wolf CM, Toka O, Conner DA, Berul CI, Eldar M, Seidman CE & Seidman JG. (2007). Calsequestrin 2 (CASQ2) mutations increase expression of calreticulin and ryanodine receptors, causing catecholaminergic polymorphic ventricular tachycardia. *J Clin Invest* 117, 1814-1823.

Sumitomo N, Harada K, Nagashima M, Yasuda T, Nakamura Y, Aragaki Y, Saito A, Kurosaki K, Jouo K, Koujiro M, Konishi S, Matsuoka S, Oono T, Hayakawa S, Miura M, Ushinohama H, Shibata T & Niimura I. (2003). Catecholaminergic polymorphic ventricular tachycardia: electrocardiographic characteristics and optimal therapeutic strategies to prevent sudden death. *Heart* 89, 66-70.

Sumitomo N, Sakurada H, Taniguchi K, Matsumura M, Abe O, Miyashita M, Kanamaru H, Karasawa K, Ayusawa M, Fukamizu S, Nagaoka I, Horie M, Harada K & Hiraoka M. (2007). Association of atrial arrhythmia and sinus node dysfunction in patients with catecholaminergic polymorphic ventricular tachycardia. *Circ J* 71, 1606-1609.

Swan H, Laitinen P, Kontula K & Toivonen L. (2005). Calcium channel antagonism reduces exercise-induced ventricular arrhythmias in catecholaminergic polymorphic ventricular tachycardia patients with RyR2 mutations. *J Cardiovasc Electrophysiol* 16, 162-166.

Sy RW GM, Klein GJ, Yee R, Skanes AC, Gula LJ, Leong-Sit P, Gow RM, Green MS, Birnie DH, Krahn AD. (2011). Arrhythmia characterization and long-term outcomes in catecholaminergic polymorphic ventricular tachycardia. *Heart Rhythm* 8, 864–871.

Tateishi H, Yano M, Mochizuki M, Suetomi T, Ono M, Xu X, Uchinoumi H, Okuda S, Oda T, Kobayashi S, Yamamoto T, Ikeda Y, Ohkusa T, Ikemoto N & Matsuzaki M. (2009). Defective domain-domain interactions within the ryanodine receptor as a critical cause of diastolic Ca^{2+} leak in failing hearts. *Cardiovasc Res* 81, 536-545.

Terentyev D, Kubalova Z, Valle G, Nori A, Vedamoorthyrao S, Terentyeva R, Viatchenko-Karpinski S, Bers DM, Williams SC, Volpe P & Gyorke S. (2008). Modulation of SR Ca release by luminal Ca and calsequestrin in cardiac myocytes: effects of CASQ2 mutations linked to sudden cardiac death. *Biophys J* 95, 2037-2048.

Terentyev D, Nori A, Santoro M, Viatchenko-Karpinski S, Kubalova Z, Gyorke I, Terentyeva R, Vedamoorthyrao S, Blom NA, Valle G, Napolitano C, Williams SC, Volpe P, Priori SG & Gyorke S. (2006). Abnormal interactions of calsequestrin with the ryanodine receptor calcium release channel complex linked to exercise-induced sudden cardiac death. *Circ Res* 98, 1151-1158.

Terentyev D, Viatchenko-Karpinski S, Gyorke I, Volpe P, Williams SC & Gyorke S. (2003). Calsequestrin determines the functional size and stability of cardiac intracellular calcium stores: Mechanism for hereditary arrhythmia. *Proc Natl Acad Sci U S A* 100, 11759-11764.

Terentyev D, Viatchenko-Karpinski S, Vedamoorthyrao S, Oduru S, Gyorke I, Williams SC & Gyorke S. (2007). Protein protein interactions between triadin and calsequestrin are involved in modulation of sarcoplasmic reticulum calcium release in cardiac myocytes. *J Physiol* 583, 71-80.

Tester DJ KL, Will ML, Ackerman MJ. (2005). Spectrum and prevalence of cardiac ryanodine receptor (RyR2) mutations in a cohort of unrelated patients referred explicitly for long QT syndrome genetic testing. *Heart Rhythm* 2, 1099-1105.

Tester DJ D, Miroslav; Carturan, Elisa; Reiken, Steven; Wronska, Anetta; Marks, Andrew R.; Ackerman, Michael J. (2007). A mechanism for sudden infant death syndrome (SIDS): Stress-induced leak via ryanodine receptors *Heart Rhythm* 4, 733-739

Thomas NL, George CH & Lai FA. (2004). Functional heterogeneity of ryanodine receptor mutations associated with sudden cardiac death. *Cardiovasc Res* 64, 52-60.

Thomas NL, Lai, F.A., George, C.H. . (2005). Differential Ca^{2+} sensitivity of RyR2 mutations reveals distinct mechanisms of channel dysfunction in sudden cardiac death *Biochem Biophys Res Commun*, 231–238

Tiso N, Salamon M, Bagattin A, Danieli GA, Argenton F & Bortolussi M. (2002). The binding of the RyR2 calcium channel to its gating protein FKBP12.6 is oppositely affected by ARVD2 and VTSIP mutations. *Biochem Biophys Res Commun* 299, 594-598.

Tiso N, Stephan DA, Nava A, Bagattin A, Devaney JM, Stanchi F, Larderet G, Brahmbhatt B, Brown K, Bauce B, Muriago M, Basso C, Thiene G, Danieli GA & Rampazzo A. (2001). Identification of mutations in the cardiac ryanodine receptor gene in families affected with arrhythmogenic right ventricular cardiomyopathy type 2 (ARVD2). *Hum Mol Genet* 10, 189-194.

Tung CC, Lobo PA, Kimlicka L & Van Petegem F. (2010). The amino-terminal disease hotspot of ryanodine receptors forms a cytoplasmic vestibule. *Nature* 468, 585-588.

Uchinoumi H, Yano M, Suetomi T, Ono M, Xu X, Tateishi H, Oda T, Okuda S, Doi M, Kobayashi S, Yamamoto T, Ikeda Y, Ohkusa T, Ikemoto N & Matsuzaki M. (1998). Catecholaminergic polymorphic ventricular tachycardia is caused by mutation-linked defective conformational regulation of the ryanodine receptor. *Circ Res* 106, 1413-1424.

Venetucci LA, Trafford AW, O'Neill SC & Eisner DA. (2007). Na/Ca exchange: regulator of intracellular calcium and source of arrhythmias in the heart. *Ann N Y Acad Sci* 1099, 315-325.

Venetucci LA, Trafford AW, O'Neill SC & Eisner DA. (2008). The sarcoplasmic reticulum and arrhythmogenic calcium release. *Cardiovasc Res* 77, 285-292.

Vyas H, Hejlik J & Ackerman MJ. (2006). Epinephrine QT stress testing in the evaluation of congenital long-QT syndrome: diagnostic accuracy of the paradoxical QT response. *Circulation* 113, 1385-1392.

Wagenknecht T, R. Grassucci, J. Frank, A. Saito, M. Inui & S. Fleischer. (1989). Three dimensional architecture of the calcium channel/foot structure of sarcoplasmic reticulum. *Nature* 338, 167-170.

Watanabe H, Chopra N, Laver D, Hwang HS, Davies SS, Roach DE, Duff HJ, Roden DM, Wilde AA & Knollmann BC. (2009). Flecainide prevents catecholaminergic polymorphic ventricular tachycardia in mice and humans. *Nat Med* 15, 380-383.

Wehrens XH, Lehnart SE, Huang F, Vest JA, Reiken SR, Mohler PJ, Sun J, Guatimosim S, Song LS, Rosemblit N, D'Armiento JM, Napolitano C, Memmi M, Priori SG, Lederer WJ & Marks AR. (2003). FKBP12.6 deficiency and defective calcium release channel (ryanodine receptor) function linked to exercise induced sudden cardiac death. *Cell* 113, 829-840.

Wehrens XH, Lehnart SE & Marks AR. (2005). Intracellular calcium release and cardiac disease. *Annu Rev Physiol* 67, 69-98.

Wehrens XH, Lehnart SE, Reiken SR, Deng SX, Vest JA, Cervantes D, Coromilas J, Landry DW & Marks AR. (2004). Protection from cardiac arrhythmia through ryanodine receptor-stabilizing protein calstabin2. *Science* 304, 292-296.

Xiao J, Tian X, Jones PP, Bolstad J, Kong H, Wang R, Zhang L, Duff HJ, Gillis AM, Fleischer S, Kotlikoff M, Copello JA & Chen SR. (2007). Removal of FKBP12.6 does not alter the conductance and activation of the cardiac ryanodine receptor or the susceptibility to stress-induced ventricular arrhythmias. *J Biol Chem* 282, 34828-34838.

Xin HB, Senbonmatsu T, Cheng DS, Wang YX, Copello JA, Ji GJ, Collier ML, Deng KY, Jeyakumar LH, Magnuson MA, Inagami T, Kotlikoff MI & Fleischer S. (2002). Oestrogen protects FKBP12.6 null mice from cardiac hypertrophy. *Nature* 416, 334-338.

Yamamoto T E-HR, Ikemoto N. (2000). Postulated role of interdomain interaction within the ryanodine receptor in Ca(2+) channel regulation. *J Biol Chem* 275, 11618-11625.

Yang Z, Ikemoto, N., Lamb, G.D. and Steele, D.S. (2006). The RyR2 central domain peptide DPc10 lowers the threshold for spontaneous Ca^{2+} release in permeabilized cardiomyocytes *Cardiovasc Res* 70, 475–485.

Yano M, Okuda S, Oda T, Tokuhisa T, Tateishi H, Mochizuki M, Noma T, Doi M, Kobayashi S, Yamamoto T, Ikeda Y, Ohkusa T, Ikemoto N & Matsuzaki M. (2005). Correction of defective interdomain interaction within ryanodine receptor by antioxidant is a new therapeutic strategy against heart failure. *Circulation* 112, 3633-3643.

Yano M, Ono K, Ohkusa T, Suetsugu M, Kohno M, Hisaoka T, Kobayashi S, Hisamatsu Y, Yamamoto T, Kohno M, Noguchi N, Takasawa S, Okamoto H & Matsuzaki M. (2000). Altered stoichiometry of FKBP12.6 versus ryanodine receptor as a cause of abnormal Ca(2+) leak through ryanodine receptor in heart failure. *Circulation* 102, 2131-2136.

Yano M, Yamamoto T, Ikeda Y & Matsuzaki M. (2006). Mechanisms of Disease: ryanodine receptor defects in heart failure and fatal arrhythmia. *Nat Clin Pract Cardiovasc Med* 3, 43-52.

5

The Effects of Lidocaine on Reperfusion Ventricular Fibrillation During Coronary Artery – Bypass Graft Surgery

Ahmet Mahli* and Demet Coskun
Department of Anaesthesiology and Reanimation, Gazi University Faculty of Medicine, Ankara, Turkey

1. Introduction

Myocardial protection with cardioplegia has resulted in significant improvement in the outcomes of cardiopulmonary bypass (CPB) in coronary artery - bypass graft (CABG) procedure. However, subendocardial damage created by ischemic injury still remains a source of morbidity and mortality associated with CABG (1). Ventricular fibrillation (VF) occurring after releasing of aortic cross-clamp in the reperfusion phase of CABG surgery (reperfusion VF) is very common (74–96 %) (1-5). This complication is considered to be related with ischemia-induced increases in reentry and automaticity as well as the possibility of reperfusion injury (6-8). Reperfusion VF may adversely affect coronary blood flow and increase ventricular wall tension, which causes a further depletion of myocardial energy reserves in an energy-depleted myocardium (2). It is estimated that reperfusion VF occurs as a result of increased myocardial wall stress and oxygen consumption besides diminished subendocardial blood flow and intramyocardial acidosis (9-12). Additional myocardial injury following defibrillation by direct current countershocks may worsen this situation (13,14). Therefore, it would be helpful for the patients' recovery after the CABG (15).

VF developing in reperfusion phase of CPB generally responds to defibrillation. Obstinate or recurrent VF increases myocardial oxygen demand, unfortunately resulting in ventricular dilatation. Furthermore, the ventricular relaxation creates irreversible myocardial injury. When heart remains in VF, it is necessary to recheck blood gases, electrolytes, and temperature. Lidocaine, a class Ib antiarrhythmic, is administered at a dose of 1 to 2 mg kg^{-1} before repeated direct current defibrillation is attempted. Occasionally, beta blockers such as esmolol and metoprolol, class II antiarrhythmics and amiodarone, a class III antiarrhythmic are added in order to treat intractable VF or ventricular tachycardia (16). A previous study reported that in patients with persistent VF during weaning from CPB in cardiac surgery for heart diseases with left ventricular hypertrophy, amiodarone was a reasonable option (17).

Lidocaine, which is a local anaesthetic in amid group, acts as an antiarrythmyhic agent and it is classified in class Ib. By binding Na^+ channels, lidocaine alters membranous conductivity

* Corresponding Author

of cations. Lidocaine decreases depolarisation plateau of phase 4 and enhances diastolic electrical flow threshold in Purkinje fibers (18,19). Lidocaine increases VF threshold, but this effect is directly related with plasma concentrations of lidocaine (20).

Although lidocaine is known to reduce VF incidence and defibrillation demand, the mechanism is not clearly understood yet. However, it is proved to be appropriate in the treatment of ventricular ectopic premature beats (18-21). In myocardial ischemic conditions, lidocaine has been shown to turn unidirectional blocking zones and slow conduction in ischemic zones to complete blocking areas (22). Another possible mechanism could be explained by inhibitory effect of lidocaine on Na^+ intake and membrane depolarisation such that cardiac arrest occurs when they are inhibited (23). As a result, the energy is kept away from electromechanical activity thus proceeding more accurate recovery for the heart. In addition to that local anaesthetics, lidocaine can block slow Ca^{++} channels and Ca^{++} channels of sarcoplasmic reticulum (24,25).

Lidocaine has previously been added to cardioplegic solutions in order to prevent reperfusion VF (see table 1). When 500 mg L^{-1} of lidocaine was added to a crystalloid solution, there was a significant decrease in the incidence of VF, but a higher percentage of atrio-ventricular (AV) block was also observed (4-12,14,26). Baraka et al. (13) showed that the incidence of reperfusion VF can be markedly reduced, from 93% to 42%, with the addition of 100 mg L^{-1} of lidocaine to a crystalloid cardioplegic solution without an increase of the incidence of AV block. Wallace and Baker (2) repeated a similar study and reported that the incidence of reperfusion VF is reduced from 63 % to 42 % with the addition of 100 mg L^{-1} of lidocaine to a crystalloid cardioplegic solution. They noted that a higher proportion of the patients who developed reperfusion VF with lidocaine cardioplegia underwent spontaneous defibrillation (30% versus 11%), even though this was not statistically significant. On the other hand, different from the above mentioned study (13), they stated that the incidence of AV block necessitating ventricular pacing to separate from CPB was significantly higher in the lidocaine treated group (44%) as compared with the control group (20%). Sellevold et al. (27) added procaine instead of lidocaine in cardioplegic solutions to be able to observe the efficiency in post-ischemic rhythm disturbances, and they showed that cardioplegia with procaine (1 mM) stabilised post-ischemic arrhythmia without any reverse effect.

Meta-analyses suggested that prophylactic lidocaine use reduces VF but increases mortality rates after acute myocardial infarction. Although its use may not be associated with increased mortality rates, the prophylactic lidocaine use, in fact, has decreased with the advent of thrombolysis, and the routine use of prophylactic lidocaine in acute myocardial infarction is not recommended (28,29). In another study, lidocaine appears to be effective in converting no more than 20% of stable ventricular tachycardias (30).

In some investigations, the possible effect of lidocaine on autonomic cardiac control in humans was studied. Aidonidis et al. (31) found that in anaesthetized dogs, there was marked attenuation of cardiac sympathetic nervous activity by lidocaine which slightly altered efferent cardiac sympathetic nervous activity in the course of acute myocardial ischemia and reperfusion, but significantly increased it during VF. Abramovich et al. (32) showed that lidocaine has a consistent and significant parasympatholytic effect on the human heart in healthy volunteers as well as in patients in the acute phase of myocardial infarction.

Authors	Lidocaine Doses	Results
Hottenrott C et al, 1974 (9) Dahl CF et al, 1974 (14) Buckberg GD and Hottenrott CE, 1975 (10) Hearse DJ, 1977 (8) Murdock D et al, 1980 (6) Kaplinsky E et al, 1981 (7) Tchervenkov CI et al, 1983 (4) Tchervenkov CI et al, 1983 (26) Khuri SF et al, 1985 (11) Lockermen ZS et al, 1987 (12) Fiore AC et al, 1990 (5)	500 mg L^{-1} (in the cardioplegic solution)	Decreasing in the incidence of VF with higher percentage of AV block than the control group
Baraka A et al, 1993 (13)	100 mg L^{-1} (in the cardioplegic solution)	Decreasing in the incidence of VF without any increasing the incidence of AV block group
Wallace SR and Baker AB, 1994 (2)	100 mg L^{-1} (in the cardioplegic solution)	Decreasing in the incidence of VF without any increasing the incidence of AV block
Praeger IP et al,1988 (41)	200 mg in bolus (before aortic declamping)	Decreasing in the incidence of VF
Kirlangitis J et al, 1990 (40)	2 mg kg^{-1} in bolus (before aortic declamping)	Decreasing in the incidence of VF
Landow L et al, 1990 (42)	1.5 mg kg^{-1} in bolus with 2 mg min^{-1} infusion rate (before aortic declamping)	No malign dysrhythmia
Juneja R et al, 1993 (43)	1.5 mg kg^{-1} in bolus with 2 mg min^{-1} infusion rate (before aortic declamping)	Nondecreasing in the incidence of VF in patients with poor left ventricular function
Rinnie T and Kaukinen S, 1998 (44)	Continuous infusion for 20 hours with a bolus dose (before aortic clamping)	Nondecreasing in the incidence of VF
Baraka A et al, 2000 (15)	100 mg in bolus (before aortic declamping)	Decreasing in the incidence of VF with higher percentage of AV block than the control

Table 1. The results of the studies about lidocaine use to reperfusion VF

Despite the theoretical advantages of lidocaine for the treatment of VF in the cardiopulmonary resusitation, it is well recognized that lidocaine can increase defibrillation threshold (33-36). Lidocaine has not been considered to have a substantial value in the majority of cases of VF because of not only its potential to increase the defibrillation threshold, but also its negative inotropic activity. Its use is probably best reserved for cases of persistently recurring VF after electrical defibrillation, particularly in association with reperfusion occurring after heart surgery (34,37,38).

Hottenrott et al. (9) showed the augmentation of coronary blood flow to a sufficient rate towards increased energy demand in normal heart and in normothermic condition. They reported that redistribution occurs to keep endocardial / epicardial blood flow proportion. However, in hypertrophied and distended hearts and if a low aortic perfusion pressure exists, coronary blood flow will not be enough to meet increased oxygen consumption and this aspect can be explained by showing diminished coronary sinus pH, increased lactate levels and K^+ concentrations. In patients with severe coronary artery stenosis, the occurrence of VFs aggravates subendocardial ischemic injury in detoriated left ventricle.

Khuri et al. (11) reported the adverse effect of VF despite venting of heart and hypothermic conditions in reperfusion state of CPB, using continuous intraoperative intramyocardial pH monitoring technique.

Dahl et al. (14) demonstrated myocardial necrosis due to defibrillation in dogs and they proved the relation between the width of pedals and the frequency of defibrillation on myocardial injury. If the pedals are small or the frequency is scarce between defibrillations, the intensity of injury will be greater.

Manolis et al. (39) compared the efficiency and safety of lidocaine and tocainide given intravenously in patients with arrhythmia following cardiac surgery. They found that the drugs were both efficient, and there was not any statistical difference between these two drugs. In their study, they had administered 100 mg lidocaine in bolus before 60 mg infusion for 15 minutes. The infusion had been continued in a dose of 1.4 mg min^{-1} and the blood level had been found to be 1-4 mg L^{-1}.

Kirlangitis et al. (40) compared the efficacy of bretylium (10 mg kg^{-1}), lidocaine (2 mg kg^{-1}) and (as placebo) saline to prevent or to reduce VF incidence during reperfusion phase after aorta declamping. VF was seen 91% with saline, 64% with lidocaine and 36% with bretylium. The need for defibrillation was found lower with lidocaine and bretylium than saline group, but among two drugs they did not find any significant differences.

Praeger et al. (41) showed that the incidence of VF was reduced to less than 33% with treatment with 200 mg of lidocaine intravenously 3 minutes before aortic declamping. In patients who had serum potassium levels that were higher than 5.1 mEq/l and treated with lidocaine before aortic delamping, the incidence of VF decreased to less than 15%.

Landow et al. (42) administered 1.5 mg kg^{-1} lidocaine in bolus with 2 mg min^{-1} infusion rate before aorta declamping. In more than 50% of the patients, lidocaine serum levels were found to be in sub-therapeutic borders, but free lidocaine levels were within therapeutic limits. During this study, they didn't realise any malign dysrhythmia. Following this study, Juneja et al. (43) performed another study using similar lidocaine doses and reported that in patients with poor left ventricular function, prophylactic lidocaine did not reduce ventricular arrhythmias after CABG surgeries.

Rinne and Kaukinen (44) studied the effect of an intravenous bolus of lidocaine given before clamping the aorta, which was followed by a continuous infusion for as long as 20 hours. They did not observe any increase in cardiac protection as evidenced by the analysis of serum troponin concentration and serum creatine kinase MB activity and by the electrocardiogram. They did not report any decrease in the incidence of reperfusion VF.

Baraka et al. (15) showed that the incidence of reperfusion VF could be significantly decreased without any increase in the incidence of AV block with the administration of a bolus of 100 mg of lidocaine by way of the pump 2 minutes before the release of the aortic cross-clamp. In this study, the better cardiac output after weaning from CPB in the lidocaine group versus the control group was noted. They suggested that the result might be explained by the significant decrease of reperfusion VF in the lidocaine group (11 % versus 70 %).

2. Conclusion

We concluded that following the CABG surgery, the incidence of reperfusion VF is quite high. During the CABG surgery, as a prophylactic measure, the administration of lidocaine at a dose of 1 to 2 mg kg^{-1} before releasing the aortic cross-clamp can decrease the incidence of reperfusion VF. However, because of the risk of AV block with using lidocaine, we believe that in patients with persistent VF and also with left venricular hypertrophy or dysfunction, the use of other anti-arrhythmic drugs would be more helpful for defibrillation.

3. References

[1] Fall SM, Burton NA, Graeber GM, Head HD, Lough FC, Albus RA, Zajtchuk R. Prevention of ventricular fibrillation after myocardial revascularization. Ann Thorac Surg 1987; 43:182-4.

[2] Wallace SR, Baker AB. Incidence of ventricular fibrillation after aortic cross- clamp release using lignocaine cardioplegia. Anaesth Intensive Care 1994; 22: 442-6.

[3] Curling PE, Nagle D, Zeidan JR, Kaplan JA. Effects of lidocaine, propranolol and bretylium on reperfusion dysrhythmias. Anesthesiology 1981; 55: A52.

[4] Tchervenkov CI, Symes JF, Wynands JE. Lidocaine as an adjunt to high potassium cardioplegia: a prospective randomized clinical trial. Surg Forum 1983; 34: 319-21.

[5] Fiore AC, Naunheim KS, Taub J, Braun P, McBride LR, Pennington DG, Laiser GC, Willman VL, Barner HB. Myocardial preservation using lidocaine blood cardioplegia. Ann Thorac Surg 1990; 50: 771-5.

[6] Murdock D, Loeb JB, Euler DE, Randal WC. Electrophysiology of coronary reperfusion and mechanism for reperfusion arrhythmia. Circulation 1980; 61: 175-82.

[7] Kaplinsky E, Ogawa S, Michelson EL, Dreifus LS. Instantaneous and delayed ventricular arrhythmias after reperfusion of acutely ischemic myocardium: Evedince for multiple mechanisms. Circulation 1981; 63: 333-40.

[8] Hearse DJ. Reperfusion of the ischemic myocardium. J Mol Cell Cardiol 1977; 9: 605-16.

[9] Hottenrott C, Maloney JV, Buckberg G. Studies of effects of ventricular fibrillation on the adequacy of regional myocardial flow. Part III. Mechanisms of ischemia. J Thorac Cardiovasc Surg 1974; 68: 634-45.

[10] Buckberg GD, Hottenrott CE. Ventricular fibrillation: its effect on myocardial flow, distribution and performance. Ann Thorac Surg 1975; 20: 76-85.

[11] Khuri SF, Marston WA, Josa M, Braunwald NS, Cavanaugh AC, Hunt H, Barsamian EM. Observations on 100 patients with continuous intraoperative monitoring of intramyocardial pH: the adverse effects of ventricular fibrillation and reperfusion. J Thorac Cardiovasc Surg 1985; 89: 170-82.

[12] Lockermen ZS, Rose DM, Cunningham JN, Lichstein E . Repefusion ventricular fibrillation during coronary artery bypass operations and ist association with postoperative enzyme release. J Thorac Cardiovasc Surg 1987; 93: 247-52.

[13] Baraka A, Hirt N, Dabbous A, Taha S, Rouhana C, el-Khoury N, Ghabash M, Jamhoury M, Sibaii A. Lidocaine cardioplegia for prevention of reperfusion ventricular fibrillation. Ann Thorac Surg 1993; 55: 1529-33.

[14] Dahl CF, Ewy GA, Warner ED, Thomas ED. Myocardial necrosis from direct current countershock. Circulation 1974; 50: 956-61.

[15] Baraka A, Kawkabani N, Dabbous A, Nawfal M. Lidocaine for prevention of reperfusion ventricular fibrillation after release of aortic crosss-clamping. Journal of Cardiothoracic and Vascular Anesthesia 2000; 14: 531-3.

[16] Shanewise JS, Hines RL, Kaplan JA. Discontinuing cardiopulmonary bypass. In: Kaplan JA, Reich DSN, Lake CL, Konstadt SN (eds). Kaplan's Cardiac Anesthesia, 5th ed. Philadelphia: Elseiver Science, WB Saunders, 2006: 1024-5.

[17] Morita Y, Mizuno J, Yoshimura T, Morita S. Efficacy of amiodarone on refractory ventricular fibrilation resistant to lidocaine and cardioversion during weaning from cardiopulmonary bypass in aortic valve replacement for severe aortic stenosis with left ventricular hypertophy. J Anesth 2010; 26: 761-4.

[18] Weld FM, Bigga JT . The effect of lidocaine on diastolic transmembrane currents determining pacemaker depolarization in cardiac purkinje fiber. Circ Res 1976; 38: 203-8.

[19] Carmeliet E, Saikawa T. Shortenings of the action potential and reduction of pacemaker activity by lidocaine, quinidine and procainamide in sheep cardiac purkinje fibers. An effect on Na and K currents? Circ Res 1982; 50: 257-72.

[20] Schinittger I, Griffin JC, Hall RJ, Meffin PJ, Winkle RA. Effects of tocainide on ventricular fibrillation threshold. Comparison with lidocaine. Am J Cardiol 1978; 42: 76-81.

[21] Tosaki A, Balint S, Szekeres L. Protective effect of lidocaine against ischemia and reperfusion-induced arrhythmias and shifts of myocardial sodium, potassium, and calcium content. J Cardiovasc Pharmacol 1988; 12: 621-8.

[22] Cardinal R, Janse MJ, van Eeden I, Werner G, dAlnoncourt CN, Durrer Dl. The effects of lidocaine on intracellular and extracellular potentials, activation, and ventricular arrhythmias during acute regional ischemia in the isolated porcine heart. Circ Res 1981; 49: 792-806.

[23] Lee AG. Model of action of local anaesthetics. Nature 1976; 262: 545-8.

[24] Almers W, Best PM. Effects of tetracaine on displacement currents and contraction of frog skeletal muscle. J Physiol 1976; 262: 583-611.

[25] Chapman RA, Miller DJ. The effects of caffeine on the contraction of the frog heart. J Physiol 1974; 242: 589-613.

[26] Tchervenkov CI, Wynands JE, Symes JF, Malcolm ID, Dobell AR, Morin JE. Electrical behavoir of the heart following high potassium cardioplegia. Ann Thorac Surg 1983; 36: 314-9.

[27] Sellevold OF, Berg EM, Levang OW. Procaine is effective for minimizing postischemic ventricular fibrillation in cardiac surgery. Anesth Analg 1995; 81: 932-8.

[28] Alexander JH, Granger CB, Sadowski Z, Aylward PE, White HD, Thompson TD, Califf RM, Topol EJ. Prophylactic lidocaine use in acute myocardial infarction: incidence and outcomes from tow international trials. Am Heart J 1999; 137: 799-805.

[29] Sadowski ZP, Alexander JH, Skrabucha B, Dyduszynski A, Kuch J, Nartowicz E, Swiatecka G, Kong DF, Granger CB. Multicenter randomized trial and a systematic overview of lidocaine in acute myocardial infarction. Am Heart J 1999; 137: 792-8.

[30] Singh BN. Acute management of ventricular arrhythmias: role of antiarrhythmic agents. Pharmacotherapy 1997; 17: 56-64.

[31] Aidonidis I, Brachmann J, Seller H, Demowsky K, Czachurski J, Kübler W. Cardiac sympathetic nervous activity during myocardial ischemia, reperfusion and ventricular fibrillation in the dog- effects of intravenous lidocaine. Cardiology 1992; 80: 196-204.

[32] Abramovich Sivan S, Bitton Y, Karin J, David D, Akselrod S. The effects of lidocaine on cardiac parasympathetic control in normal subjects and in subjects after myocardial infarction. Clin Auton Res 1996; 6: 313-9.

[33] Baskett PJF. Advances in cardiopulmonary resusitation. Br J Anaesth 1992; 69: 182-93.

[34] Weaver WD, Fahrenbruch CE, Johnson DD, Hallsrom AP, Cobb LA, Copass MK. Effect of epinephrine and lidocaine therapy on outcome after cardiac arrest due to ventricular fibrillation. Circulation 1990; 82: 2027-34.

[35] Ujhelyi MR, Schur M, Frede T, Bottorff MB, Gabel M, Markel ML. Mechanism of antiarrhythmic drug-induced changes in defibrillation threshold: role of potassium and sodium channel conductance. J Am Coll Cardiol 1996; 27: 1534-42.

[36] Ujhelyi MR, Sims JJ, Miller AW. High- dose lidocaine does not affect defibrillation efficacy: implication for defibrillation mechanisms. Am J Physiol 1998; 274: 1113-20.

[37] Lake CL, Kron IL, Mentzer RH, Crampton RS. Lidocaine enhances intraoperative ventricular fibrillation. Anesth Analg 1986; 65: 337-41.

[38] Fujita Y, Endoh S, Yasukawa T, Sari A. Lidocaine increases the ventricular fibrillation threshold during bupivacaine-induced cardiotoxicity in pigs. Br J Anaesth 1998; 80: 218-22.

[39] Manolis AS, Smith E, Payne D, Rastegar H, Cleveland R, Estes NA 3d. Randomized double-blind study of intravenous tocainide versus lidocaine for suppression of ventricular arrhythmias after cardiac surgery. Clinical Cardiology 1990; 13: 177-81.

[40] Kirlangitis J, Middaugh R, Knight R, Goglin W, Helsel R, Grishkin B, Briggs R. Comparison of bretylium and lidocaine in the prevention of ventricular fibrillation after aortic cross-clamp release in coronary artery bypass surgery. J Cardiothorac Anesth 1990; 4: 582-7.

[41] Praeger IP, Kay RH, Moggio R, Somberg E, Pooley R, Sarabu M, Sanshaia V, Kubai K, Kumar V, Reed GE. Prevention of ventricular fibrillation after aortic declamping during cardiac surgery. Clinical Investigation 1988; 15: 98-101.

[42] Landow L, Wilson J, Heard SO, Townsend P, VanderSalm TJ, Okike ON, Pezzella TA, Pasque M. Free and total lidocaine levels in cardiac surgical patients. J Cardiothorac Anesth 1990; 4: 340-7.
[43] Juneja R, Mehta Y, Trehan N. Prophylactic lidocaine hydroclorid dose not reduce ventricular arrhymias after CABG in patients with poor left ventricular function. Indian Heart J. 1993; 45: 483-7.
[44] Rinnie T, Kaukinen S. Does lidocaine protect the heart during coronary revascularisation. Acta Anaesthesiol Scand 1998; 42: 936-40.

6

Tachycardia as "Shadow Play"

Andrey Moskalenko
The Institute of Mathematical Problems of Biology RAS
Russia

1. Introduction

Despite major scientific, medical and technological advances over the last few decades, a cure of tachycardia remains elusive. For example, the most of ventricular tachycardias (VT), including ventricular fibrillation, rank among life-threatening arrhythmias; but, in accordance with the recent multicenter investigations (CAST, ESVEM, CASCADE etc), treatment of the ventricular tachycardias using antiarrhythmic drugs of all classes leads to positive results in 58.5% of cases. In other words, the situation in its very essence indicates that the antiarrhythmic treatment is commonly prescribed nearly at random. In this context, investigation of ventricular arrhythmias must be continued in the most intensive manner, including the search for new diagnostically valuable features of cardiovascular signals.

Meanwhile, how odd it is that we should have taken the trouble of fighting tachycardia despite all the enormous progress in medicine knowledge! What we must understand is the plausible reason of this failure in treating tachycardia. The history of science gives us a lot of resembling examples convincing us that the actual state of affairs suggests a self-evident necessity of drastic alteration of the scientific paradigm that forms the basis of modern cardiology. Indeed, when all the enormous progress in modern diagnostic aids is accompanied by prescribing antiarrhythmic treatment nearly at random, we are made think seriously about adequacy of modern diagnostic aids. In other words, does modern diagnostics routine allow one to discern what should be discerned when choosing among cardiac remedy? Judging from the facts of our failure in treating tachycardia, we should conclude, that it is doubtful. Therefore, the difficulties that we encounter in our attempts to distinguish between different kinds of tachycardia correctly seem to remain to present day.

But what is the problem? We should bear in mind that the procedure of making a medical diagnosis, as "a general problem of function estimation based on empirical data" (Vapnik, 1999), consists of two tasks. The first one is creation of adequate classification, which should be free from fallacious distinction (a distinction without a difference) as well as from fallacious identification (assigning of two essentially different things to the same class of things based on a mere assumption or insufficient or erroneous grounds). To form classes (with or without the use of *a priori* reliable information on the statistical law underlying the problem) is the essence of the first part of making diagnosis, with the decision boundaries being constructed, that all the data can be separated into these classes. The second task of making diagnosis, in fact, consists in carrying out some diagnostic routine that allows one to assign an observed occurrence to one of the previously fixed classes. This bipartite procedure of making medical diagnosis is common for both human performance and performance of various learning machines in solving the problem of recognition.

Investigation of how precisely modern diagnostic routines assign patients to one of the previously fixed classes of cardiac disorders, which are customary in the framework of a current conception, lies away from the subject of this chapter. Included among the results of this study were a number of examples that, in author's opinion, prejudice against adequacy of customary classification of tachycardia.

But in the beginning, it shows itself to the best advantage to recollect some of the basic principles of cardiology, making them be a subject of a small speculation.

1.1 Can electrocardiography be omnipotent?

For more than a century both classification and distinction of tachycardias have been grounded mainly on observation results of electrocardiography, the technique for recording the electrical activity of the heart. Clinical diagnostics in cardiology includes a lot of invasive as well as non-invasive procedures, but only few of them, such as electrocardiography, offers the possibility to characterize the dynamics of the cardiovascular system over time, from minutes to hours and days. Since being offered by Willem Einthoven, electrocardiography has been captivating doctors with its facility to register easily and objectively the events related to cardiac activity. Although later technological advances brought about better and more portable ECG devices, much of the terminology used in describing an ECG originated from Einthoven. This is just he who assigned the letters P, Q, R, S and T to the various deflections, and described the electrocardiographic features of a number of cardiovascular disorders, which still remain in wide use. However the questions of what events exactly are registered, when recording ECG, and how exactly these events are related to functioning of the heart, recur time and again according to growing our knowledge of what exactly should been understood as functioning of the heart.

What do we observe indeed, when examining ECG? The theory implies (Titomir & Kneppo, 1994) that even detailed electrocardiographic mapping avails to restore only the allocation of excitation process on surfaces of the heart, but not through the heart walls. Even the modern non-invasive electrocardiographic imaging (Ramanathan et al., 2004), ascending to the summit of electrodynamics, allows watching in real time the excitation process only on epicardium; nevertheless, there is need in many cases to know accurate excitation ways through the myocardium to provide heart patients with timely, accurate diagnoses. So, electrocardiography, the most engaging technique for observation of the heart, actually seems to be similar as if actor's personal character were guessed in shadow play flitted across a screen, does it not? Generally speaking, the ECG is a kind of shadowgram. Being in ignorance of this negative trait of the electrocardiography is resulting in a total misconception about examining ECG.

Inasmuch as physicians have been aspiring to knowing accurate excitation ways through the myocardium, the clinical cardiac electrophysiology began in the early 1970s with such a goal. And? Though electrophysiology laboratories improved both cardiac diagnostics and treatment, cardiac death remains a leading medical problem. However the cardiologic data were analysed, the results remained consistent: a cure of tachycardia requires improvement. Further investigations lead to the conviction that even very precise information about ways of excitation process in the myocardium is scanty for adequate diagnosis of cardiac disorders because, for example, cardiac disorders are likely to differ essentially in their etiology, while being similar in the ways of excitation spread. Hence, examining pictures of electrical activity of the heart obtained with electrocardiography, electrocardiographic imaging or electrophysiology mapping, doctors practise some sorts of divination and guess-work on the basis of shadow play nevertheless.

To improve the guess-work and to make it science-based mathematical approaches for ECG analysis were suggested in abundance. For example, some of the recent developments are described in (Loskutov & Mironyuk, 2007; Wessel et al., 2007). In general, there is an apparent tendency for science to become more and more mathematical. Moreover, biochemical and even genetic methods have been recently united, with the other appropriate diagnostic tools to improve making precise diagnosis of tachycardia sort. For instance, a congenial form of the long-QT syndrome, LQT3, which is consistent with the clinical presentation of bradycardia-related arrhythmogenic episodes during sleep or relaxation, was detected by genetic methods (Noble, 2002a). It is noted (Crampin et al., 2004) that studies of human disease using microarray for gene expression are increasingly common in cardiovascular research and medicine. In spite of that, it is rather undoubtful that there are many thousands of genic combinations that can result (under one or another living conditions) in a phenotype with high risk of sudden cardiac death. Thus, cardiologists become more and more powerful in detailed description of the heart but can't seem to find a good solution for arrhythmic sudden death prediction and prevention.

All these facts lead us to the comprehension, that mechanisms of tachycardia are much more intricate than one used to consider them in the frames of the physiology of the 20th century. Drawing our analogy between electrocardiography and shadow pantomime still further, we ought to admit the possibility of quite objective evaluation of several actor's properties (such as, probably, their height or some other body traits) by observing their shadows flitted across a screen. The traditional electrocardiography keeps its positions in medicine since it gives likewise convenient possibility of swift and quite objective evaluation of several characteristics relative to cardiac performance. Some of medical questions can already be answered by visual inspection of the ECG paper strips themselves, e.g. whether the electrical excitation in different parts of the heart (sinus node, atrium, atrioventricular node, and ventricle) is normal or not. In some cases, location of arrhythmia origin as well as several morphologic disturbances, such as atrioventricular block, WPW syndrome, atrioventricular dissociation and injury currents after myocardial infarction can be visually identified on the ECG; however, this is nearly all reliable information which one should search, when using traditional examination of the ECG. "The ECG is, unfortunately, an unreliable indicator of potential arrhythmogenicity," a noted scientist explains the problem (Noble, 2002a). "Similar changes in form of the QT interval and T waveform can be induced by very different molecular and cellular effects, some benign, others dangerous." Other authors (Wessel et al., 2007) state very decidedly: "There exists no 'golden parameter' whose measurement is able to reliably describe and estimate all risks. From time to time there is an excessive enthusiasm of some scientists claiming that their new developed parameter is better than previously used ones. However, none of the known risk predictors probably is or can ever serve as an omnipotent outcome determinant." The last statement is referred to beat-to-beat analysis, but I am sure that the same is valid also for ECG analysis as a whole.

Thus, if ten years ago we did dare say about electrocardiography that there was "sufficient grounds to expect that the role of this method in differential diagnosis of cardiac arrhythmias will increase in future" (Moskalenko et al., 2001), now this thought appears to be rather doubtful. Admittedly, present-day mathematical approaches to analysis of time series (the ECG is a typical time series) gives birth to hopes to elicit information about intimate details of the functioning of the heart from the ECG. The mathematical approaches are considered bellow, but it is helpful to make more exact some details concerned with functioning of the heart before discussing these mathematical approaches.

1.2 What should the activity of the heart and the action of the heart mean?

Some time ago, I came up against the problem of appropriate translation of several basic ideas, which spread among the Russian scientists, into English. During my endeavours to solve it I realized that the puzzle lies far outside linguistic problems, but rather consists in essential difference of conceptual models of living creatures. Moreover, multitudinous literal adoption, when translating from English into Russian and vice versa, resulted with time in fanciful muddle of terms. One of such a pseudo-linguistic problems was discussed not long ago (Elkin & Moskalenko, 2009) in connection with basic mechanisms of cardiac arrhythmias. In that case, the matter concerned fallacious use of the term "spiral wave" instead of "reverberator [1]", which seems to be more correct when considering a two-dimensional autowave vortex (for instance, a vortex of excitation in myocardium).

The terms such as "electrical function of the heart", "cardiac performance", "cardiac functioning" etc. are widely used in scientific literature although there are not any clear definitions of them. For the purpose of this preamble, it appears to be very helpful to emphasize the importance of distinguishing the phenomena that are associated with action of the heart [2], according to scientific and medical literature of Russia, from the phenomena that are reckoned among appearance of cardiac activity [3]. As a matter of fact, the Russian scientific doctrine is grounded, in many respects, upon the ideas that were evolved by P.K. Anokhin, P.V. Simonov, K.V. Sudakov and others who developed the theory of functional systems in the frames of cybernetic description of living things. Conceptually, the theory is close to control theory as well as to such relatively novel branches of science as biophysics, computational biology, and synergetics. In brief, the term "action" should be used to refer to events that can be characterised by target function in cybernetic way of description, while the term "activity" is appropriate for the other cases.

Hence, the terms "(any) cardiac activity" or "(any) activity of the heart" should be used only for designation of any aimless functioning of the heart. On the other hand, "the action of the heart" should be comprehended as functioning of the heart that is directed to maintenance of physiological homeostasis, which is the target function in this case. Obviously, the action of the heart can be put into effect only due to a quantity of control loops and guidance loop[4],

---

[1] Some authors (Winfree, 1991) applied the term "rotor" to make distinction with "spiral wave", but the term is not in current use because of overload of its meaning. Both spiral wave and reverberator are sorts of re-entry, the main mechanism of tachycardia.

[2] In Russian: "сердечная деятельность"; here translated as "action of the heart" in accordance with English-Russian Dictionary by Professor V.K. Mueller, 24-th Revised Edition; Moscow, "Russky Yazyk", 1995, p. 35 and p. 511.

[3] In Russian: "активность сердца"; "the electrical activity of the heart" ≡ "электрическая активность сердца".

[4] Notice that the control is used to maintain a desired output of the system under control, while the guidance is intended for shifting the system from a state A to a state B.

which all together organize one and indivisible cardiovascular system. Electrical phenomena, that accompany the functioning of the heart and can be recorded by electrocardiography, are nowise satisfying the target of the cardiovascular functioning, because they are but side effects of the autowave function of the heart (Elkin & Moskalenko, 2009). In English scientific and medical literature, the electrical phenomena to accompany the functioning of the heart are referred to as "the electrical activity of the heart" in a good accordance with the remarks above.

Though there are still some technical difficulties in distinguishing between these two concept nodes (aimed and aimless functioning) and though the language structures referred to them can be discussed as yet, nevertheless, it is very important for methodical purpose to keep in mind the necessity of such distinguishing. It is important because the distinguishing modifies a conceptual position of a cardiologist and can consequently change his or her evaluation of the symptoms. For example, the "new" cardiologic conception allows an assertion to make that the atrioventricular node reentrant tachycardia (AVNRT), which is a re-entrant rhythm within the atrioventricular (AV) node, should be considered in a number of cases as a variant of normal cardiac rhythm. Actually, the AVNRT is shown by recent investigations (Kurian et al., 2010) to be possible merely due to specific heterogeneity of AV node, which is peculiar to the human because of its genetic causes. But according to well-known theory of biological evolution, the peculiarity would be eliminated ages and ages ago by mechanism of natural selection, if the heterogeneity of AV node were harmful for our ancestry. Nevertheless, we are very successful in observing the reverse: the hereditary trait was fixed by the natural selection. Hence, the supposition seems to be quite valid that the AVNRT was a variant of normal cardiac rhythm in that cases, when our remote ancestors required (for very quick running, for instance) developing the cardiac rhythm more rapid than the one that can be supplied by the sinoatrial node. Is it reasonable then to suppose that this hypothetic ancient mechanism of cardiac adaptation to extremely high load remains hitherto not to be rudimentary or atavistic, but plays still an important role as a potential mechanism of cardiac adaptation for human being? Since publishing this hypothesis (Elkin & Moskalenko, 2009), some facts for its support have been revealed. For example, a very interesting case has been reported to me recently by professor Ardashev [5] (in personal communication). At the time of scheduled medical examination of Russian Olympic team, the AVNRT was revealed in a racing cyclist during cardiac stress test. There were no patient complaints in this case, the cyclist felt himself very well and demonstrated remarkable results in the sport. Nevertheless, the objective data of electrocardiography were thought to be more important, and the man was operated to prevent a high risk of sudden cardiac death. There were no patient complaints after the ablation, this simple operation in our time, but the sportsman became incapable of sustaining his previous level of physical exertion and had to leave great sport. In my opinion, the case indicates how solicitous a cardiologist should be about such patients. Our adequate comprehension of cardiac functioning must be achieved more prompt, when doctors become more attentive to medical practice of this sort.

The case reported in the previous paragraph improves the conviction, that even the most solid data about the path of excitation spread in myocardium are just data about "shadow

[5] Prof. Andrey V. Ardashev, M.D., Ph.D.; Director of Cardiac electrophysiology and arrhythmia service, 83 Clinical Hospital of Federal Biomedical Agency of Russia; official web-site: http://ardashev-arrhythmia.ru/

play" ascertained exactly. The correct distinguishing of normal cardiac rhythm from pathological one, which appears to be similar visually and statistically, requires something greater than knowing the precise excitation path in the heart. We need something much more skilful than simple data-analysis of any existent type because the novel skilful data-analysis must give us the ability to differ whether the functioning of the heart observed corresponds to the target function of the organism or conversely leads the biological system away from it. In the example above, the tachycardia seems to be a sort of adequate response of the organism to the requirements of its environment. To make adequate diagnosis, we need a complete model of situation, which consists of an adequate model of the patient and an adequate model of the surroundings in which he or she has resided for a sufficiently long period of time.

"The large complexity of cardiovascular regulation, with its multiplicity of hormonal, genetic and external interactions, requires a multivariate approach based on a combination of different linear and nonlinear parameters. <...> Biological control systems have multiple feedback loops and the dynamics result from the interplay between them. <...> Considering these rather system-theoretical characteristics, the development of nonlinear and also knowledge-based methods should lead to a diagnostic improvement in risk stratification. <...> A further aim, therefore, is, to go a qualitatively new step: the combination of data analysis and modeling" (Wessel et al., 2007). A cardiologist will be likely to gain the adequate diagnostic capacity of distinguishing the normal action of the heart from pathological one only, when having such a skilful knowledge-based model, realized either in computer or in the cardiologist's brain.

1.3 Magic? Chaotic cardiology? Or cardiophysics?

The discussion above reveals faultiness of the cardiologic paradigm, which is constructed owing to the epoch-making discoveries made by the greatest physiologist of the 19th and 20th centuries. The faultiness appears to be caused by our rather simple comprehension of how biological systems work, which arose from the historic specificity of scientific knowledge evolution. During 17–19th centuries the science development is known to be mainly grounded on the notions of determinism, with great advantage in applied mechanics to constitute their historical basis. It resulted in permeating the conception, which is referred to as mechanistic approach now, into many fields of science. Nor has medicine escaped the common lot, since all modern physiology is per se a manifestation of mechanistic approach in biology, as it was discussed formerly (Elkin & Moskalenko, 2009). In accordance with scientific tradition, the phenomena observed in physiology are explained as a result of different mechanical movements. The movement of ions through membrane of a biological cell in order to explain the action potential is a good example of the approach. Prevalent endeavours of modern cardiologists to treat cardiac disorders by adjusting membrane channels using one or another drug is another such example.

But, there have been gathered a lot of observations by the end of the 20h century that remain out the conceptual framework prescribed by the language of physiology. The time for new conceptual generalization has come. Physicists and mathematicians managed to find that processes to occur in "purely physical" systems (for example, in laser or even just in boiling water) are similar, in some sense, to those observed by physiologists in excitable biological tissues. Little by little, a new comprehension arose, that such phenomena, observed in biological tissues, as excitability, conductivity, all-or-nothing response, adiaphoria etc. are inherent not only to biological objects, but they widely happen in nonliving material as well. Notice that it is not a sort of drawing an analogy, but exactly a new valid generalization of scientific knowledge stored until now. The generalization entailed developing a new, more universal, language, namely the biophysical language. The new language enables not only rendering properly the description of all that was depicted before in the frames of physiology, but also representing, in unified terms, a wide range of experimental results which were hardly designated by the old language of physiologists.

The penetration of new scientific ideas in the old cardiology can be exemplified in developing the conception of autowave function of the heart (Elkin & Moskalenko, 2009). Clear perception that autowave rather than electric properties of the heart give the base for the normal cardiac functioning seems to be really of great importance. Cardiac electrical activity, which was initially conceived by physiologists as the main cause of cardiac functioning, is rather similar to "shadows" of respective autowave processes. Physiologists used to think that the normal action of the heart is provided by conduction of ion channels of myocardial cells, but indeed it is provided by normal values of some integral myocardial parameters that characterize the heart as active medium. Different combinations of conduction of different ion channels can result in the same values of the integral parameters, and, therefore, some medical influence upon any sort of ion channels is likely to result in changing the integral myocardial parameters away from its values optimal for organism under given conditions. Further, cardiac abnormalities should be divided into two groups: those that are related with disorders of the cardiac autowave function and those that result from injuries of control and guidance loop in the integral cardiovascular system.

In addition to remarkable progress in biophysics, another important conceptual breakthrough of science was performed in the field that now is referred to as nonequilibrium thermodynamics, "physics of becoming" (Prigogine, 1980) or synergetics. "For centuries, humankind has believed that the world with all its form and structure was created by supernatural forces. In recent decades science has shaken these beliefs with the discovery of the exciting possibility of a self-created and self-creating world – of self-organization. Synergetics endeavours to reveal the intimate mechanisms of self-organization. The transitions from chaos to order, the nature of self-organization, the various approaches to it and certain philosophical inferences are outlined. Synergetics thus represents a remarkable confluence of many strands of thought, and has become a paradigm in modern culture" (Bushev, 1994). A significant role in this new conception pertains to the bifurcation theory as well as to the chaos theory. As to cardiology, there has been originated a modern discipline, computational biology, which applies the newest achievements of modern physics and mathematics. Note that all these modern studies are grounded, in many respects, on the dynamical systems theory, an area of applied mathematics used to describe the behaviour of complex dynamical systems. Much of modern research of dynamical systems is focused on the study of their chaotic behaviour. Despite initial insights in the first half of the 20th century, chaos theory became formalized as such only after mid-century, when it first became evident for some scientists that linear theory, the prevailing system theory at that time, simply could not explain the observed behaviour of certain experiments. Finite dimensional linear systems are well-known nowadays to be never chaotic; for a dynamical system to display chaotic behaviour, it has to be either nonlinear, or infinite-dimensional. Biological systems are complex and nonlinear, and, therefore, demonstrate complex and nonlinear behaviour, which may be chaotic, in many cases. The heart appears to be the same (Loskutov et al., 2009; Zhuchkova et al., 2009).

All these modern disciplines lead to the conclusion that often adequate comprehension of a complex system requires analysing not the observed values, but some of its integral characteristics, which can be mathematically obtained as a combination of a number of the observed. If speaking the language of mysticism [6], the most important things occur on invisible plane supporting the visible one. In the dynamical systems theory, that invisible plane corresponds to phase space (state space) and parameter space of a dynamical system. Details of using the spaces were described elsewhere (Prigogine, 1980; Winfree, 1991; Loskutov et al., 2009). When a cardiologist attempts to analyse features of tachycardia observed on the ECG, the human mind appears to be unfit to observe the movement performed by the dynamical system corresponding to the patient under medical inspection. As a result, we have a very strange state of affairs: natural faculty of human mind does not allow correct diagnosis to be made in most of tachycardia cases. The results of analysing phase and parameter spaces of a patient seem only to give a good opportunity to clarify whether the cardiac phenomena observed correspond to the normal activity of the heart or some case of cardiac disorders happens.

Chaotic attractor is a good illustration of how important ideas of modern physics are for cardiology. Whether any sort of chaotic attractors correspond to the normal cardiac action, is a very good question.

Other crucial phenomena that must certainly be taken into account when treatment for a cardiologic patient is provided are caused by so-called "bifurcation memory", which has attracted special attention of investigators since recently (Feigin & Kagan, 2004; Ataullakhanov et al., 2007; Moskalenko & Elkin, 2009). The bifurcation memory is considered (Feigin & Kagan, 2004) "within the framework of the general problem, when bifurcation situations generate in state space bifurcation tracks that isolate regions of unusual transition processes (phase spots)." Unusual behaviour of systems is attributed to the existence of the specific regions in phase space, the phase spots, where controllability of a dynamic system decreases dramatically. "Ships with high manoeuvring capabilities, aircraft and controlled underwater vehicles designed to be unstable in steady-state motion are dynamic systems of this class and are important for applications" (Feigin & Kagan, 2004). Recent evidence suggests that similar phenomena can be found in the heart (Elkin & Moskalenko, 2009; Moskalenko & Elkin, 2009). The results of investigating the bifurcation memory in a cardiac model are presented and discussed below.

To gain a better insight into all these intricate things, the newest mathematical achievements as well as modern supercomputers should be widely adopted. "Mathematical modelling is widely accepted as an essential tool of analysis in the physical science and engineering, yet many are still sceptical about its role in biology. <...> It is however already clear that incorporation of cell models into tissue and organ models is capable of spectacular insights. <...> The potential of such simulations for teaching, drug discovery, device development,

[6] The point of Mysticism is that we humans have the capacity – a non-rational capacity – to identify with and to experience that invisible plane. It is possible, according to Mysticism, because in our deepest being, we belong to that invisible plane. Thus, a cardiologist probably uses such a non-rational capacity when guessing at the ECG, does he not?

and, of course, for pure physiological insight is only beginning to be appreciated" (Noble, 2002b). Integrative physiology of the 21st century is set to become highly quantitative and, therefore, one of the most computer-intensive disciplines (Crampin et al., 2004; Noble, 2002a). Although, for historical reasons, the focus has been to study these events through experimental and clinical observations, mathematical modelling and simulation, which enable analysis at multiple time and spatial scales, have also complemented these efforts. "One of the intriguing opportunities presented by the availability of high resolution imaging and anatomically based computational models is that of the patient-specific modelling. That is, the generic model of the heart or lungs can be adjusted to match MR images of the heart or helical scan CT images of the lungs. Coupled with measurements of both gene sequence and physiological function for that individual, the realization of patient-specific, model-based clinical diagnosis becomes more feasible" (Crampin et al., 2004).

Thus, we ought to conclude that the 21st century seems to yield a new discipline, which is referred to as cardiovascular physics or cardiophysics (since it combines cardiology with novel achievements of physics). The cardiophysics is expected to solve the problems of prediction and prevention of sudden arrhythmic death.

1.4 Polymorphic and monomorphic tachycardias: A distinction without differences?

For about two last decades, it has been used to distinguish monomorphic and polymorphic ventricular tachycardias. The term "polymorphic" in cardiology refers to those ventricular arrhythmias that are characterised by the structure (morphology) of the QRS complexes continuously varied with time (Kukushkin et al., 1998). While a monomorphic ventricular tachycardia (MVT) is considered to distinguish itself by stable morphology of the QRS complexes in combination with constant value of the RR-intervals, a polymorphic one (PVT) is characterised by unstable morphology of the QRS; however, it remains still not fully clear how often and how profoundly the subsequent QRS complexes must be altered (Kukushkin & Medvinskii, 2004). Moreover, because electrocardiographic signals in PVT are of irregular shape, the very entity of PVT is not defined unambiguously in the known classifications of arrhythmias: its definition frequently overlaps with definitions of other types of cardiac rhythm disorders – see more elaborately in (Moskalenko et al., 2001). PVT is believed to precede ventricular fibrillation (VF) and sudden cardiac death. It has been stated (Kukushkin & Medvinskii, 2004) that the stability of QRS morphology is reflected in the notion "degree of ECG polymorphism (variability)" and qualitatively corresponds to the extent of reentry nonstationarity. Discussion about etiology and mechanisms of PVT and VF remains after 160 years of inquiry due to exceedingly difficult methodological obstacles (Kukushkin & Medvinskii, 2004; Kurian & Efimov 2010). Despite this entire muddle, danger of arrhythmic death is linked by tradition with deepness of impression that polymorphic shape of the ECG creates in the mind of a cardiologist. Summarizing all these facts, we must conclude that some doubts are cast upon attempts to distinguish different types of cardiac disorders on base of practically identical set of signs. Should polymorphic shape of the ECG be apprehended as "shadow play", when essentially different cardiac disorders cast similar "shadows" on the ECG or when the same cardiac disorders appears on the ECG as noticeably different "shadows"? The remainder of the chapter is dedicated to studying the problem of how polymorphic shape of the ECG is significant for making adequate diagnosis.

2. Methods of the investigation: The Russian style in "affairs of the heart"

Setting down quantitative criteria (Kukushkin et al., 1998) for identifying the electrocardiogram type correspondent to polymorphic shape of the ECG (polymorphic, monomorphic, or quasi-monomorphic [7]), which relied on the amplitudes and frequencies of the recorded signal, was likely the first attempt of accurate estimation of how polymorphic the shape of the ECG is. Mathematical approach for quantitatively assessing the amount of polymorphism present in electrocardiograms was proposed three years later (Moskalenko et al., 2001; Moskalenko et al., 2008). This approach was referred to in an earlier paper as normalized-value analysis of electrocardiographic variability (NVAEV, or "ANI-method" in Russian notation).

2.1 The main idea of the ANI-method

The ANI-method belongs to nonlinear and knowledge-based methods of time series analysis. Similar to a number of other methods of time series analysis (for example, Singular Spectrum Analysis, SSA), the first step of the ANI-method consists in transformation of the one-dimensional time series (the ECG in our case) into the trajectory matrix by means of a delay procedure. On the next step (instead of making the singular value decomposition, as it is in SSA), the normalized measure is calculated for each couple of columns of the trajectory matrix that is recognized as the nearest neighbours in some special sense. In such a way, a mathematical measure of "instant ECG variability" is obtained for each point of the source time series. Then some of average characteristics, so-called indices of ECG variability, are calculated in addition.

In the beginning, the new method was developed for automation of customary activities performed by a cardiologist assessing the ECG recorded during tachycardia in order to reckon the tachycardia among monomorphic or among polymorphic sets of an arrhythmia. To perform the assessing, one needs, in accordance with the known classifications of arrhythmias, to find adjacent arrhythmic cycles in the ECG (adjacent cycles of cardiac activation during arrhythmia), then to compare them in pairs, and finally to construct an assessment summarizing locally a few adjacent arrhythmic cycles. Thus, developers of such an automatic tool find themselves relatively free in their choice of key steps of the tool, namely: 1) a criterion for search, 2) a rule for the comparison procedure, and 3) a rule for the summarizing procedure.

In the course of designing the tool, we tried several ordinary approaches, and then an optimal combination of the key steps was empirically picked out. Of course, there is no good reason sufficient for insisting that the current realisation of the ANI-method is the most appropriate for solving the cardiologic problems which it is designed for. Therefore, any of the three key steps of the algorithm referred to as the ANI-method is likely to be replaced by a more appropriate one in order to improve the tool. Developing better

---

[7] According to the authors (Kukushkin et al., 1998), arrhythmia is considered monomorphic if the changes in the frequency and the amplitude of the corresponding ECG is smaller then 15 and 30%, respectively. Quasi-monomorphic is an arrhythmia that is "close to monomorphic". In other words, such a quasi-monomorphic arrhythmia is similar to a monomorphic one, being visually examined, but these two differ in a quantitative sense. The others are considered to be polymorphic.

algorithms for analysis of electrocardiographic polymorphism may become a goal of future studies.

Anyway, the most important idea lying in the basis of the ANI-method is the decision to refuse flatly making any precise comparison between successive arrhythmic ventricular complexes on the ECG. Instead of precise comparison, an arbitrary ECG segment (reference sample) of length less than the length of the arrhythmic cycle is wittingly chosen as a pattern under consideration in order to be compared with the homologous phase segment of the successive (adjacent) arrhythmic ventricular complexes. The comparison must be reiterated with other pairs of such homologous segments while a statistically significant quantity of the comparison results is collected for each part of the ECG under study. The arbitrary ECG segment is also referred to as a sampling window (SaW), which width is taken equal 50-70% of the average arrhythmic cycle length. In practice, we chose the segment length (sampling window width) to be comparable with the shortest width of the QRS of the biological species under studying under control conditions (normal sinus rhythm), and the comparison is repeated for each point of the sampled ECG. In our experience, when errors of the comparison are present, their effects on the final result of quantitatively assessing polymorphic shape the ECG are often offset, at least in part. In other words, the fortuitous errors of such a comparison reciprocally compensate each other due to averaging the comparison results collected.

So, the new approach to analysis of arrhythmic ECG is free of the need to identify individual QRS complexes, because the ANI-method assesses the variability by numerically comparing adjacent segments of the ECG. The entire electrocardiogram or any of its fragments is described with two parameters, of which one is an index of ECG variability and the other specifies how this index changes with time. These two parameters are useful in assessing the arrhythmic polymorphism within one ECG and in comparing different electrocardiograms. Notice that, with the ANI-method for assessing the dynamics of changes in the ECG, there is no need to recognize individual peaks. Therefore, it is reasonable to expect that the variability indices will be useful in assessing real polymorphic electrocardiograms, especially when individual QRS complexes are difficult or impossible to identify.

After realising the current version of the ANI-method, some attempts to understand its mathematical sense were made. By this time, there are two variants of mathematical description given for the ANI-method. Both are adduced just below.

2.1.1 Formalism by Medvinskii

The first variant of mathematical description of the ANI-method was proposed by A. Medvinskii in a form appropriate for a discrete signal analysis (Moskalenko et al., 2001) and is given briefly here.

The procedure of comparison is implemented for each moment of time, which yields the local characteristic of electrocardiographic variability (instant ECG variability index I_i). This index is a tool for numerically comparing segment i corresponding to the current position of the SaW with segment j, the first segment most closely resembling segment i in the subsequent recording. The segment j is supposed to be the homologous phase segment for the segment i. Formally, the procedure of their comparison is as follows. For any segment of the electrocardiogram, vector F is defined:

$$F_k = \left(f_k, f_{k+h}, \dots, f_{k+(p-1)h}\right),$$

where f_n is the signal amplitude at time n; n varies from k to $k + (p - 1)/h$, where p is the dimension of the so-called embedding space, and h is the embedding step. The distance between the ith and jth vectors is determined by the norm:

$$r_{ij} = \left|\mathbf{F}_i - \mathbf{F}_j\right|. \tag{1}$$

Note that, for periodic signals, $r_{ij} = 0$ if $|i - j| = mT$, where $m = 0, 1, 2, 3$, etc. For aperiodic signals, the smaller the difference between the ith and the jth segments, the smaller the r_{ij}.

Segments i and j are separated by a time interval τ_i: $\tau_i = j - i, j > i$. Seeking the jth segment and determining the τ_i value are based on the assumption that j is a unique function of i. If τ_i were known, it would be possible to assess the similarity between the two segments using norm (1) in the p-dimensional embedding space. Therefore, we postulate:

$$I_i \equiv \frac{1}{S_i} r_{i(i+\tau_i)}, \tag{2}$$

where S_i is the peak-to-peak amplitude of the electrocardiographic signal in the sampling window corresponding to time i.

To automatically seek a segment most closely corresponding to the current SaW and separated from it by the shortest interval, we systematically scan an electrocardiogram segment of length T_{ScW} (where ScW is an abbreviation for scanning window) using step size h. Every next segment within the scanning window is compared with the current sample by any technique (for example, a technique based on the use of an autocorrelation function or the norm in the embedding space). In simple cases in which the QRS complexes are identifiable, τ_i is equal to the inter-QRS interval, irrespective of the used technique. When the QRS complexes are difficult to identify, as in real polymorphic ventricular tachycardia, τ_i is formally set into correspondence with the position of the norm minimum. In other words, we assume that the r_{ij} minimum determines the segment j position in the scanning window. In this case, expression (2) reads

$$I_i = \frac{1}{S_i} \min_{k \in (i,i+L)} (r_{ik}) \tag{3}$$

This approach considerably saves the time for computing I_i by combining the search for a segment homologous to the current sample with their comparison. The scanning window width L is chosen to be as wide as the greatest width of normal QRS in the biological species under study.

For further analysis of electrocardiograms or their fragments of arbitrary lengths, it is useful to construct some integral characteristics of electrographic variability. Also, one of the simplest solutions is applied to construct the summarizing assessment. In our analysis, we use (i) the mean value of the I_i function, or the electrocardiographic variability index V_1, and (ii) the coefficient of variation of the I_i function, V_2. So, Index V_1 represents an average evaluation of the unlikeness of ECG segments inside the studied fragment and the index V_2

is its variation. To monitor the electrocardiogram changes with time, we calculate the variability index V_{1i} and the coefficient V_{2i} in some fixed-width window, (the averaging window, AW), corresponding to time i. Shifting the AW along the time axis, we obtain a trajectory in the (V_{1i}, V_{2i}) parameter space, which enables one to visualize the detailed ECG dynamics. Note that the properties of the end segment of the ECG whose length is equal to the averaging window width are uncertain; therefore, the AW should not be too wide. On the basis of the definition of ventricular tachycardia, we chose the width of the averaging window to be six QRS widths. We assume everywhere that, unlike V_{1i} and V_{2i}, V_1 and V_2 characterize segments that are considerably longer than the averaging window width.

2.1.2 Formalism by Elkin

An analytical form of mathematical description for the ANI-method was suggested by Yu. Elkin in 2005 and is published here for the first time.

According to Yu. Elkin, the ANI-method is a computational algorithm that could be analytically described as follows.

Let us define a function:

$$R(t,T)=\left[\int_{t}^{t+T_{SaW}}(\varphi(\tau+T)-\varphi(\tau))^2 d\tau\right]^{1/2}, \tag{4}$$

where T_{SaW}, the width of the SaW, is a fixed value, which is a subject to adjustment (the T_{SaW} is taken equal 50-70% of the average arrhythmic cycle length, as it was mentioned above).

The procedure of seeking the next homologous phase segments is executed within the scanning window, ScW, with its width confined to an area of expectation to find the adjacent arrhythmic cycle. At each instant of time t, a segment is supposed to be the adjacent homologous phase segment for the current sampling window, SaW, if the segment is situated at the distance $T_0(t)$ such, that

$$R(t,T_0(t))=\min_{T_{SaW}\le T\le T_{ScW}}(R(t,T)) \tag{5}$$

For the ECG under consideration, the comparison of the homologous phase segments is repeated continuously with some constant time step Δt_0, without binding to any phase of an arrhythmic ventricular complex. The comparison of the pair recognized to be the adjacent homologous phase segment is carried out by the formula:

$$I(t)\equiv\frac{1}{S(t)}R(t,T_0(t)) \tag{6}$$

The function $T_0(t)$ is referred to as quasi-period, so long as, for a cyclic process, it corresponds to a quantity that is analogous to the period of a periodic process; for a periodic signal, $T_0(t)$ is exactly equal to its period.

Further, the ECG variability indices V_1 and V_2 can be produced for any fragment of $I(t)$. The functions $V_1(t)$ and $V_2(t)$ can be yielded with the help of shifting the AW along the time axis.

2.1.3 ANI -2003

It is noteworthy that the current implementation of the NVAEV (Medvinsky et al., 2003), referred to as ANI-2003, is improved by preliminary normalization of time series within the ScW, in order to increase the stability of the algorithm. The normalization is performed by substituting the sample mean or sample deviation into the formula for standard score. All results presented bellow are obtained with use of the ANI-2003.

3. Results and discussion

We studied pseudo electrocardiograms (pseudo-ECGs) obtained from *in vitro* studies of ventricular arrhythmias ("physiological ECG") as well as from numerical simulations ("numerical ECG").

Each "physiological ECG" represented a time series constructed by weighted summation of separate electrocardiograms obtained by multielectrode mapping of excitation propagation during an arrhythmia obtained from the isolated wall of the ground squirrel right ventricle. The experimental model and the procedure for constructing the pseudo-ECG were described in detail elsewhere (Sarancha et al., 1997; Kukushkin et al., 1998).

For calculation of "numerical ECGs" we used the Aliev-Panfilov mathematical model of heart tissue (Aliev & Panfilov, 1996):

$$\frac{\partial u}{\partial t} = \Delta u - ku(u-a)(u-1) - uv,$$

$$\frac{\partial v}{\partial t} = \varepsilon(u,v)(-u - ku(u-a-1)),$$

$$\varepsilon(u,v) = \varepsilon_0 + \frac{\mu_1 v}{u + \mu_2}.$$

The parameters in the equations were adjusted (Aliev & Panfilov, 1996) to accurately reflect cardiac tissue properties ($k = 8.0$; $\mu_1 = 0.2$; $\mu_2 = 0.2$; $a = 0.15$; $\varepsilon = 0.01$). In our simulations, the parameter μ_2 was equal to 0.3 or 1.3, with the parameter a being varied from 0.12 to 0.19. Note that the parameter a specifies the threshold of excitation. The simulations were carried out in 2D excitable media (128 elements along each dimension) with von Neumann boundary conditions. The details of the simulations and the procedure for constructing the pseudo-ECGs in the simulations were described in detail elsewhere (Moskalenko & Elkin, 2007; Moskalenko & Elkin, 2009).

3.1 Tachycardia of the lacetic type

The reverberator, a typical autowave phenomenon in two-dimensional excitable media, can be described simplistically as a half of a plane wave curved around its break point. The break point is also called the tip of the reverberator. Reverberator behaviour is commonly sketched in the terms of movement of its tip. Autowave reverberators are known to be the main cause of different kinds of tachycardia. As long as the dynamics of the reverberators rides on myocardium state, the myocardium state can be estimated, perhaps, by details of their dynamics.

Formerly, three types of reverberator tip movement in homogeneous two-dimensional medium were known. These are 1) uniform circular movement, 2) meander, i.e. two-periodic movement, with the tip moving along a curve similar to cycloid (epicycloid or hypocycloid), and 3) hyper-meander, i.e. a 'complex' or maybe 'chaotic' movement whose wave tip trajectory could not be described in terms of two periods. Recently we found (Moskalenko & Elkin, 2009) a new autowave behaviour, which we called the lacet, – namely, the transformation of reverberator motion from a two-periodic meander into one-periodic circular rotation due to spontaneous deceleration of reverberator drift (Fig. 1). The lacet is perhaps a phenomenon of so called bifurcation memory.

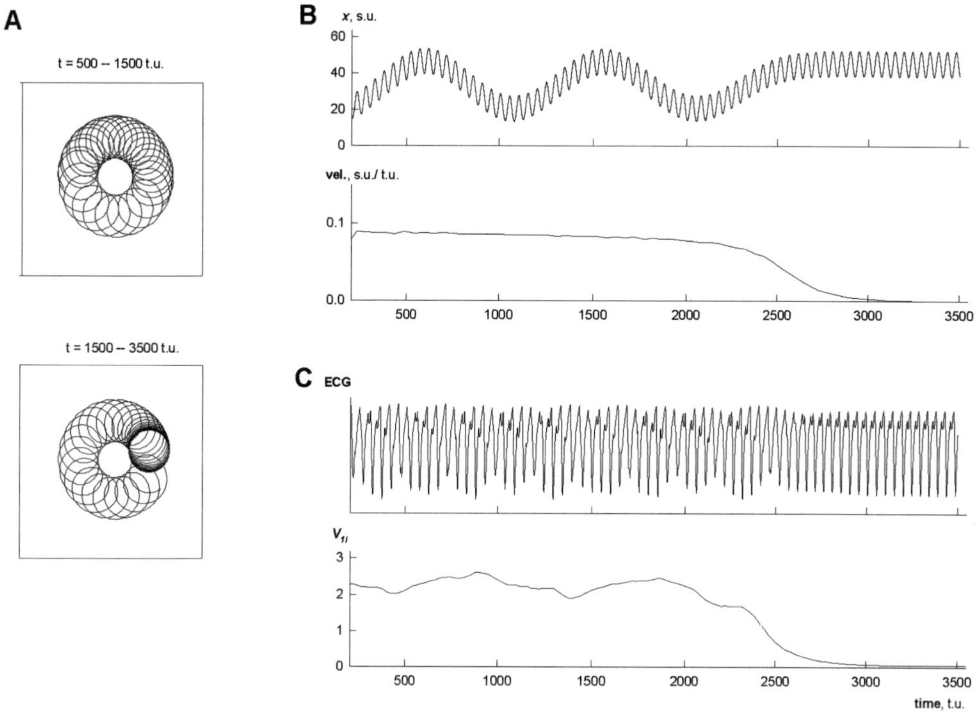

Fig. 1. The transition from polymorphic to monomorphic tachycardia of the lacetic type in the Aliev-Panfilov model at a = 0.1803. **A**. The trajectory of the reverberator tip in the case of the vortex drift deceleration (the lacet type of the vortex motion). For the convenience, the trajectory is segregated into two pictures because some different parts of the trajectory overlap. **B-C**. From top to bottom: the dynamics of the *x* coordinate of the reverberator tip, the dynamics of velocity of the instant centre of the autowave vortex, the ECG, and index of the ECG variability, $V_1(t)$. All the graphs have the same horizontal scale.

It was demonstrated in computational simulation (Moskalenko & Elkin, 2007; Elkin & Moskalenko, 2009) that the lacet in the myocardium coincides with spontaneous transition from polymorphic to monomorphic arrhythmia in the ECG dynamics. Also, it was shown by the example of the lacet (Moskalenko, 2010) that the information revealed in ECG with the ANI-2003 corresponds sufficiently to velocity of the reverberator drift. Fig. 1 represents these results. The comparison of the velocity of reverberator drift and ECG dynamics described with $V_1(t)$ shows that there is perfect coincidence between them.

By visual inspection of the ECG paper strips, there is no way to distinguish a tachycardia caused by an ordinary autowave vortex from a tachycardia of the lacetic type. Observing the ECG on Fig. 1 during but the first 2000 time units, cardiologist will certainly think it to be just typical re-entrant tachycardia, because there is no obvious difference between ECG shapes of these different sorts of tachycardia. Moreover, even the transition from polymorphic to monomorphic type of tachycardia, being spontaneous, appears to be similar to the transition caused by anchoring the autowave vortex in an obstacle (cardiac veins, for instance). But as a matter of fact, the dynamic system, the heart, is in the state of bifurcation memory, and, consequently, therapeutic treatment in this case is likely to result in unpredictable effect, since controllability of the system has decreased dramatically.

Thus, the result demonstrates that two different types of tachycardia produce similar "shadows" on the ECG. Therefore, more sophisticated methods to analyse cardiac activities are required so that the adequate treatment could be prescribed.

3.2 Is monomorphic tachycardia indeed monomorphic?

The dependence of some ECG characteristics on the excitation threshold was studied by mathematical modelling of cardiac arrhythmia in a 2D homogeneous excitable medium (Moskalenko & Elkin, 2007). The authors of the model used here (Aliev & Panfilov, 1996) state that normal excitability corresponds to $a = 0.150$. In the present work we have observed monomorphic tachycardia at this parameter value as well as at those higher and lower. In other words, monomorphic tachycardias can arise both at elevated and at lowered excitability (Fig. 2).

This result appears to be very important in the medical aspect. It indicates that re-entrant monomorphic ventricular tachycardia may require different treatment depending on the sign of the deviation of excitability from the norm. Currently, physicians do not attempt to distinguish such cases. If further studies prove that these results can be extended to clinical ECGs, the more accurate diagnosis would make possible more expedient therapy.

For monomorphic re-entrant tachycardias, indices V_{1i} and V_{2i} also behave unexpectedly. Comparing the cases of monomorphic pseudo-ECGs in Figs. 3, one can find that the trajectories of the "physiological ECGs" and the trajectories of the "numerical ECGs" have significantly different locations, with the ECGs shape having no evident visual differences. It is interesting that the "numerical ECGs" are more "deterministic" than the "physiological ECGs" in monomorphic cases. We explain these results in the following manner. In both our natural and numerical experiments, monomorphic arrhythmias were caused by a 2D autowave vortex. Therefore, it is reasonable that the "numerical ECGs" have no stochastic component and are estimated to be more regular. However, the difference may also be supposed to result from more chaotic behaviour of real myocardium. A further study could assess the participation of stochastic and chaotic components in producing the difference.

Note, however, that changes in V_1 are usually correlated fairly well with changes in V_2 when it related to polymorphic "physiological ECGs", but there is no correlation observed in the "numerical ECGs" Research into the nature of this fact will shed new light on the mechanisms of polymorphic tachycardias. It is also important to address the issue of whether the changes in the myocardial excitation patterns are correlated with the changes in the trajectories in the (V_{1i}, V_{2i}) parameter plane.

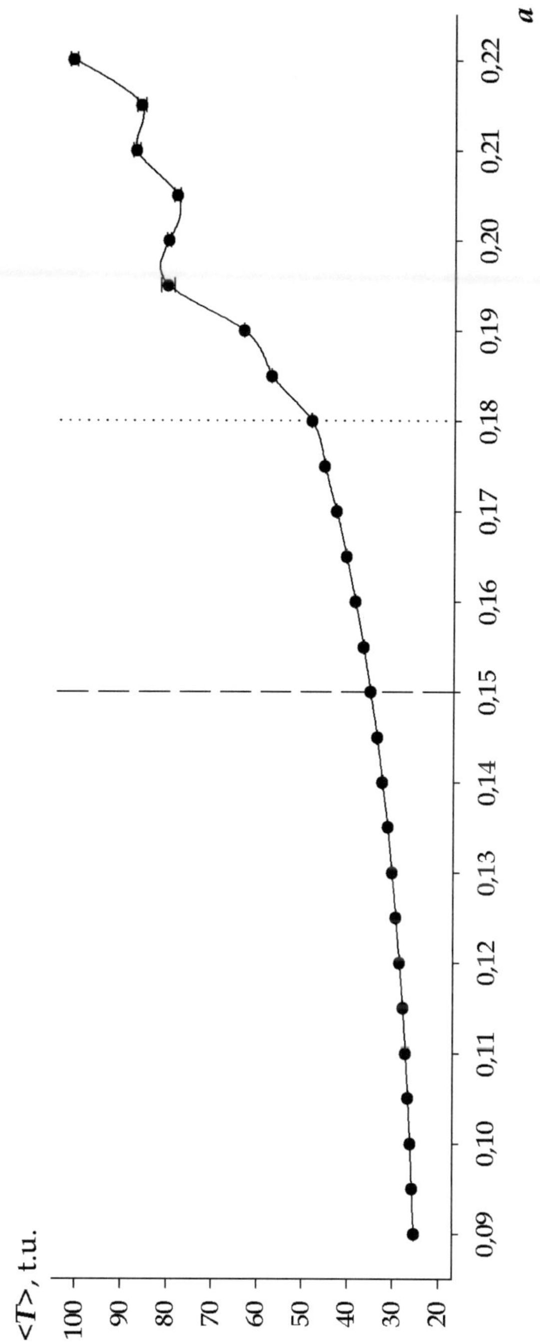

Fig. 2. Averaged ECG quasi-period (conventional units) as a function of the excitation threshold (parameter a in the Aliev-Panfilov model) for monomorphic and polymorphic tachycardias caused by a single autowave reverberator. $a = 0.150$ corresponds to normal excitability, and $a = 0.18036 \pm 0.00007$ corresponds to the bifurcation boundary.

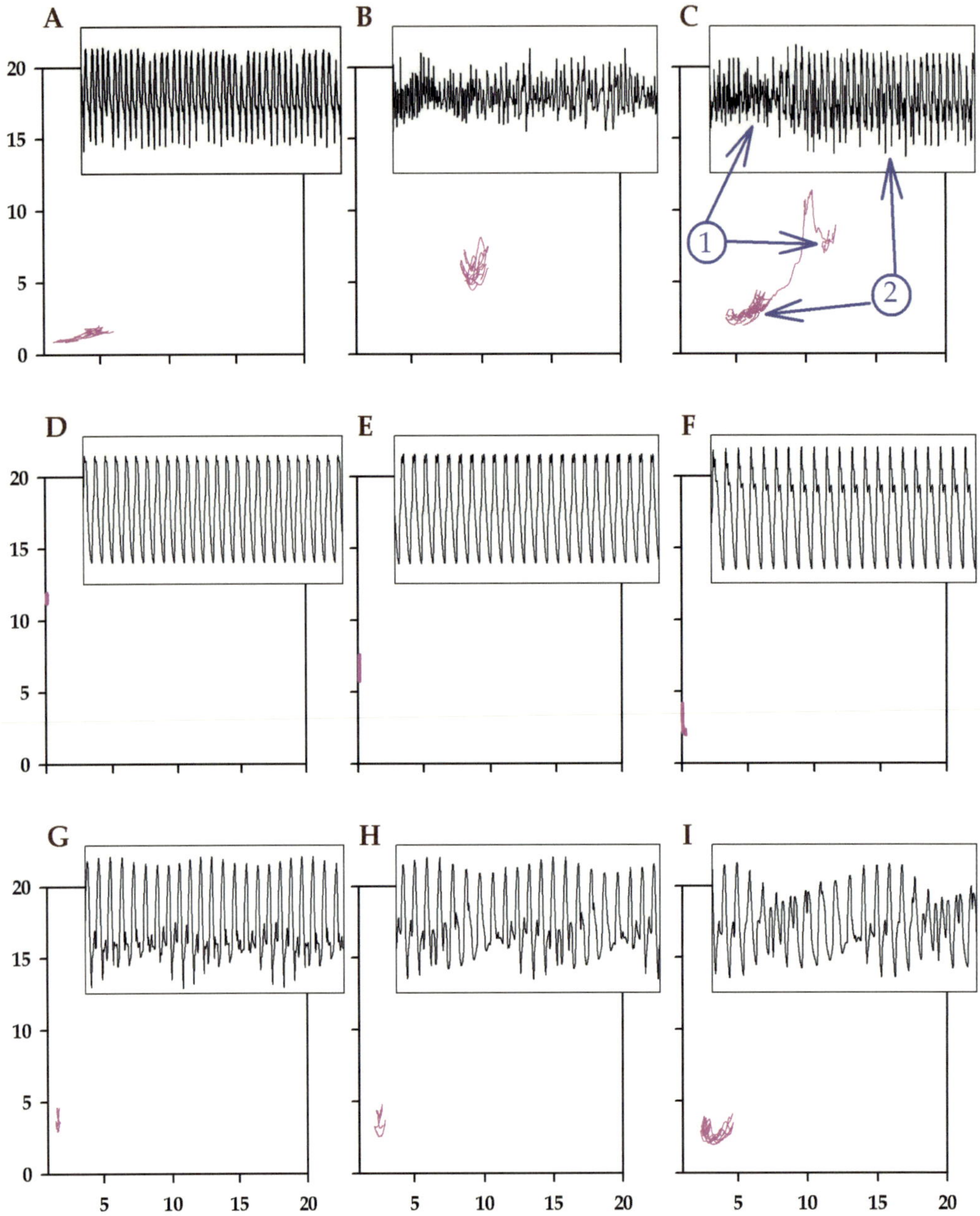

Fig. 3. The trajectories in the (V_{1i}, V_{2i}) parameter plane for both "physiological" (upper row) and "numerical" ECGs (the others). Everywhere V_{1i}, is abscissa and V_{2i} is ordinate. Each ECG fragment shown on the insert in the upper right corner corresponds to 5000 ms. The middle row contains monomorphic ECGs, whereas lower row demonstrates polymorphic ones. For the middle row, μ_1 is equal to 0.3, and a is equal to 0.15; 0.16; 0.17 from (D) to (F), respectively. For lower row, μ_1 is equal to 1.3, and a is equal to 0.16; 0.17; 0.18 from (G) to (I), respectively.

3.3 The same tachycardia observed from various standpoints

Just as one is accustomed to watch that different dispositions of an object against a source of light produce sometimes very different shapes of the object shadow, the same should be expected for the ECG, if it is something like shadow, should it not? This hypothesis can be confirmed in a very simple experiment, the scheme and the results of which are presented in Fig 4. The numerical experiment demonstrates that one is able to obtain a desirable arrhythmic shape by choosing appropriate positions of the ECG recorders. The same experimental tachycardia arrived at the same time under the electrocardiographic guise of polymorphic arrhythmia similar to *torsade de pointes* in one lead and under the guise of nearly monomorphic arrhythmia in another lead. In this experiment, both electrocardiographic guises are engendered by a single autowave reverberator moving in meander manner, which is analogous as if human hands would concurrently produce a shadow of a rabbit on one wall and a shadow of a wolf on another. Could you manage it?

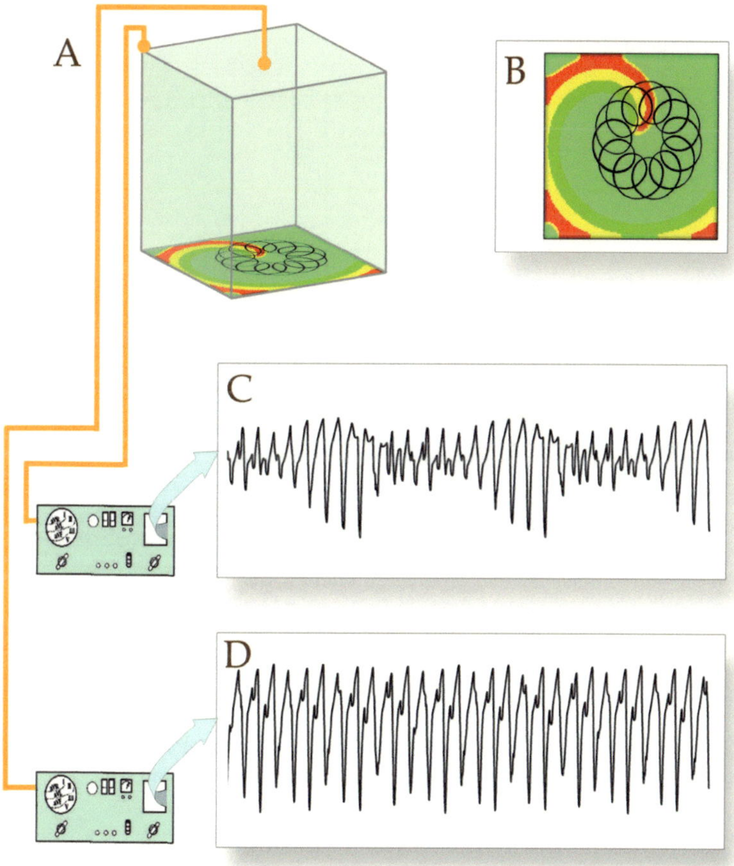

Fig. 4. Arrhythmic ECG shapes produced concurrently in different unipolar leads and engendered by a single autowave reverberator moving in meander manner during the same experimental tachycardia in model excitable medium. **A** – scheme of the numerical experiment. Insert: **B** – a trajectory of reverberator tip; **C** and **D** – ECGs, recorded over a corner and over the centre of the medium, respectively. Scale is the same for both ECGs.

On the other hand, the similar ECG shapes can be caused by totally different arrhythmic sources. For instance, the following mechanisms are reported to be a cause of polymorphic tachycardia (Kukushkin et al., 1998): abnormal automaticity, focal triggered activity from after-depolarization, drift of a single re-entry, multiple re-entries or the excitation-wave overlap. Thus, it is doubtful that visual analysis of an ECG could in common case lead to the correct conclusion about the nature of the tachycardia, because an ECG seems to be just a "shadow" produced by one or another of the totally different arrhythmic sources.

3.4 Is the degree of ECG polymorphism any informative?

To tell the difference between more and less polymorphic ECGs, the term "degree of ECG polymorphism" was introduced (Kukushkin & Medvinskii, 2004). According to primordial concept (Kukushkin et al., 1998), "arrhythmia was deemed monomorphic if the changes in the frequency and the amplitude of the pseudo-ECG during it did not exceed 15 and 30%, respectively". Since being developed, the ANI-method has given a more detailed scale for measuring the degree of ECG polymorphism.

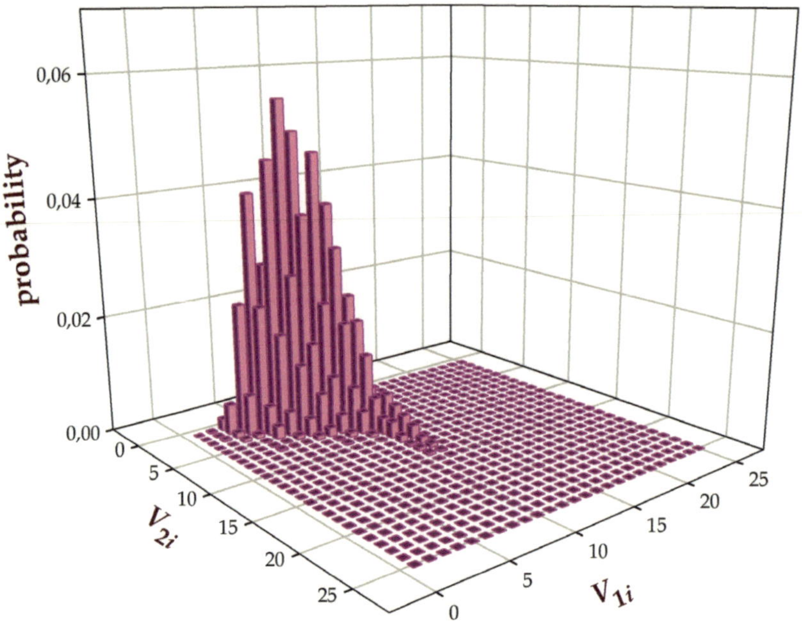

Fig. 5. Generalized histogram of "physiological ECGs", obtained from 12 physiological experiments and mapped onto the (V_{1i}, V_{2i}) parameter plane.

One of exciting questions is: do different degrees of ECG polymorphism conform to different classes of polymorphic tachycardia? In other words, how many modes have the probability distribution of tachycardias with different degree of ECG polymorphism? In order to answer the question, more than 600 "physiological ECGs" were analysed with the use of the ANI-2003. These were obtained from 12 experiments. The total duration of the ECGs was above 50 minutes and they put together more that twenty thousands arrhythmic cycles. The results are presented here for the first time (Fig. 5). One can see that the generalized histogram, which presents an estimation of the probability distribution of the "physiological ECGs" in the

(V_{1i}, V_{2i}) parameter plane, appears to be unimodal. Even if it is assumed to be polymodal, the different classes of tachycardia lie so compactly that they can hardly be segregated

The "physiological ECGs" were obtained (Moskalenko, 2009) in an experimental model study *in vitro* of ventricular tachycardia in the presence of different concentrations of lidocaine, a sodium channel blocker raising the membrane excitability threshold, which has been in broad clinical use as a local anesthetic and as an antiarrhythmic. Data were obtained with 10, 20, 30 40, 50, and 100μM. The incidence of arrhythmia with a certain degree of polymorphism was assessed by plotting the ECG distribution with respect to V_{1i}. The efficacy of the antiarrhythmic influence can be evaluated by considering the probability of arrhythmia for which V_1 exceeds a certain value V^*:

$$P(V_1 > V^*) = [1 - F(V^*)] \tag{7}$$

where $F(V_1)$ is the distribution function.

A control experiment demonstrated that the myocardial specimen itself, in the absence of lidocaine, remains quite stable over at least 8 h, producing monomorphic kinds of tachycardia all the time. Though the histograms became somewhat broader with time, the modal value remained the same and the probabilities of polymorphic arrhythmia were practically zero. Only extrasystolia (3-7 oscillations) could be evoked at 40 or 50μM and no arrhythmia could be evoked at 100μM, i.e., lidocaine produced a clear antiarrhythmic effect; these ECG data were not further processed. Note that in antiarrhythmic therapy, lidocaine has been commonly administered in doses creating a blood concentration over 50μM. At 30μM, lidocaine admitted some arrhythmia (19 cases of max. 3-s duration; in two cases spontaneous cessation was not registered). Upon visual inspection, these ECGs appeared more monomorphic than the reference ones. Administration of 10 and 20μM lidocaine did not change the duration of arrhythmias (recording up to 20 s) and did not change appreciably the ECG patterns (in visual comparison with the initial reference).

However, in the histograms obtained upon ECG variability analysis (Fig. 6) one can see that 10μM and especially 20μM lidocaine increased the probability of polymorphic arrhythmia, whereas 30μM produced an opposite effect. When lidocaine was washed off at the final stage of the experiment, the histogram tended to revert to the initial form, but restoration was only partial, which can be explained by incomplete drug removal.

The results obtained with the induced-VT model confirm the usual "antiarrhythmic" effect of lidocaine at conventional "therapeutic doses," but reveal enhanced ECG polymorphism at lower drug concentrations. Since control specimens remained stable, this "paradoxical" influence should be attributed to the direct action of small doses of lidocaine, rather than to its poor efficacy at low levels against increasing inhomogeneity of myocardium. These experimental results are in nice accord with the earlier theoretical consideration (Efimov et al., 1995) of myocardial vortices in the Beeler–Reuter model as well as another theoretical study (Winfree, 1991) with a simpler FitzHugh–Nagumo model. In accordance with either theoretical work, intermediate levels of sodium conductance could produce drift of the excitation vortex, which corresponds to polymorphic VT. Thus, the findings for lidocaine reported here can likely be applied to other drugs of this class. Both theoretical works as well as this experimental work indicate that there is a nonlinear dependence of ECG polymorphism degree on myocardial excitability (and in this way on the concentration of sodium channel blockers): while myocardial excitability is reduced, the polymorphism degree is low first, then it increases and then becomes low again. This nonlinear dependence is in contradiction with the conventional medical conception according to which a monomorphic VT is much better than a polymorphic one. In other words, one should consider the therapeutic efficacy of sodium channel blockers as its pseudo-antiarrhythmic efficacy because the blockers at their so-called "therapeutically accepted levels" really make myocardium rather lifeless.

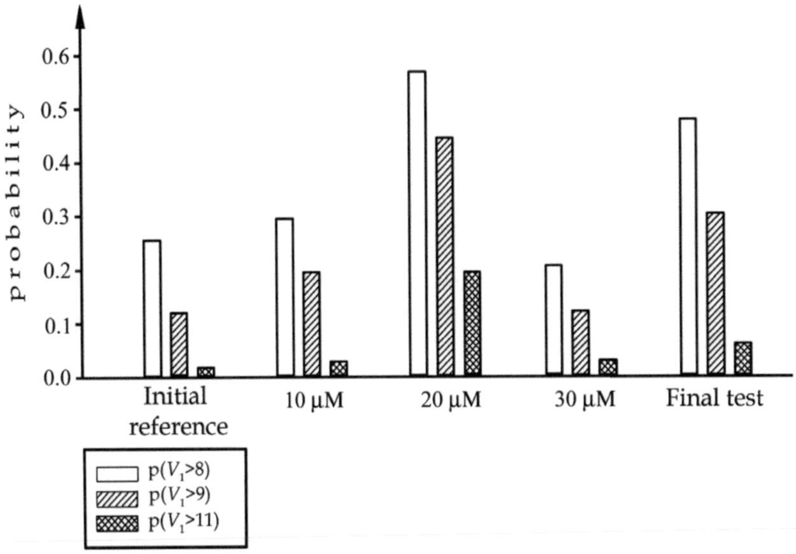

Fig. 6. The probability of appearance of the experimental ECG with different values of degree of polymorphism in the presence of different concentrations of lidocaine. Note again that the more value of V_1, the more degree of ECG polymorphism. The labels along the horizontal axis indicate the stage of experiment.

4. Discussion and conclusions

To disprove a theory, a single fact contradicting the theory is enough, but thousands facts are scanty to prove it. What new and good has this study been able to demonstrate?

First of all, the conclusion should be made, that monomorphic tachycardias appear to be rather mixed group of cardiac arrhythmias, which ought to be distinguished in very accurate manner in order to prescribe adequate treatment for cardiac disorders. The results presented here show that taking into account attractive resemblance of consecutive electrocardiographic shadows solely seems to be insufficient for good diagnostics.

Second, inasmuch as the phenomena of bifurcation memory in real myocardium are expected to be revealed, many cases of unsuccessful treatment of cardiac disturbances are likely to result from the phenomena. Within the scope of traditional electrocardiography, however, making diagnosis of bifurcation disorders in the heart seems to be doubtful.

Third, supposition about linear dependence of therapeutic effect on concentration of a medicament looks naive. Evidently, application of new techniques for monitoring "invisible" phase space of the heart would improve our capacity of using flexible and sophisticated schemata of medical treatment of cardiac diseases. Noble states: "There will probably therefore be no unique model that does everything at all levels. In any case, all models are only partial representations of reality. One of the first questions to ask of a model therefore is what questions does it answer best" (Noble, 2002b). So, appropriate collection of cardiac models is believed to improve both diagnostics and treatment.

In this investigation, the aim was also to assess the importance of polymorphic shape of the ECG in diagnostics of cardiac disorders. By painting a picture with metaphors and analogies, one create a visual image of one's concept; in doing so, one ensure that it sticks with one's prospect better than would a litany of industry- or science-specific terms. "Shadow play" appears to be a good suitable metaphor for understanding some problems of cardiology more deeply. As it was demonstrated in numerical study, there is no ground to believe, that degree of ECG polymorphism indicates severity of cardiac disease for certain. The only thing we can say without any doubt is that the electrical phenomena of the cardiac action attributed, in accordance with the most widely held current opinion, to different types of VT can be obtained in reality from a single patient concurrently. Thus, we should conclude that, in some cases, disgustful ugliness of consecutive electrocardiographic shadows during so-called polymorphic tachycardia is not likely to be as awful as the impression produced on a cardiologist by it. Besides, the customary classification of tachycardia should be improved.

This chapter has given an account of and the reasons for the widespread use of novel achievements of mathematics and physics for solving problems of cardiology. The results of this research support the idea that adequate diagnostics of cardiac disturbance should be grounded rather on observation of events on the "invisible" phase space of the heart than on raw sings in the electrocardiograms, which should be considered most likely to be a sort of intriguing "shadows" of the real cardiac action.

In this study, we have shown that the technique for ECG analysis referred to as ANI-2003 could provide cardiologists with a sensitive clinical tool for identifying life-threatening arrhythmias. The estimates derived from virtual ECGs in this study reveal some unexpected details of ventricular arrhythmia dynamics, which probably will be useful for diagnosis of cardiac rhythm disturbances. The data presented here pertain sometimes to "latent" polymorphism, revealed by the ANI-method while conventional ECG inspection did not reveal any important signs. The dependence of the trajectory location on ECG polymorphism defines a partial order in the (V_{1i}, V_{2i})-space. The result is a new detailed quantitative description of polymorphic ECGs. Note that one cannot know the number of latent transitions in the ECG recorded during polymorphic ventricular tachycardia or ventricular fibrillation, but one can use the ANI-method to estimate it. The evidence from this study suggests that this method may prove useful in laboratory screening for new antiarrhythmics as well as in clinical testing to optimize the treatment regimen.

As concerns further investigations, studying influence of bifurcation memory phenomena on the cardiac action will lead to a better insight in the nature of cardiac diseases. Trying to understand nonlinear nature of cardiac arrhythmias, a cardiologist is expected to improve a cure for pathological tachycardia. Correct distinguishing between normal and pathological tachycardia seems to remain the most challenging problem for modern cardiology. Deeper comprehension of mechanisms of different sorts of both ventricular tachycardia and fibrillation is still required. Further work should explore also how re-entrant and focal arrhythmias could be distinguished by their ECGs. All these are good tasks for modern cardiovascular physics. Besides, further work needs to be done to establish whether the ANI-method is helpful for real clinical tasks.

5. Acknowledgment

Author is thankful for Dr. E. Shnol, Dr. Yu. Elkin, Dr. N. Wessel, Prof. A. Loskutov, and Prof. A. Ardashev for interesting discussion of important aspects of modern cardiovascular physics.

The partial support of Russian Foundation for Basic Research is acknowledged (the project 11-07-00519).

6. References

Aliev, R., Panfilov, A. (1996) A simple two-variable model of cardiac excitation. *Chaos, Solutions & Fractals*, Vol.7, No.3, pp. 293-301, ISSN 0960-0779

Ataullakhanov, F., Lobanova, E., Morozova, O., Shnol', E., Ermakova, E., Butylin, A. & Zaikin, A. (2007). Intricate regimes of propagation of an excitation and self-organization in the blood clotting model. *Physics – Uspekhi*, Vol.50, No.1, pp. 79–94, ISSN 1063-7869

Bushev, M. (1994). Synergetics: *Chaos, Order, Self-Organization*, World Scientific Pub Co Inc., ISBN: 978-9810212865

Crampin, E.J., Halstead, M., Hunter, P., Nielsen, P., Noble, D., Smith, N. & Tawhai, M. (2004). Computational physiology and the physiome project, *Experimental Physiology*, Vol.89, No.1, pp. 1-26, ISSN 0958-0670

Efimov, I., Krinsky, V. & Jalife, J. (1995). *Chaos, Solutions & Fractals*, Dynamics of rotating vortices in the Beeler-Reuter model of cardiac tissue. Vol.5, No.3/4, pp. 513–526., ISSN 0960-0779

Elkin, Yu. & Moskalenko, A. (2009). Basic mechanisms of cardiac arrhythmias, In: *Clinical Arrhythmology* (Russian), A.V. Ardashev, (Ed.), pp. 45-74, MedPraktika-M, ISBN 978-5-98803-198-7, Moscow

Feigin, M. & Kagan, M. (2004). Emergencies as a manifestation of effect of bifurcation memory in controlled unstable systems. *International Journal of Bifurcation and Chaos*, Vol.14, No.7, pp. 2439–2447, ISSN 0218-1274

Kukushkin, N. & Medvinskii, A. (2004) Ventricular tachycardias: and mechanisms. *Vestnik aritmologii* (in Russian), No.35, pp.49–55, ISSN 1561-8641

Kukushkin, N., Sidorov, V., Medvinskii, A., Romashko, D., Burashnikov, A., Baum, O., Sarancha, D., & Starmer, F.C. (1998). Slow excitation wave and mechanisms of polymorphic ventricular tachycardia in an experimental model: Isolated walls of the right ventricles of the hearts of rabbit and ground squirrel. Biophysics, Vol.43, No.6, pp. 995–1010, ISSN 0006-3509

Kurian, T. & Efimov I. (2010) Mechanisms of fibrillation: neurogenic or myogenic? Reentrant or focal? Multiple or single? Still puzzling after 160 years of inquiry. *J Cardiovasc Electrophysiol.*, Vol.21, No.11, pp. 1274-5, ISSN: 1540-8167

Kurian, T., Ambrosi, C., Hucker, W., Fedorov, V. & Efimov I. (2010). Anatomy and Electrophysiology of the Human AV Node. *Pacing Clin. Electrophysiol.*, Vol.33, No.6, pp. 754-62, ISSN: 0147-8389, 1540-8159

Loskutov, A. & Mironyuk, O. (2007). Time series analysis of ECG: A possibility of the initial diagnostics. *International Journal of Bifurcation and Chaos*, Vol.17, No.10, pp. 3709-3713, ISSN 0218-1274

Loskutov, A., Shavarov, A., Dolgushina, E. & Ardashev, A. (2009). Cardiac tissue as active media: Invariant characteristics of the theory of dynamical systems and heart rate variability. In: *Clinical Arrhythmology* (Russian), A.V. Ardashev, (Ed.), pp. 1085-1103, MedPraktika-M, ISBN 978-5-98803-198-7, Moscow

Medvinsky, A., Rusakov, A., Moskalenko, A., Fedorov, M., Panfilov, A. (2003). The study of autowave mechanisms of electrocardiogram variability during high-frequency arrhythmias: the result of mathematical modelling. Biophysics, Vol.48, No. 2, pp. 297–305, ISSN 0006-3509

Moskalenko, A. & Elkin, Yu. (2007) Is monomorphic tachycardia indeed monomorphic? *Biophysics*, Vol.52, No.2, pp. 237-240, ISSN 0006-3509

Moskalenko, A. & Elkin, Yu. (2009). The lacet: a new type of the spiral wave behaviour. *Chaos, Solitons & Fractals*, Vol.40, No.1, pp. 426-431, ISSN 0960-0779

Moskalenko, A. (2009). Nonlinear effects of lidocaine on polymorphism of ventricular arrhythmias. *Biophysics*, Vol.54, No.1, pp. 47-50, ISSN 0006-3509

Moskalenko, A. (2010) Nonlinear and nonstationary ECG analysis of spontaneous transition from polymorphic to monomorphic arrhythmia in a mathematical model of cardiac tissue dynamics. *Proceedings of the International Biosignal Processing Conference*, pp. 084:1-4, Berlin, Germany, July 14-16, 2010

Moskalenko, A., Kukushkin, N., Starmer, C.F., Deev, A., Kukushkina, K. & Medvinsky, A. (2001). Quantitative analysis of variability of the electrocardiograms typical of polymorphic arrhythmias. *Biophysics*, Vol.46, No.2, pp. 313-323, ISSN 0006-3509

Moskalenko, A., Rusakov, A. & Elkin, Yu. (2008). A new technique of ECG analysis and its application to evaluation of disorders during ventricular tachycardia. *Chaos, Solitons & Fractals*, Vol.36, No.1, pp. 66-72, ISSN 0960-0779

Noble, D. (2002a). Modelling the heart – from Genes to Cells to the Whole Organ. *Science*, Vol.295, pp. 1678-1682

Noble, D. (2002b). Modelling the heart: Insights, failures and progress. *BioEssays*, Vol.24, pp. 1156-1163, ISSN 0265-9247

Prigogine, I. (1980). *From Being to Becoming: Time and Complexity in the Physical Sciences*, W.H Freeman & Co., ISBN: 978-0716711079, San Francisco.

Ramanathan, Ch., Ghanem, R.N., Jia, P., Ryu, K. & Rudy, Y. (2004). Noninvasive electrocardiographic imaging for cardiac electrophysiology and arrythmia. *Nature Medicine*, Vol.10, pp. 422-428, ISSN 1078-8956

Sarancha, D., Medvinsky, A., Kukushkin, N., Sidorov, V., Romashko, D., Burashnikov, A., Moskalenko, A., Starmer, C.F. (1997). A system for the computer visualization of the propagation of excitation waves in the myocardium. *Biophysics*, Vol.42, No.2, pp. 491–496, ISSN 0006-3509

Titomir L.I. & Kneppo P. (1994). *Bioelectric and Biomagnetic Fields. Theory and Applications in Electrocardiology*, CRC Press, ISBN 978-0849387005, Boca Raton.

Vapnik, V. N. (1999) *The Nature of Statistical Learning Theory* (2nd edition), Springer, ISBN: 0387987800

Wessel, N., Malberg, H., Bauernschmitt, R. & Kurths J. (2007). Nonlinear methods of cardiovascular physics and their clinic application. *International Journal of Bifurcation and Chaos*, Vol.17, No.10, pp. 3325-3371, ISSN 0218-1274

Winfree, A.T. (1991).Varieties of spiral wave behavior: An experimentalist's approach to the theory of excitable media. *Chaos*, Vol.1, No.3, pp.303-334, ISSN 1054-1500

Zhuchkova, E., Radnayev, B., Vysotsky, S. & Loskutov, A. (2009). Suppression of turbulent dynamics in models of cardiac tissue by weak local excitations. In: *Understanding Complex Systems*, S.K. Dana, P.K. Roy, J. Kurths. (Eds.), pp. 89-105, Springer, Berlin

7

Metabolic Modulators to Treat Cardiac Arrhythmias Induced by Ischemia and Reperfusion

Moslem Najafi and Tahereh Eteraf-Oskouei
Faculty of Pharmacy and Drug Applied Research Center,
Tabriz University of Medical Sciences, Tabriz
Iran

1. Introduction

Cardiac arrhythmias are one of the important problems in coronary ischemia/reperfusion (I/R) therapy and constitute a major risk for sudden cardiac death after coronary artery occlusion (Pourkhalili et al., 2009). Arrhythmias occur in up to 25% of patients treated with digitalis, 50% of anesthetized patients, and over 80% of patients with acute myocardial infarction (AMI) (Hume & Grant, 2007). Although reperfusion is the only way to restore blood flow of coronary arteries and prevent the myocardium from suffering from necrosis, it will lead to the occurrence of life-threatening arrhythmias which containing premature ventricular beats (PVBs), ventricular tachycardia (VT) and ventricular fibrillation (VF) (Wei & Yang, 2006). There are few safe and effective antiarrhythmic drugs for use in patients with ischemic heart diseases (IHD). Class I antiarrhythmic agents such as quinidine, flecainide, propafenone, and procainamide have the potential to cause proarrhythmia and hemodynamic collapse in the setting of IHD and should be used with caution. The use of beta-adrenergic receptor blockers and calcium channel blockers such as diltiazem and verapamil may be limited by side effects such as heart rate slowing and blood pressure drop (Dhalla et al., 2009). Therapeutic strategies currently used for primary prevention of VF, VT, or cardiac arrest remain controversial as few trials have shown a survival benefit. In addition, sudden cardiac death caused by I/R-induced arrhythmias is a warning to the development of new antiarrhythmic agents (Pourkhalili et al., 2009). Pharmacological protection of the heart from I/R-induced damage has been investigated by academic and industrial scientists for a considerable period of time. A central aim of research directed towards the science and pharmacology of I/R injury is the discovery of drugs that can be used in human to prevent ischemic cardiac injury and its sequelae (Black, 2000).

This chapter reviews and describes the pharmacology of some important "metabolic agents" that suppress arrhythmias by metabolism modulating in cardiac cells.

2. Energy metabolism in the aerobic heart

The high energy demand of the heart is met by utilizing a variety of carbon substrates, including free fatty acids (FFAs), carbohydrates, amino acids and ketone bodies. FFAs and carbohydrates are the major substrates from which heart derives most of its energy (Sambandam & Lopaschuk, 2003; Calvani et al., 2000). Under normal aerobic conditions, 50–70% of the total energy is obtained from fatty acids, while the majority of the rest is obtained from carbohydrates (mainly glucose and lactate) (Sambandam & Lopaschuk, 2003). The carbon substrates are all converted to acetyl coenzyme A (acetyl-CoA) and enter the citric acid (Krebs) cycle whereby they produce the high-energy phosphate molecule adenosine triphosphate (ATP) which powers both contractile and noncontractile functions (McBride & White, 2003). The citric acid cycle also generates the electron accepting molecule nicotinamide adenine dinucleotide (NADH), which produces additional ATP molecules by interacting with the electron transport chain inside the mitochondria. These 3 macronutrients possess different metabolic pathways to generate acetyl-CoA molecules. Glycogen is converted to glucose, which is then converted to pyruvate in the cytoplasm. Pyruvate enters the mitochondria and is converted to acetyl-CoA by pyruvate dehydrogenase (PDH). Conversely, fatty acids are converted to fatty acyl-CoA and then undergo several metabolic steps before being converted to acetyl-CoA by the β-oxidation pathway. The principal difference between the 2 pathways of energy production is the amount of oxygen required to produce a given amount of ATP. With fatty acid oxidation, 32 grams of oxygen will yield 5.5 ATP molecules while glucose oxidation produces 6.3 molecules of ATP (McBride & White, 2003). The rate of fatty acid oxidation is mainly regulated by the concentration of free fatty acids in the plasma, the activity of carnitine palmitoyl transferase-I (CPT-I), and the activity of a series of enzymes that catalyze the multiple steps of fatty acid β-oxidation. Fatty acid oxidation strongly inhibits glucose and lactate oxidation at the level of PDH (Sabbah & Stanley, 2002).

3. Myocardial ischemia and reperfusion injury

Myocardial ischemia is one of the major causes of death in nowadays cardiac diseases (Wei & Yang, 2006). Among the heart diseases, I/R-induced arrhythmias contribute to episodes of sudden death (Gandhi et al., 2009). Reperfusion of myocardium subjected to a transient ischemia rapidly induces ventricular arrhythmias including PVBs, VT and VF in both animals and human (Lu et al., 1999).

3.1 Myocardial function and energy production during ischemia

Myocardial ischemia is a condition that exists when there is a reduced coronary blood flow, and results in a decrease in the supply of oxygen and nutrients to the heart (Suleiman et al., 2001). Due to restricted oxygen supply to the myocardium during ischemic period, both fatty acid and carbohydrate oxidation decreases and ATP production is impaired. Glycolysis, a minor source of ATP in the aerobic heart, becomes a more significant source of energy during ischemia. In the severely ischemic myocardium, production of H^+ from hydrolysis of glycolytically derived ATP is the major contributor to acidosis (Sambandam & Lopaschuk, 2003; Suleiman et al., 2001; Calvani et al., 2000). In particular, lactic acid accumulates, leading to an increase in intracellular Na^+ and Ca^{2+} (Suleiman et al., 2001). The accumulation of fatty acids and their intermediates during myocardial ischemia as well as metabolic and ionic changes provoke a reduction of myocardial function and also have been shown to be deleterious to the recovery of myocardial function of the reperfused heart (Ford, 2002).

3.2 Myocardial function and energy production during reperfusion

Functional recovery upon reperfusion is largely dependent upon the duration of the ischemic period; the longer the period, the more likely the heart is to undergo irreversible damage. Consequences of reperfusion injury include cardiac arrhythmias, myocardial stunning and loss of intracellular proteins (Suleiman et al., 2001). Numerous mechanisms for the increase in tissue injury after reperfusion have been proposed including oxidative stress (Gandhi et al., 2009), the generation of oxygen-derived free radicals (Wei & Yang, 2006), calcium overload (Wei & Yang, 2006; Lu et al., 1999), and dysfunction of myocardial energy metabolism (Wei & Yang, 2006).

4. Metabolic pharmacology

As mentioned previously, the myocardium preferentially uses fatty acids for an energy source because the chemical bonds of fatty acid molecules have higher energy content and are capable of producing more ATP molecules per molecule of fatty acid consumed. Since the inhibition of β-oxidation could permit the heart to produce ATP at lower oxygen tensions, it is plausible that an inhibitor of β-oxidation could prevent damage to the myocardium when subjected to ischemia (McBride & White, 2003). The principal goal of the metabolic modulator approach is to decrease the rate of fatty acid oxidation by the heart and increase the oxidation of pyruvate derived from glucose, glycogen, and lactate (McCormack et al., 1998). Switching the source of acetyl CoA from fatty acids toward pyruvate results in: greater ATP yield and amelioration of the buildup of potentially harmful fatty acid metabolites, and should also act to decrease lactate and hydrogen ion production under low flow conditions and during postischemic reperfusion (McCormack et al., 1998).

5. Pharmacology of some important metabolism modifiers

5.1 L-carnitine (L-Car)

5.1.1 Structure

Carnitine, a name derived from the Latin *caro* or *carnis* (flesh), was discovered in muscle extracts in 1905. Soon after, the chemical formula $C_7H_{15}NO_3$ was accepted, and in 1927, its structure, a trimethylbetaine of γ-amino-β-hydroxybutyric acid, was identified and published (Fig 1). In 1962, the configuration of the physiological enantiomer was determined, and in 1997 confirmed as L(-) or R-(-)-3-hydroxy-4-N,N,N-trimethylaminobutyrate (Sweetman, 2002; Kerner and Hoppel, 1998; Rebouche and Seim, 1998).

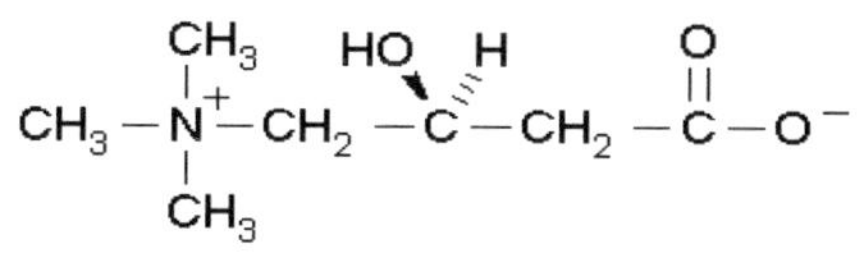

Fig. 1. Chemical structure of carnitine.

5.1.2 Pharmacokinetics

Oral doses of L-Car are absorbed slowly and incompletely from the small intestine via a stereoselective active transport system located in the intestinal mucosa of the duodenum and ileum (Sweetman, 2002). L-Car transport does not appear to occur below the ileum in the large intestine. The transport system can concentrate L-Car, resulting in a 10 to 100 fold gradient between the extracellular and intracellular compartments. Additionally, a passive diffusion of L-Car has also been demonstrated in the intestine. Peak plasma levels of free and total carnitine occurs 3-5 hours after oral administration. The normal total plasma carnitine concentrations for healthy men and women are 59 μmol/L and 51 μmol/L, respectively (Bach et al., 1983). It does not appear to bind to plasma proteins (Rebouche, 2004; Sweetman, 2002). The plasma half-life of L-Car has been estimated to range from 2-15 h in humans. Although carnitine is largely eliminated via renal excretion, it is highly conserved by the kidney. L-Car is freely filtered at the renal glomerulus and greater than 90 percent of the filtered load is reabsorbed in the proximal kidney tubules and returned to the circulation when plasma carnitine levels are normal or low. L-Car given orally may undergo degradation in the gastrointestinal tract, leading to the formation of metabolites such as trimethylamine-*N*-oxide and γ-butyrobetaine (Sweetman, 2002).

5.1.3 Pharmacodynamics

L-Car facilitates oxidation of long-chain fatty acids (LCFAs) and is involved in trapping acyl residues from peroxisomes and mitochondria. It participates in metabolism of branched chain amino acids (Lango et al., 2001). Supplementation of the myocardium with L-Car results in an increased tissue carnitine content which restores carnitine losses and lessens the severity of ischemic injury. It also improves the recovery of heart functions during reperfusion. The beneficial effects of L-Car on heart function recovery from ischemia cannot be justified by this drug stimulating fatty acid oxidation only. Fatty acids, high in plasma during reperfusion, may provide 90 % of ATP production in the absence of L-Car treatment, whereas in its presence a marked increase in glucose oxidation is observed, without changes in total ATP production. Thus, these results suggest that the drug tends to restore the balance between fatty acid and glucose oxidation. L-Car is thought to increase glucose oxidation by relieving PDH inhibition caused by the elevated intramitochondrial acetyl-CoA/CoA ratio. This effect also results in an increased synthesis of malonyl-CoA, the physiological inhibitor of CPT-1, the first committed enzyme in overall fatty acid oxidation. Increased glucose oxidation is beneficial for cardiac cells because of a lower conversion of pyruvate into lactate, a metabolic step contributing to acidification of the intracellular compartment. Finally, L-Car have been proposed to mitigate the noxious effects of oxygen free radicals in the reperfused hearts and to render cardiac cells more resistant to I/R damage by stabilizing cellular membranes (Lango et al., 2001, Calvani et al., 2000).

5.1.4 Uses of L-Car in cardiovascular health and diseases

A decreased carnitine concentration in the heart was observed in patients who died of myocardial infarction (MI). In patients with AMI, a four fold increase was observed in free carnitine elimination and almost a two-fold increase in the elimination of short chain carnitine esters by kidney (Lango et al., 2001). There is some evidence that L-Car supplementation may exert a cardioprotective role. Benefit in patients with cardiomyopathies,reduction of infarct size and prevention of arrhythmias in patients with MI,increased exercise tolerance in patients with angina,and protection from the cardiotoxicity of the anthracycline antineoplastics have all been described in patients given

L-Car supplementation (Lango et al., 2001). Arsenian et al. demonstrated a decrease in mortality and incidence of circulatory failure in a group of patients with AMI, who were administered 3 g of L-Car along with solution of glucose, insulin, potassium and magnesium (Arsenian et al., 1996). L-Car supplementation in patients with congestive heart failure (CHF) for 12 weeks significantly improved the exercise tolerance of patients with effort angina. Studies involving about 2500 patients with coronary artery disease (CAD) treated with L-Car for a year also showed a reduced incidence of angina, a decreased need of cardiac drugs and a greater effort tolerance (Naguib, 2005). Placebo-controlled studies performed in patients with stable chronic effort angina suggest that L-Car given acutely (40 mg/kg, iv) or chronically (1–3 g daily for a month) improves exercise capacity and the electrocardiographic manifestations of ischemia (Ferrari et al., 2004). L-Car does not have hemodynamic effects in healthy volunteers or patients with CAD. However, an improvement of individual maximal aerobic power is demonstrated in healthy subjects and athletes after chronic treatment with L-Car (4 g daily over a period of 2 weeks) (Ferrari et al., 2004). In a randomized, double-blind, placebo controlled, multicenter study called the Levocarnitine Ecocardiografia Digitalizzata Infarto Miocardico (CEDIM) trial was performed to evaluate the effects of L-Car administration on long-term left ventricular dilatation in patients with AMI. Placebo or levocarnitine (9 g iv daily for the first 5 days and then 6 g orally daily) was administered for 12 months. The primary end points of the trial were left ventricular volumes and ejection fraction, at 12 months after the emergent event, assessed by two-dimensional echocardiography. Treatment with the active compound resulted in a significant reduction of left ventricular dilatation. The percentages of both end-diastolic and end-systolic volumes were reduced significantly in the L-Car-treated group. No modification of left ventricular ejection fraction was observed. The incidences of death, congestive heart failure, and/or ischemic events were less in the L-Car-treated groups (Ferrari et al., 2004). Administration of L-Car, combined with other treatments, also proved effective in the treatment of childhood cardiomyopathy (Szewczyk and Wojtczac, 2002). Oral L-Car (3–4 g daily) normalizes plasma total cholesterol or triglyceride levels (or both) and increases high-density lipoprotein (HDL)–cholesterol in patients with type II and type IV hyperlipoproteinemia over a 2-month period (Ferrari et al., 2004). Oral L-Car (4 g daily for 21 days) improves the maximal walking distance of patients with intermittent claudication caused by peripheral arterial disease (Ferrari et al., 2004). Decreased level of free and total carnitine in diabetes, with a simultaneous increase in concentrations of long-chained acyl-CoA and long-chain carnitine esters has been shown. Some correlation has been also demonstrated between the left ventricular contraction index and long-chain acyl-carnitine concentration in the myocardium during reperfusion in patients after mitral valve replacement. These data suggest, in line with the results of experimental studies that carnitine and its derivatives protect human ischemic heart against oxidative stress not only by modifying carnitine acyl-transferase activity and metabolic effect, but by other mechanisms as well (Lango et al., 2001).

5.1.5 Experimental and clinical findings on beneficial effects of L-Car against cardiac arrhythmias

A prolonged L-Car therapy in patients with angina pectoris was associated with a considerable decrease in the frequency of ventricular arrhythmias (Lango et al., 2001).

Rizzon et al. noticed a statistically significant decrease of the frequency of ventricular arrhythmia in a group of patients with AMI who were administered 100 mg of L-Car/kg. Although the studied groups of patients were small, L-Car administration to patients with ischemic heart disease appears to be a promising therapy of ischemia-induced arrhythmia as potentially addressed to restoring of membrane rest-potential (Rizzon et al., 1989). Cardiac electrophysiology after L-Car administration (30 mg/kg over 3 min) did not show any changes either in the conductivity time or in refraction period. The cycle duration in the sinus node was shortened by 5%, while the arterial blood pressure remained unchanged (Lango et al., 2001). Results of some experimental studies showed protective effects of L-Car against I/R- induced injuries and cardiac arrhythmias. In a study, we tested the effects of 0.5, 2.5 and 5 mM/L of L-Car on cardiac arrhythmias in the ischemic reperfused isolated rat heart in Langendorff setup. At the ischemic phase, number, duration and incidence of VT were decreased by doses of 2.5 and 5 mM/L L-Car ($p<0.05$). In addition, L-Car by doses of 2.5 and 5 mM/L reduced the number of VT ($p<0.05$) at the reperfusion phase. The total number of ventricular ectopic beats (VEBs: Single+Salvos+VT) also were reduced in treated groups by 0.5-5 mM/L of L-Car versus the control group ($p<0.05$). However, duration of reversible VF (Rev VF) was decreased only by 5 mM/L L-Car (Najafi et al., 2005). In another study, the effects of pre-ischemic administration of 0.5, 2.5 and 5 mM/L of L-Car were investigated in isolated rat hearts. Interestingly, the results showed that short time pre-ischemic administration of L-Car (10 min before induction of 30 min regional ischemia) had concentration dependent arrhythmogenic effects on both ischemia and reperfusion-induced arrhythmias (Najafi et al., 2008). The authors hypothesized that pre-ischemic using of L-Car for an inadequate time can be harmful for the heart because of incomplete metabolism of fatty acids and more accumulation of their intermediates (Najafi et al., 2008). They concluded that L-Car produced a protective effect against reperfusion arrhythmias only when it is perfused for the whole period of the experiment. This protective action was reversed by concomitant using of etomoxir (palmitoylcarnitinetransferase-1 inhibitor), suggesting that the efficacy of L-Car is due to its mitochondrial action, but is probably not solely attribute to an increase in fatty acid oxidation (Najafi et al., 2008). Cui et al. investigated the effects of L-Car on the incidence of reperfusion-induced VF during 30 min global ischemia followed by 120 min reperfusion. Their results showed that different concentrations of L-Car failed to reduce the incidence of VF (Cui et al., 2003). Suzuki et al. reported intravenous pre-treatment of the ischemic dog heart by L-Car (100 mg/kg) reduced the grade of ventricular arrhythmias. They suggested that the administration of L-Car might be beneficial to prevent serious arrhythmias in ischemic heart disease, presumably by restoring the impaired free fatty acid oxidation (Suzuki et al., 1981). Recently, we reported that pre-ischemic administration of L-Car could precondition the heart as evidenced by its ability to lower the infarct size markedly ($p<0.001$) and improved postischemic ventricular functional recovery. L-Car reduced left ventricular end diastolic pressure (LVEDP) elevation at the reperfusion phase. Heart rate (HR) and coronary flow rate (CFR) did not show significant changes in treated groups as compared to the control. Among the three different concentrations, L-Car (2.5 mM) was found to be optimal for preconditioning purpose (Najafi et al., 2010a). It was also found in this study that pre-ischemic administration of L-Car in ischemic/reperfused hearts preconditions the hearts by reduction of left ventricular lactate content (Najafi et al., 2010a).

5.1.6 Uses of L-Car in other human diseases

As well as cardiovascular health and diseases, L-Car is administered to treat many other human diseases such as primary carnitine deficiency syndromes or secondary carnitine deficiency/insufficiency states (Ferrari et al., 2004). Primary carnitine deficiency results from inborn defects in specific proteins or carnitine transferases. Therapy with carnitine in primary deficiency states is considered to have a rational basis. Secondary causes of carnitine deficiency include inherited metabolic defects in fatty acid β-oxidation, mitochondrial myopathy, prematurity, carnitine deficiency in the diet, dialysis therapy, etc. The value of carnitine for these conditions is controversial (Sweetman, 2002; Szewczyk et al. 2002; Kerner & Hoppel, 1998).

5.1.6.1 Infant nutrition

Preterm infants require carnitine for life-sustaining metabolic processes. When infants were supplemented with 2.2 mg of L-Car/100 ml in the bovine milk formula, their plasma carnitine and acylcarnitine levels were similar to those observed in the breast-fed group (Naguib, 2005).

5.1.6.2 Immune system and AIDS

The effect of long-term L-Car supplementation on CD4 and CD8 absolute counts, rate, and apoptosis was studied in HIV-infected subjects, who were treated with daily infusions of L-Car (6 g) for 4 months. CD4 and CD8 are specific types of lymphocytes; their absolute counts are decreased in patients with AIDS, resulting in compromised immune function. At the end of the study, L-Car was found to substantially increase the rate and absolute counts of CD4 and, to a lesser degree, of CD8 lymphocytes (Ilias et al., 2004; De Simone & Tzantzoglou, 1993). In this case, the antioxidant activity of L-Car may be responsible for the observed changes in apoptosis because increases in free radical oxidative stress can accelerate this process (Moretti et al., 1998).

5.1.6.3 Brain health

L-Car has been considered of potential use in senile dementia of Alzheimer's because of its ability to enhance energy production and to restore aged cell membranes (Naguib, 2005). In brain tissue, the carnitine shuttle mediates translocation of the acetyl moiety from mitochondria into the cytosol and thus probably contributes to the synthesis of acetylcholine (Szewczyk & Wojtczac, 2002). Positive clinical effects of L-Car administration were also observed in brain ischemia (Lango et al., 2001) and hypoglycemia induced by insulin overdose (Hino K. et al. 2005). In addition, L-Car protects motor neuron cells from ischemic spinal cord injury (Akgun et al., 2004).

5.1.6.4 Physical performance

In addition to enhancing β-oxidation of LCFAs in skeletal muscle, L-Car may also benefit exercise performance by decreasing muscle glycogen depletion, shifting energy sources to the highly efficient aerobic glucose metabolic pathways, replacing decreased L-Car that has shifted to acylcarnitine during exercise, lowering content of toxic acyl groups and increasing of muscle blood flow secondary to vasodilation (Lango et al., 2001; Brass, 2000). Beneficial effect of L-Car in healthy subjects in an attempt to improve athletic performance is controversial (Sweetman, 2002). However, it is used as legal dope in sports (Szewczyk & Wojtczac, 2002).

5.1.6.5 Other uses

L-Car treatment significantly improved symptoms in chronic fatigue syndrome (CFS) patients without side effects (Naguib, 2005). There is some suggestion that L-Car supplementation may be benefit in alleviating chemotherapy-induced fatigue (Sweetman, 2002). L-Car supplementation has been approved by the FDA not only for the treatment but also for the prevention of carnitine depletion in dialysis patients. Regular L-Car supplementation in hemodialysis patients can improve their lipid metabolism, protein nutrition, antioxidant status and anemia requiring large doses of erythropoietin. It also may reduce the incidence of intradialytic muscle cramps, hypotension, asthenia, muscle weakness and cardiomyopathy (Bellinghieri et al., 2003). Chronic hemodialysis produces cardiac damage caused by anemia, hypertension and overhydration. L-Car in a long-term supplementation has been shown to be beneficial to the function of erythrocytes in hemodialysed patients. Additionally, supplementing improves measures of vitality and overall self-perceptions of general health and quality of life in hemodialysed patients and the typical dialysis-associated muscle symptoms (Lango et al., 2001; Kazmi et al., 2005). Sodium valproate is a commonly used as an antiepileptic agent that has been reported to inhibit the biosynthesis of carnitine (Farkas et al., 1996) and reduce carnitine plasma concentrations via its ability to bind L-Car. Researchers have suggested that the incidence of idiosyncratic fatal hepatotoxicity caused by sodium valproate results from impaired β-oxidation of fatty acids in the liver. Valproate has also been shown to impair the tissue uptake of carnitine. Ataxia, hyperammonemia, lethargy, nausea and stupor characterize both carnitine deficiency and sodium valproate hepatic toxicity. In 1996, the pediatric neurology advisory committee recommended supplemental L-Car for younger patients who are taking sodium valproate, carbamazepine, phenytoin or phenobarbital. In addition, L-Car (i.v.) is considered as a treatment of choice to prevent potentially fatal liver dysfunction associated with valproate overdose (LoVecchio et al., 2005; Lango et al., 2001). L-Car alleviates the cardiotoxic effect of adriamycin. Adriamycin is highly toxic to nonmalignant tissues due to the generation of reactive oxygen species (ROS) (Szewczyk & Wojtczac, 2002). In diabetes, L-Car supplementation causes a decrease in triglyceride synthesis, a drop in the cellular free fatty acids (FFAs) uptake, and the removal from organism of excessive long-chain carnitine esters, as well as increase in glycolysis, oxidation of pyruvate, and improvement in neuronal transmission (Mingrone, 2004; Lango et al., 2001). Moreover, protective effects of L-Car against I/R-induced apoptosis were shown by immunohistochemical detection method in rat cardiomyocytes (Najafi et al., 2007).

5.1.7 Adverse effects of L-Car

Gastrointestinal disturbances such as nausea, vomiting, diarrhea, abdominal cramps (Sweetman, 2002), heart-burn, dyspepsia, seizures, blurred vision and headache (Lango et al., 2001) have been reported following the administration of L-Car. Unpleasant body odor that is similar to that of rotten fish has also been noticed in some patients (fish odour syndrome), possibly due to the formation of the metabolite trimethylamine (Lango et al., 2001). There are no reports to date of serious side effects caused by L-Car (Sweetman, 2002; Lango et al., 2001). Patients with severe renal impairment should not be given high orally doses of L-Car for long periods, because of the accumulation of the metabolites trimethylamine and trimethylamine-N-oxide. Diabetic patients administered carnitine while receiving insulin or hypoglycemic drugs should be monitored for hypoglycemia (Sweetman, 2002).

5.2 Acetyl-L-carnitine (ALC)

ALC belongs neither to the vitamin nor the amino acid category. It is chemically similar to carnitine, but is more efficient. While it is synthesized by the liver from lysine and methionine, adequate amounts of vitamins C, B_3, and B_6, plus iron, lysine, and methionine are needed in the diet for this to occur (David, 2000). It is also synthesized in the human brain and kidney by the enzyme ALC transferase (Furlong, 1996). Its main body stores are skeletal and cardiac muscles. It is found along with free plasma carnitine and other acyl-esters of varying chain length (Goa & Brogden, 1987).

5.2.1 Structure of ALC

ALC is an ester of the trimethylated amino acid, L-carnitine (David, 2000) with following structure (molecular formula: C9H17NO4•HCl) (Budavari, 2001)

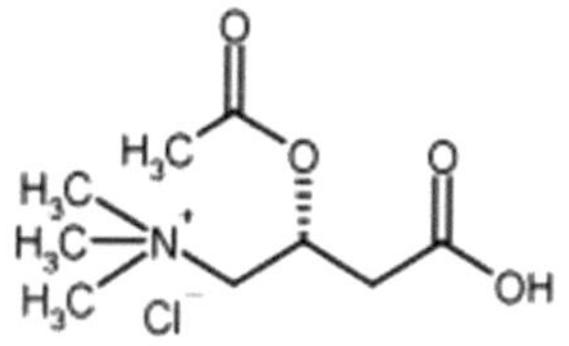

Fig. 2. Chemical structure of ALC. HCl.

5.2.2 Pharmacokinetics of ALC

ALC is administered orally or intravenously and is then absorbed in the jejunum by simple diffusion (Marcus & Coulston, 1996; Parnetti et al., 1992). Bioavailability of ALC is thought to be higher than L-Car. The results of in vitro experiments suggest that ALC is partially hydrolyzed upon intestinal absorption (Gross et al., 1986). Both IV and oral administration result in a corresponding increase in cerebrospinal fluid (CSF) concentrations of ALC, indicating it readily crosses the blood-brain barrier. ALC undergoes little metabolism and is subsequently excreted in the urine via renal tubular reabsorption (Marcus & Coulston, 1996; Parnetti et al., 1992). Though ALC is an ester of the L-Car, nutritional carnitine deficiencies have not been identified in healthy people without metabolic disorders, suggesting that most people can synthesize enough L-Car (Rebouche et al., 2006). Even strict vegetarians show no signs of carnitine deficiency, despite the fact that most dietary carnitine is derived from animal sources (Lombard et al., 1989).

5.2.3 Mechanism of action of ALC

ALC is an ester of carnitine and plays a fundamental role in normal mitochondrial function, being a transport molecule for free fatty acids and an important acetyl group donor in high energy metabolism and free fatty acid β-oxidation (Malaguarnera et al., 2008; Bremer, 1990;

Colucci & Gandour, 1988). Results of some studies show that ALC stabilizes the inner mitochondrial membrane and reverses the decline in activity of a number of mitochondrial translocases and of cytochrome c oxidase thus maintaining energy levels of the cells and stabilizing mitochondrial translocase activity (Qureshi et al., 1998; Paradies et al., 1994). ALC is known to have antioxidant effects by increasing intracellular coenzyme Q10 levels, which accounts for the increase in glutathione reductase activity and high levels of reduced glutathione. The augmentation in antioxidant defense system by ALC finally leads to quenching of free radicals and reduction in reactive oxygen species and lipid peroxidation (Barhwala et al., 2007). ALC could inhibit oxidant-induced DNA single-strand breaks in human peripheral blood lymphocytes (Liu et al., 2004).

5.2.4 Uses of ALC in cardiovascular health and diseases

Like L-Car, ALC enhances fatty acid transport for ATP production in the mitochondria of both skeletal and heart muscles, thereby affording protection from free radical damage (Furlong, 1996; Di Giacomo et al., 1993). Additionally, it may improve cardiolipin levels in the aged heart, a substance which maintains crucial membrane factors in cardiac mitochondria and thus ensures efficient phosphate transport for energy. In a rat mitochondrial model, it was shown that ALC administered to aged animals returned cardiolipin levels to that of young ones (Paradies et al., 1999; Furlong, 1996). Cerebral and peripheral circulation are apparently affected differently by administration of ALC. Ten patients with recent cerebral vascular accidents were given ALC intravenously which resulted in acute enhancement of cerebral blood flow to areas of ischemia via sensitive tomography assessments. In evaluation of patients with peripheral arterial occlusive disease, two studies show that the effect of carnitine esters on improved walking distance was due to metabolic vs. hemodynamic changes and that Propionyl L-carnitine (PLC) was clearly superior to L-Car in this effect. These studies demonstrate the ability of carnitine esters to positively influence tissue energetics which may prove beneficial in a chronic administration model (Paradies et al., 1999; Furlong, 1996).

5.2.5 Findings on beneficial effects of ALC against cardiac arrhythmias

In an experimental study, we focused on the pharmacological effects of ALC on I/R-induced cardiac arrhythmias and infarct size in isolated rat heart when it was used during 30 min regional ischemia followed by 30 min reperfusion. The results of this study showed that ALC produces antiarrhythmic effects against regional I/R-induced arrhythmias such as VEBs, VT and VF. Perfusion of ALC produced significant reduction in the number of VEBs, number and duration of ischemic VT, and duration and incidence of reversible VF by 0.375, 0.75 and 1.5 mM ($p<0.05$ for all) and total VF in ischemia time with mentioned concentrations ($p<0.05$). At the reperfusion phase, number of VT and VEBs were decreased by all concentrations of ALC, but they weren't statistically significant. In addition, VT duration and incidence of total VF were significantly lowered by 0.375, 1.5 and 3 mM of ALC ($p<0.05$). Our findings also demonstrated that ALC caused marked and potent protective activity against I/R injuries as reduction of infarct size in this model of study (Najafi et al., 2010b). In another study, Cui et al. investigated the effects of ALC on incidence of reperfusion-induced VF and infarct size after 30 min global ischemia in isolated rat heart.

Their results showed that perfusion of 0.5 and 5 mM of ALC for 10 min before the induction of global ischemia (not regional ischemia) failed to reduce the incidence of VF. Their results also demonstrated significant reduction in infarct size only by the concentration of 5 mM ALC (Cui et al., 2003). Our results are consistent with the results of Cui et al. in the case of infarct size reduction quality only. However, in contrast to their results, all the used concentrations of ALC in our model significantly reduced infarct size even the lowest concentration (0.375 mM). In addition, our results showed that ALC not only lowered VF incidence in reperfusion time, but also decreased the number and duration of VT, number of VEBs, duration and incidence of total VF in both ischemia and reperfusion time, and incidence of reversible VF in both ischemia and reperfusion phase, when it was used throughout I/R. We suggested that the existence of some methodological differences between the above studies (i.e. type of ischemia and duration of ALC perfusion into the heart) caused different results by low concentrations of ALC. However, other studies, such as the work done by Rosenthal et al (2005), have also demonstrated the same differences that ALC does not promote clinically measurable neuroprotection if administration is significantly delayed following restoration of spontaneous circulation. Thus, in order to maximize the chances of effective neuroprotection, they postulate that for optimal neuroprotective benefit, ALC should be administered as shortly as possible following resuscitation, most definitely within 30 min of reperfusion (Rosenthal et al., 2005). It seems that the potential cardioprotective mechanisms of action of ALC are very similar to those of L-Car (the parent compound of ALC).

5.2.6 Uses of ALC in other diseases

5.2.6.1 Cerebral metabolism

ALC can cross the blood–brain barrier through the γ-amino butyric acid (GABA) uptake system (Burlina et al., 1989). In studies on short-term treatment with ALC in aged rats, the molecule was found to improve some behavioural and biochemical parameters and normalize the age-related impairment in membrane phospholipids metabolism (Aureli et al., 1990), and shown to reduce the sphingomyelin and cholesterol accumulation in the aged rat brain (Aureli et al., 1994a). ALC treatment was also reported to enhance brain energy metabolism and to decrease lactate levels following transient cerebral ischemia (Aureli et al 1994b). In addition, ALC is involved in acetyl group trafficking among different intracellular compartments, and to be a precursor of different lipogenic acetyl CoA pools in rat brain (Ricciolini et al., 1997). Studies on the effects of ALC on cerebral metabolism reported a significant increase in brain phosphocreatine levels, which was associated with a reduction in tissue content of lactic acid and inorganic phosphate (Aureli et al., 1990). ALC administration immediately after 20 min of severe cerebral ischemia has also been demonstrated to induce a faster recovery of cerebral ATP and a strong decrease in tissue lactic acid levels during early post-ischemic reperfusion in the rat (Aureli et al., 1994b). The reduction in cerebral glucose oxidative metabolism associated with the increase in newly synthesized glycogen, suggests that treatment with ALC may modulate cerebral substrate oxidation. Researches showed that the relative flux through pyruvate carboxylase and pyruvate dehydrogenase pathways was not affected by ALC. These findings appear to suggest an overall metabolic effect of ALC on both neurons and glial cells (Tommaso et al., 1998).

5.2.6.2 Aging processes and Alzheimer's dementia

ALC was reported to ameliorate the spatial memory performance of rats exposed to neonatal anoxia (Dell et al., 1997) and improvement of spatial memory. In aged rats it could be achieved only in intermediate but not in good or poor classes of spatial learning performance (Taglialatela et al., 1996). Data shows that improvement could be achieved for novel but not for familiar environments (Caprioli et al., 1995). In the Alzheimer's disease (AD), brain is under extensive oxidative stress and evidenced by significant protein oxidation, lipid peroxidation, and DNA oxidation and is characterized by deposition of amyloid β (Aβ) peptide (Butterfield et al., 2003). Aβ induces lipid peroxidation in ways that are inhibited by free radical antioxidants (Butterfield & Lauderback, 2002). ALC improves neuronal energetic and repair mechanism, decreases the level of lipid peroxidation in the aged rat brain (Kaur et al., 2001), is involved in mitochondrial metabolism (Hagen et al.,1998), and may have antioxidant properties (Poon HF at al., 2006; Kaur J et al., 2001). However, the precise mechanism of action by which ALC may be neuroprotective in aging and neurodegeneration, is not known.

5.2.6.3 Chemotherapy-evoked neuropathic pain

Neurotoxicity is the dose-limiting side effect for chemotherapeutics in the taxane and vinca alkaloid classes, and in many cases the nerve damage is accompanied by a chronic painful peripheral neuropathy (Cata et al., 2006; Dougherty et al., 2004). Impaired mitochondrial function suggests that there might be an energy deficit that compromises the neuron's ability to operate ion transporters. This would lead to membrane depolarization and the generation of spontaneous action potentials. Recent evidence suggests that treatment with ALC, an agent known to ameliorate mitochondrial dysfunction (Virmani et al., 2005; Zanelli et al., 2005), prevents and reverses chemotherapy-evoked pain in rats (Flatters & Bennett GJ, 2006; Ghirardi et al., 2005a, b).

5.2.6.4 Diabetic neuropathy

Studies show that prevention and correction of the metabolic, functional, and structural abnormalities characterizing the neuropathy in the diabetic rat after ALC administration. In addition, the same treatment showed a promoting effect on suppressed nerve fiber regeneration in diabetic rats. In addition, ALC treatment appears to have a sustained beneficial effect on vasoactive prostanoid analogues, possibly counteracting the deleterious effects of decreased endoneurial blood flow in diabetic nerve (Sima et al., 1996).

5.2.6.5 HIV infection

HIV-infected patients on nucleoside analogue therapy commonly experience peripheral neuropathy as an adverse effect of the medications. Patients taking stavudine, zalcitabine or didanosine may have to discontinue therapy as a result. Some studies have suggested ALC as well as recombinant human nerve growth factor may be beneficial in managing this condition (Moyle & Sadler, 1998).

5.2.6.6 Fatigue

Patients with chronic fatigue syndrome show reduced exercise tolerance, and post exercise fatigue induced by minimal physical activity, suggesting decreased muscle function, is considered as one of the causes of this syndrome (Jones et al., 2005). Abnormal mitochondria have been observed in muscle of some elderly patients with fatigue, suggesting some underlying abnormalities in muscle mitochondrial energy production (Behan et al., 1991). The ALC treatment reduced significantly both physical and mental fatigue and improved physical activity and cognitive status (Malaguarnera et al., 2007). The improvement of energetic metabolism in myocardial tissue and in muscular-skeletal tissue is probably the factor that reduces the presence and the severity of physical fatigue in treated subjects. Also researches show that ALC is better tolerated and more effective than amantadine for the treatment of multiple sclerosis-related fatigue (Tomassini et al., 2004).

5.2.6.7 Immune enhancement

ALC has been found to be a powerful immune enhancer. This is due to its ability to promote the health of the nervous system, which in turn governs the activity of the immune system (Scarpini et al., 1997).

5.2.6.8 Effect on cataract

Cataract accounts for most cases of treatable blindness worldwide. Hence, it is important to identify factors that contribute to cataractogenesis with a view to developing novel therapeutic and preventive strategies. It has previously shown that ALC exhibits anticataractogenic activity in an in vitro and in vivo model of selenite cataractogenesis by maintaining antioxidant enzymes at near normal levels and by controlling lipid peroxidation (Geraldine et al., 2006). These observations suggest a novel use for ALC as a possible cataract-preventing drug (Elanchezhian et al., 2009).

5.2.6.9 Male infertility

L-Car and ALC are highly concentrated in the epididymis and are important for sperm metabolism and maturation. In a double-blind, cross over trial of 100 infertile patients, receiving either L-Car or placebo, a significant improvement in sperm quality was observed in the L-Car group. In addition, combination therapy with both L-Car and ALC was given to 60 infertile men and similar outcomes were observed (Movassaghi & Turek, 2008).

5.2.7 Adverse effects of ALC

ALC may cause gastrointestinal disorders and a change in body odor, which can be reduced or eliminated with lower dosages. Less frequent side effects include diarrhea, abdominal pain, nausea, and vomiting (David et al., 2000). ALC may interfere with thyroid metabolism. In individuals with seizure disorders, an increase in seizure frequency and severity has also been reported. ALC also increase agitation in some Alzheimer's disease patients (Hendler & Rorvik, 2001). Overdosing can produce severe muscle weakness, though some have experienced only mild diarrhea with doses as high as 26,000 mg /day (David et al., 2000). With long-term (one year) administration, the most common adverse reactions noted have been agitation, nausea, and vomiting (Spagnoli et al., 1991).

5.3 Propionyl-L-carnitine (PLC)

PLC is a natural short-chain derivative of L-Car and it has a higher transport rate into the myocardium than L-Car (Sayd-Ahmed et al., 2000).

5.3.1 Structure of PLC

PLC is chemically similar to carnitine, but is more efficient (Ferrari et al., 2004). Chemical structure of PLC is shown in fig. 3 (molecular formula: C10H19NO4).

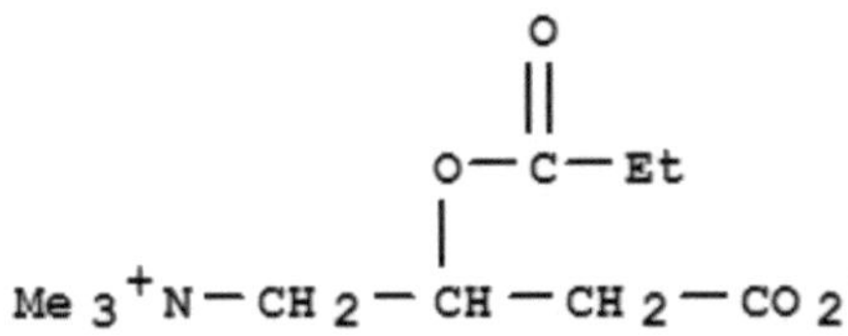

Fig. 3. Chemical structure of PLC

5.3.2 Pharmacokinetics of PLC

PLC is formed via carnitine acetyltransferase from propionyl-CoA, a product of methionine, threonine, valine, and isoleucine, as well as of odd-chain fatty acids (Ferrari et al., 2004). PLC has higher affinity for the plasma membrane transport system. It is more lipophylic and penetrates myocytes faster than L-Car (Lango et al., 2001). Pharmacokinetic studies demonstrated that, in humans, plasma concentration of PLC increases following intravenous administration and then decreases to baseline values within 6 to 24 h. This life span varies with dosage (Ferrari et al., 2004). The plasma concentrations of endogenous PLC in placebo-treated subjects averaged 1.28 nanomol/ml, over the 24 h period of observation. Intravenous PLC has a short elimination half-life (1 h), a small volume of distribution (18 l) and a clearance of about 11 l/h; the renal clearance of PLC increases as the intravenous dose of PLC hydrochloride is increased; and, based on urinary excretion data, L-Car is a major metabolite of intravenously administered PLC hydrochloride. The corresponding value for the estimate of creatinine clearance, which is assumed to be equal to GFR, was 6.08 l/h. Because PLC does not bind to plasma proteins, these data indicate extensive tubular reabsorption of PLC (about 95%). The renal handling of PLC in humans involves saturable tubular reabsorption. The results of in vitro studies have found that PLC is stable to hydrolysis in whole blood, but readily undergoes hydrolysis to L-Car on exposure to hepatic and renal homogenates. The L-Car formed from PLC was likely to have been converted to ALC, resulting in the observed increases in the plasma and urinary levels of the acylated product (Pace et al., 2000).

5.3.3 Mechanism of action of PLC

PLC is an energy source, and it stimulates the Krebs cycle as a precursor of succinyl-CoA, decreases oxidative stress in various systems, and improves cardiac dysfunction in rodent models (Vermeulen et al., 2004). It is now generally agreed that I/R injury in the heart is associated with accumulation of long chain acylesters. The increase of long chain acylesters and depletion of free L-Car in the myocardium have been suggested to damage the cardiac cell membrane and impair the electrical and contractile activities of the heart. It has been shown that PLC administration improves the recovery of mechanical function of the ischemic-reperfused hearts. PLC administration to rats with pressure-overload heart hypertrophy and volume overload heart hypertrophy has been reported to improve cardiac function. Furthermore, PLC was found to exert beneficial effects on myocyte performance and ventricular dilatation in rats subjected to MI (Sethi et al., 1999). PLC increases plasma and cellular carnitine content, thus enhancing FFA oxidation in carnitine-deficient states, as well as increasing glucose oxidation rates. During the reperfusion of previously ischemic hearts, PLC stimulated glucose oxidation and significantly improved the functional recovery. This supported the theory that carnitine's beneficial effects on ischemic myocardium are the result of its ability to overcome the inhibition of glucose oxidation that is induced by increased levels of fatty acids (Ferrari et al., 2004). PLC enhances the propionyl group uptake by myocardial cells. This is important because propionate can be used by mitochondria as an anaplerotic substrate, thus providing energy in the absence of oxygen consumption. Note that propionate alone cannot be administered because of its toxicity. Because of the particular structure of the molecule with a long lateral tail, PLC has a specific pharmacologic action that is independent of its effect on muscle metabolism; this result in peripheral dilatation, positive inotropic effects and coronary vasodilatation with reduced oxygen extraction. It is clear that typical inotropic agents, such as digitalis, calcium, and adrenergic compounds, cause a decline in the phosphocreatinine (PCr)/Pi ratio; this suggested that they place the heart in a supply/demand imbalance. This was not the case for PLC. Thus, all of the cardiovascular actions of PLC can be attributed to its pharmacologic properties rather than to its role as a metabolic intermediate. Energy metabolism remained unchanged despite the increase in myocardial performance (Ferrari et al., 2004). It seems that PLC improved skeletal muscle metabolism in patients with idiopathic dilated cardiomyopathy by increasing pyruvate flux into the Krebs cycle and decreasing lactate production. This effect, which occurs in the absence of major hemodynamic and neuroendocrine changes, may underlie the ability of PLC to increase exercise performance in patients with CHF. It was reported that, when PLC was given to patients with severe heart failure (NYHA IV), it was able to reduce the increase in tumor necrosis factor-α (TNF-α) and, in particular, its soluble receptor that is elevated in CHF, and that is responsible for intracellular signaling of the effects of TNFα. An increased TNF was implicated in the skeletal muscle changes of patients with CHF (Ferrari et al., 2004). Similar to L-Car, PLC have also been proposed to alleviate the noxious effects of oxygen free radicals in the reperfused hearts and to delineate cardiac cells more resistant to I/R damage by stabilizing cellular membranes (Calvani et al., 2000). Endothelial cellular membranes are better protected by PLC against Fe2 and Fe3 ions induced peroxide production, the protection being possibly due to ion chelating (Lango et al., 2001). Finally, attenuating defects in the sarcolemmal membrane may be the other mechanism of PLC and thus may improve heart function in CHF due to MI (Sethia et al., 1999).

5.3.4 Uses of PLC in cardiovascular health and diseases

PLC has shown efficacy in the treatment of a number of cardiovascular disorders including ischemic heart disease, CHF and hypertrophic heart disease. PLC efficacy on cardiac performance is greater than that observed with L-Car (Calvani et al., 2000). Because of PLC's characteristics, it was hypothesized that it could provide adjuvant benefit over standard therapy by specifically improving impaired metabolism of skeletal and heart muscle in patients with CHF (Ferrari et al., 2004). The effects of PLC in a number of models of CHF are particularly evident under conditions of high-energy demand that is induced by increases in workload. Therefore, it seems likely that PLC is able to correct some metabolic steps of the process that leads to heart failure. Besides its effect on the heart, PLC could be helpful in CHF for a specific action on peripheral heart muscle. In CHF, exertional fatigue is not simply the result of skeletal muscle under perfusion. In most patients, there is a decrease in flow responses to exercise as a result of an abnormality of arterial vasodilatation, evidenced by a failure of leg vascular resistances to decrease during exercise. The use of PLC improves the walking capacities of patients with peripheral arterial disease, suggested that PLC could specifically improve metabolism and function of skeletal muscle in patients with CHF. There are several studies on the effects of PLC in peripheral artery disease (Ferrari et al., 2004). PLC hemodynamic effect was evaluated in patients with CAD with normal LV function. When PLC was intravenously administered at 15 mg/kg, it improved the stroke volume and reduced the ejection impedance as a result of decreased systemic and pulmonary resistances and increased arterial compliance. Total external heart power improved with a proportionally smaller increase in the energy requirement; this suggested that PLC has a positive inotropic property. PLC increased the performance of the aerobic myocardium independent on changes of peripheral hemodynamics or coronary flow when administered chronically to the animals several days before the isolation of the heart (Ferrari et al., 2004). PLC used in doses of 15 mg/kg caused a slight decrease in peripheral vascular resistance in patients with stable coronary disease, but due to a simultaneous increase in stroke volume, no decrease in arterial blood pressure was observed. A similar dose administered to patients with ischemic heart disease caused in a short time (5 min) a 43% increase in lactate uptake by myocardium and increase in stroke volume by 8% (Lango et al., 2001). The protective effect of PLC in perfused rat hearts is dose-dependent and also depends on the time of administration, provided it is administered before post-ischemic reperfusion begins. From the accumulated results, it seems that positive biological effects observed after PLC are more evident than those after L-Car administration. Better penetration into myocytes and supplying a substrate for the citric acid cycle can explain this observation in short-term supplementation (Lango et al., 2001). In isolated rat hearts that were subjected to global low-flow ischemia, the group that was treated with PLC exhibited significantly greater recovery of all hemodynamic variables during reperfusion. In a similar preparation, 1 mmol PLC had no protective effect, whereas 5.5 and 11 mmol improved the recovery of cardiac output. The beneficial effect is greater than that of L-Car on a molar basis. PLC was also found to directly improve postischemic stunning. Specific experimental studies were conducted on the efficacy of this agent with respect to CHF. In particular, treatment with PLC (50 mg/kg, intra-arterially) for 4 days significantly improved the hemodynamics of pressure overloaded (by constriction of the abdominal aorta) in conscious rats. In another study, papillary muscles were isolated from rats that had been treated with 180 mg/kg PLC for 8 weeks, starting from weaning. Aortic constriction was performed at 8 weeks of age and lasted for 4 weeks. The papillary muscles of untreated animals showed increased time-to-peak tension and a reduced peak rate of tension rise and delay. PLC normalized all of these parameters. In an infarct model of CHF, chronic administration of PLC (60 mg/kg orally given for 5 months) positively influenced ventricular remodeling; it was equally as effective as the ACE inhibitor, enalapril (1 mg/kg orally), in limiting the magnitude of LV dilatation estimated by pressure-volume curves. PLC limited the alterations in ventricular chamber stiffness that was induced by infarction at low and high filling pressures. In isolated myocytes obtained from infarcted rats, PLC increased peak systolic calcium, peak shortening, and velocity of cell shortening to a greater extent than in normal cells (Ferrari et al., 2004).

5.3.5 Experimental and clinical findings on beneficial effects of PLC against cardiac arrhythmias

The antiarrhythmic effect of PLC was evaluated in the guinea-pig isolated heart; arrhythmias were induced with hypoxia followed by reoxygenation and by digitalis intoxication. PLC 1 μm, was found to be the minimal but effective antiarrhythmic concentration against reoxygenation-induced VF. The antiarrhythmic action of L-PC on reoxygenation-induced arrhythmias is not correlated with its direct electrophysiological effects studied on normoxic preparations. No antiarrhythmic effect was observed against digitalis induced arrhythmias. D-Propionyl carnitine and propionic acid did not exert antiarrhythmic effects. During hypoxia and reoxygenation, PLC consistently prevented the rise of the diastolic left ventricular pressure, and significantly reduced the release of the cardiac enzymes creatine kinase (CK) and lactic dehydrogenase (LDH) (Barbieri et al., 1991).

5.3.6 Uses of PLC in other human diseases

5.3.6.1 Cisplatin induced nephrotoxicity

It is well known that Cisplatin induced nephrotoxicity is the most important dose-limiting factor in cancer chemotherapy. Cisplatin therapy is usually associated with cardiotoxicity including electrocardiographic changes, arrhythmias, myocarditis, cardiomyopathy and congestive heart failure. Combinations of Cisplatin with other anticancer drugs as methotrexate, 5-fluorouracil, bleomycin and doxorubicin are associated with lethal cardiomyopathy. PLC has potential protective effect against Cisplatin-induced cardiac damage with no interfere with the antitumor activity of anticancer drugs. PLC mechanism of action in this case may be due to membrane stabilization by the L-Car portion of PLC with the consequent decrease in release of cardiac enzymes or due to its antioxidant activity (Al-Majed et al., 2006).

5.3.6.2 Sickle-cell anemia

Sickle-cell anemia erythrocytes are under oxidative stress which contributes to some modifications observed in these cells. PLC by antioxidant activity is able to stabilize damaged cell membranes and is also able to decrease the formation of thiobarbituric acid reactive substances. Thus it may be beneficial in maintaining the normal shape of sickle-cell anemia erythrocytes at low oxygen tension and in decreasing the peroxidative damages which accumulate during the life of red blood cells (Ronca et al., 1994).

5.3.6.3 Peripheral arterial disease

PLC stimulates energy production in ischemic muscles by increasing citric acid cycle flux and stimulating pyruvate dehydrogenase activity. Also PLC improves coagulative fibrinolytic homeostasis in vasal endothelium and positively affects blood viscosity. Improvements in maximum walking distance (MWD) correlated positively with increased mitochondrial oxidative ATP synthesis in patients with intermittent claudication. Oral PLC therapy was associated with significant improvements in quality of life in patients with a baseline MWD < 250m (Wiseman et al., 1998). In comparison with pentoxifyllin, PLC had the better effect in the treatment of critical ischemia (Milio et al., 2009; Signorelli et al., 2001). In patient with Leriche-Fontaine stage II peripheral arterial disease of lower limbs LPC showed improvement on circulatory reserve of the ischemic limb without any effect on heart rate and arterial blood pressure. The effect of LPC on the hyperemic response to stress, mainly on halftime of hyperemia, was possibly due to a drug-induced increase of ATP utilization by the ischemic tissues (Corsi et al., 1995).

5.3.6.4 Chronic fatigue syndrome

The symptoms of chronic fatigue syndrome by treatment of PLC showed considerable improvement in 63% of the patients (Vermeulen et al. 2004).

5.3.7 Adverse effects of PLC

PLC may cause some transient and mild gastrointestinal side effects. These adverse effects include nausea, vomiting, abdominal pain, cramps and diarrhea. PLC also may cause seizures in susceptible individuals because of its close structural resemblance to L-Car. Some patients with pre-existing seizure disorders have reported an increase in the number or frequency of seizures upon using PLC. A study mentions that L-Car, a chemical component of PLC, is a peripheral antagonist of the action of thyroid hormones on the body. This means that the circulating L-Car in the blood opposes the action of the thyroid hormones at their site of action. For patients suffering from decreased thyroid function, this could aggravate their condition. PLC could cause other rare side effects such as a body odor, fishy smell of urine and stool and increased appetite. Such adverse effects are more common upon administration of doses as high as 3 grams of PLC. Decreasing the dose usually eliminates these untoward side effects (Nnama, 2010).

5.4 Ranolazine

5.4.1 Structure of ranolazine

Ranolazine is a substituted piperazine compound similar to Trimetazidine (Morin et al., 2001). It is a racemic mixture and chemically described as 1-piperazine acetamide, *N*-(2, 6-dimethyl phenyl)-4-[2-hydroxy-3-(2-methoxyphenoxy) propyl]. Its empirical formula is C24H33N3O4 with following chemical structure (Bhandari & Subramanian, 2007):

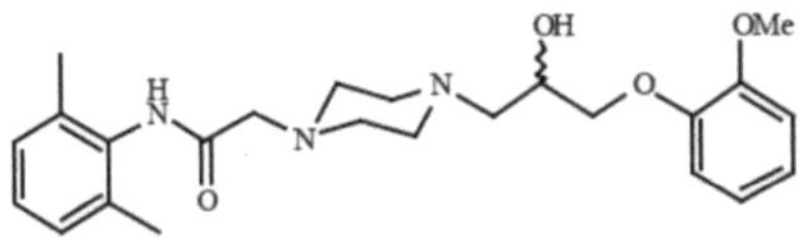

Fig. 4. Chemical structure of ranolazine.

5.4.2 Pharmacokinetics of ranolazine

Peak plasma concentrations (Cmax) are observed within 4-6 hours of administration with extended-release tablets. In case of oral solution or immediate release (IR) capsule, Cmax is achieved in an hour. After administration of radiolabelled ranolazine, 73% of administered dose was excreted in urine with <5% excreted unchanged in both urine and feces. Bioavailability of ranolazine is 35-50% and food does not interfere with its absorption. It is primarily metabolized by cytochrome P450 (CYP) 3A enzyme. Pharmacokinetics of ranolazine is not affected by sex, but existence of marked gender difference in ranolazine pharmacokinetics in rats has been demonstrated. Pharmacokinetics is unaffected in the presence of concomitant illnesses like CHF and diabetes mellitus. Dose adjustments are required in renal failure (Bhandari & Subramanian, 2007).

5.4.3 Mechanism of action of ranolazine

Ranolazine is a partial fatty acid oxidation (pFOX) inhibitor that directly inhibits fatty acid β-oxidation and thus reduces inhibition of PDH by fatty acid oxidation (Sabbah & Stanley, 2002). This metabolic switch increases ATP production per mole of oxygen consumed, reduces the rise in lactic acid and acidosis, and maintains myocardial function under conditions of reduced myocardial oxygen delivery. This mechanism of action of ranolazine may explain its antiischaemic action, in the absence of any hemodynamic effects (without reduction of heart rate or blood pressure or increases of coronary blood flow) in human and animal models (Zacharowski et al., 2001; Cairns, 2006). In addition, blockade of a late sodium current that facilitates calcium entry may play a role in the action of ranolazine (Hume & Grant, 2007). Reducing reactive oxygen species (ROS) concentration by decreasing lipid oxidation could be another possible mechanism of action of ranolazine (Bhandari & Subramanian, 2007).

5.4.4 Experimental and clinical findings on beneficial effects of ranolazine in cardiovascular diseases

Ranolazine has shown cardiac antiischemic and antianginal activity in several in vitro and in vivo animal models and clinical trials (Morin et al., 2001). Results of a study demonstrated that ranolazine behaves as a weak β1- and β2-adrenoceptor antagonist in the rat cardiovascular system (Létienne et al., 2001). In dogs with experimentally-induced heart failure, acute intravenous administration of ranolazine, improved LV ejection fraction as well as other indexes of LV performance. In contrast, ranolazine had no effect on LV function in normal dogs, suggesting that this agent was devoid of any classical cAMP-mediated positive inotropic effects. Ranolazine also improved LV systolic function without increasing coronary blood flow or myocardial oxygen consumption. These studies suggest that pharmacologically switching the oxidative fuel of the heart away from fatty acids towards carbohydrate can improve mechanical efficiency of the failing heart (Sabbah et al., 2002). Previously, we demonstrated that ranolazine reduced number and incidence of VT and the time spent for reversible VF in the ischemic-reperfused isolated rat heart (Najafi & Eteraf Oskouei, 2007). Dhalla et al. tested the effect of ranolazine on ventricular arrhythmias in an ischemic model using two protocols. In protocol 1, anesthetized rats received either vehicle or ranolazine (10 mg/kg, iv bolus) and were subjected to 5 min of LAD occlusion and 5 min of reperfusion with electrocardiogram and blood pressure monitoring. In protocol 2, rats received either vehicle or three doses of ranolazine (iv bolus followed by infusion) and 20 min of LAD occlusion. With both protocols, occurrence and duration of VT and incidence of VF significantly reduced in ranolazine-treated rats. Ranolazine also reduces experimental ST segment elevation and myocardial infarct size and enhances function of stunned myocardium in the peri-infarct area (Dhalla et al., 2009). In isolated canine ventricular myocytes and arterially perfused left ventricular function, ranolazine have shown to produce antiarrhythmic activity along with antianginal actions. Ranolazine produces ion channel effects similar to those observed after chronic exposure to amiodarone. Although ranolazine have shown to cause modest prolongation of the QT interval and action potential duration, but this prolongation is not associated with early after depolarization, triggered activity or polymorphic ventricular activity. Torsades de pointes arrythmias were not observed spontaneously and even on stimulation at concentration as high as 100 micromol/L. Rather, ranolazine is found to possess significant antiarrhythmic activity and suppress the arrhythmogenic effects of other QT-prolonging drugs (Bhandari & Subramanian, 2007). After several clinical trials, ranolazine was approved in the United States and Europe for the treatment of chronic angina pectoris (Dhalla et al., 2009). Because ranolazine prolongs the QTc, the FDA approval is limited to patients who have not responded to other antianginal drugs, and its use in combination with amlodipine, beta-blockers, or long-acting nitrates is recommended. The daily dose should be limited to 1,000 mg and precautions are advised regarding QTc prolongation (Cairns, 2006). Clinical trials also demonstrate the ability of ranolazine to decrease the incidence of VT, supraventricular tachycardia, and ventricular pauses. These antiarrhythmic effects likely arise from the ability of ranolazine to inhibit the late Na^+ current. The antiischemic and antiarrhythmic effects of ranolazine are not mutually exclusive, as they occur at similar concentrations (Lopaschuk et al., 2010). Non-insulin-dependent diabetes mellitus is characterized by elevated fatty acids (FA) levels due to diminished action of insulin in inhibiting FA release from adipocytes. FA may contribute to hyperglycemia by stimulating gluconeogenesis in the liver in the post absorptive state. It also attenuates glucose disposal in skeletal muscle in the fed state. FA oxidation inhibitors may be helpful in controlling hyperglycemia by reducing glucose production in humans. Protective role of the metabolic agents in diabetes with ischemic cardiomyopathy with trimetazidine have been demonstrated. However, the potential usefulness of ranolazine in diabetic patients is expected, but clinical trials are still awaited (Bhandari & Subramanian, 2007).

5.4.5 Adverse effects of ranolazine

The most common adverse effects are dizziness, nausea, asthenia and constipation. Postural hypotension, syncope, headache, dyspepsia and abdominal pain are also reported. Ranolazine should not be administered along with CYP3A inhibitors like ketoconazole, verapamil, diltiazem etc. Ranolazine itself is a weak inhibitor of CYP3A and increases Cmax for simvastatin. By inhibiting P-glycoprotein, it increases plasma concentration of digoxin. Ranolazine should be avoided in liver disease, hypokalemia, or if there is a personal or family history of Long QT syndrome (Bhandari & Subramanian, 2007).

5.5 Trimetazidine

Trimetazidine is likely to stimulate carbohydrate oxidation by directly inhibiting the β-oxidation of fatty acids and secondarily activating PDH (Hara et al., 1999).

5.5.1 Structure of trimetazidine

Trimetazidine [(1-(2,3,4-trimethoxy-benzyl)-piperazine dihydrochloride] with molecular formula: C14H22N2O3 (Fig. 5) is a well-established drug which has been extensively used since 1961 in the treatment of ischemia in angina pectoris and during heart surgery (Tanaka et al., 2005; Ancerewicz et al., 1998).

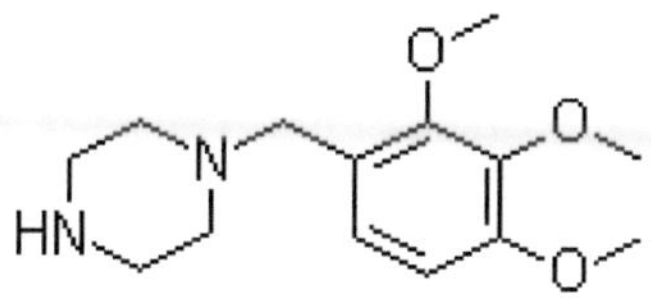

Fig. 5. Chemical structure of trimetazidine.

5.5.2 Pharmacokinetics of trimetazidine

Trimetazidine is absorbed through the intestinal mucosa with a Tmax of 5.4 hours. The Cmax is 89 microgram/L. The bioavailability is 87%, slightly inferior with trimetazidine modified release than with the immediate-release formulation, explaining the increase in the dose of trimetazidine. The bioavailability is not influenced by food. The steady state is reached 2 to 3 days after starting the treatment. The volume of distribution, unaffected by the modified-release formulation, is 4.8 L/kg which means good tissue diffusion. Protein binding affinity is low (16%), with equal binding to albumin and alpha-glycoprotein. No uptake of trimetazidine in red blood cells was observed. The major drug related component observed in plasma and urine was unchanged trimetazidine. In addition to the parent drug, 10 metabolites were detected in urine. Seven routes of metabolism have been identified in man: 2 phase I oxidation and 5 phase II conjugation routes. Trimetazidine and its metabolites are predominantly eliminated in urine. A small proportion of trimetazidine is excreted in the faeces (about 6% of the administered dose). The renal trimetazidine clearance is 350 ml/min and is independent of the urine and plasma concentration of the drug, whereas it is correlated with renal creatinine clearance. That is why the elimination half-life is shorter in the healthy patients as compared with the elderly patients (7 and 12 hours, respectively). Trimetazidine can be safely prescribed without adapting the dose in elderly patients and in case of renal insufficiency (if creatinine clearance remains above 15 ml/min) (http://www.cipladoc.com/therapeutic/pdf_cipla/trivedon_mr.pdf).

5.5.3 Mechanism of action of trimetazidine

Trimetazidine has been shown in numerous trials to be a moderately effective prophylactic antianginal agent. The exact mechanism of antiischemic effect of trimetazidine remains controversial, but its efficacy cannot be accounted for on the basis of purely hemodynamic changes (Horowitz et al., 2010). Trimetazidine has no negative inotropic or vasodilator properties. It is thought to have direct cytoprotective actions on the myocardium (Kantor et al., 2000). The experimental finding that trimetazidine inhibits the enzyme long-chain 3-ketoacyl-CoA thiolase (3-KAT) has led to its being categorized as a partial fatty acid oxidation inhibitor (Horowitz et al., 2010) and a stimulation of glucose oxidation (Kantor et al., 2000). Recent clinical studies have supported this suggestion, demonstrating that trimetazidine inhibits myocardial fatty acid oxidation and augments glucose utilization. Importantly, trimetazidine is also free of the potential to induce tissue phospholipids accumulation with associated toxicity (Horowitz et al., 2010). The relatively low potency of trimetazidine as a carnitine palmitoyltransferase-1 inhibitor makes the mechanism of inhibiting of long-chain fatty acid oxidation and increasing myocardial oxygen utilization, and explains its therapeutic antiischemic effect (Kennedy et al., 1998). Trimetazidine is clinically utilized as an antianginal therapy throughout Europe and in over 90 countries. By inhibiting fatty acid β-oxidation, trimetazidine causes a reciprocal increase in glucose oxidation, thereby decreasing the production of H^+ arising from glycolysis uncoupled from glucose oxidation. Interestingly, in the setting of pressure-overload cardiac hypertrophy, where the rates of fatty acid β-oxidation are depressed, trimetazidine confers cardioprotection independently of alterations in fatty acid β-oxidation. Rather, trimetazidine attenuates the elevated rates of glycolysis and increases glucose oxidation to limit the production of H+ attributed to glucose metabolism. The inhibition of glycolysis coupled with the increase in glucose oxidation, or the partial inhibition of fatty acid β–oxidation and the parallel stimulation of glucose oxidation, can limit ischemia-induced disturbances in myocardial ionic homeostasis. Specifically, the improved coupling of glucose metabolism attenuates intracellular acidosis as well as Na^+ and Ca^{2+} overload during ischemia and subsequent reperfusion and improves the recovery of post ischemic cardiac function. Trimetazidine also affects on cardiac myocyte Ca^{2+} handling that can limit ischemic myocardial injury, including reductions in Ca^{2+} current, prevention of elevated$[Ca^{2+}]i$, and preservation of SR Ca^{2+}-ATPase activity that may limit or prevent cytosolic Ca^{2+} overload. Therefore, the metabolic effects of trimetazidine are permissive to increasing cardiac efficiency by sparing ATP hydrolysis from being utilized to correct ionic homeostasis, and making it available to fuel contractile work (Lopaschuk et al., 2010). Trimetazidine also enters brain tissues in low concentrations. Since oxygenated free radicals are believed to play a major role in both I/R injury and neurodegenerative diseases (Alzheimer and Parkinson's disease), it was suggested that trimetazidine might possess antioxidant properties (Ancerewicz et al., 1998).

5.5.4 Experimental and clinical findings on beneficial effects of trimetazidine in cardiovascular diseases

Trimetazidine is efficacious in the treatment of angina, MI and heart failure. The antiischemic effects of trimetazidine in the treatment of angina include an increased time to 1-mm ST segment depression and decreased weekly nitrate consumption disease (Lopaschuk et al., 2010). Trimetazidine has also been shown to significantly improve exercise-induced anginal symptoms in patients with CAD without eliciting any of the classic antiischemic effects of traditional therapies such as a decrease in heart rate, coronary vasodilation, or a decrease in arterial blood pressure (Sabbah & Stanley, 2002). In acute MI, the cardioprotective effects of trimetazidine are evident as a reduction in reperfusion arrhythmias and a more rapid resolution of ST segment elevation. The addition of trimetazidine to treatment regimens also improves NYHA functional class, LV end-diastolic volume, and ejection fraction in patient with heart failure and ischemic cardiomyopathy, as well as idiopathic dilated cardiomyopathy. Thus, the partial inhibition of fatty acid β-oxidation, via the reversible, competitive inhibition of 3-KAT attenuates several consequences of various forms of ischemic heart disease (Lopaschuk et al., 2010). It was reported that trimetazidine therapy was associated with QTc interval shortening in patients with ischemic heart failure (Zemljic et al., 2010). In the ischemic cardiomyopathy, despite treatment with conventional agents, a high proportion of patients continue to have symptoms and a substantial proportion shows progressive contractile dysfunction leading to LV enlargement and heart failure. Thus, there is a need for new treatments for ischemic cardiomyopathy that apply mechanisms other than those already addressed by conventional agents. There are many evidences suggesting that in patients with ischemic cardiomyopathy, LV dysfunction progress in consequence of alterations in substrate metabolism. Trimetazidine, which acts on myocardial metabolic pathways, appears to protect the heart from the deleterious effects of ischemia, and it has been shown to enhance LV contractility in patients with stunned or hibernating myocardium. Trimetazidine has been shown to improve symptoms and LV ejection fraction and to have a beneficial effect on the inflammatory profile and endothelial function in these patients. These results suggest that trimetazidine is a useful adjunct to the current treatments for the patients with ischemic cardiomyopathy (Bertomeu-Gonzalez et al., 2006). Muscle's metabolic and vascular effects of trimetazidine add new interest in the use of trimetazidine in type 2 diabetic patients with ischemic cardiomyopathy (Monti et al., 2006). It has shown improvement in LV function, symptoms, glucose metabolism and endothelial function in such patients (Bhandari & Subramanian, 2007). Despite beneficial uses, trimetazidine can induce some adverse effects including parkinsonism, gait disorder and tremor (Martí Massó et al., 2005).

5.6 Etomoxir

5.6.1 Structure of etomoxir

Etomoxir {2-[6-(4-chlorophenoxy)hexyl]oxirane-2-carboxylate} is an irreversible inhibitor of carnitine palmitoyl transferase I (CPT-I) that was initially introduced as a potential anti-diabetic agent based on its hypoglycemic effects (Lee et al., 2004, Lopaschuk et al. 2010).

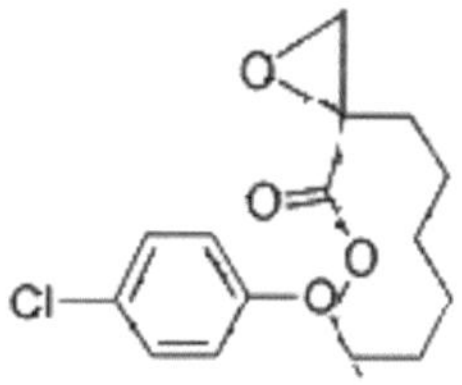

Fig. 6. Chemical structure of etomoxir.

5.6.2 Mechanism of action of etomoxir

Etomoxir inhibits CPT-I, the key enzyme involved in fatty acid uptake by the mitochondria (Baetz et al., 2003), and alters the balance between myocardial fatty acid β-oxidation and glucose oxidation. It leads to reduced fatty oxidation rates, increased glucose oxidation rates and improved myocardial energy efficiency. Although etomoxir has been investigated as a treatment for heart failure, it has not yet been studied as an antianginal agent (Lam A & Lopaschuk, 2007).

5.6.3 Experimental and clinical findings on beneficial effects of etomoxir in cardiovascular diseases

In experimental models of I/R, etomoxir improves the recovery of ventricular function following ischemia. In palmitate-perfused ischemic rat hearts, etomoxir reduced oxygen consumption during ischemic recovery and also prevented depression of myocardial function. In pressure-overloaded, hypertrophic, and failing rat hearts, etomoxir led to an improvement in indices of left ventricular dysfunction (Lee et al., 2004). In isolated rat hearts, perfusion of etomoxir-enriched K/H solution significantly decreased the incidence of ischemic VT and the time spent for reversible VF (Najafi & Eteraf Oskouei, 2007). This cardioprotective effect is also afforded to the postischemic diabetic heart and may suggest the possible clinical utility of etomoxir in patients with diabetic cardiomyopathy. The protective effects of etomoxir in the postischemic period are accompanied by increased rates of myocardial glucose oxidation and an increased production and utilization of ATP for contractile work due to the stimulation of the cardiac PDH complex (via the Randle cycle). Although clinical experience with etomoxir is very limited, its potential beneficial effects on heart function have been assessed in a small (15 patients) uncontrolled, open-label study of patients with NYHA class II heart failure. Following 3 months of etomoxir treatment (80 mg), there was an improvement in LV ejection fraction, cardiac output at peak exercise, and clinical status; however, this trial was not able to assess the long-term safety of etomoxir treatment. More recently, etomoxir for the recovery of glucose oxidation (ERGO) study had to be stopped early as several patients with NYHA class II-class III heart failure in the treatment group were found to have elevated liver transaminase enzyme levels. This adverse effect may be related to the irreversible inhibition of CPT-1 in response to etomoxir, an effect that may allow toxicity to manifest from its excessive accumulation. This study did not detect any significant improvement in the etomoxir group (40 and 80 mg) as compared with placebo (likely due to limited power); however, there was a trend to increased exercise time (Lopaschuk et al. 2010).

5.7 Dichloroacetate (DCA)

DCA is a PDH activator (Liu et al., 2002) and stimulates carbohydrate oxidation through direct inhibition of PDH kinase and reduces fatty acid oxidation through inhibition of fatty acid uptake by mitochondria (Hara et al., 1999).

5.7.1 Structure of DCA

DCA is a compound with formula $CHCl_2COOH$ and below chemical structure (Fig. 7). (http://en.wikipedia.org/wiki/Dichloroacetic_acid).

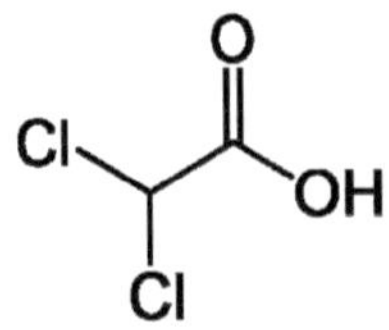

Fig. 7. Chemical structure of DCA.

5.7.2 Pharmacokinetics of DCA

DCA is completely absorbed following oral dosing and about 20% is bound to human plasma proteins. In all species examined, the first dose is cleared from plasma more rapidly than subsequent doses, although the mechanism for this effect is unknown. Glyoxylate is an intermediate in DCA metabolism, and oxalate and CO2 are terminal end products. Neither glyoxylate nor oxalate stimulates PDC activity. However, because the actions of DCA in humans often persist for several days after its clearance from plasma, it is possible that other reactive intermediates of DCA accumulate intracellularly at active sites and bind covalently to target proteins, or that DCA (or a metabolite) induces enzymes responsible for its pharmacodynamic effects. DCA is excreted with little of the dose unchanged (Stacpoole et al., 1998).

5.7.3 Mechanism of action of DCA

DCA exerts multiple effects on pathways of intermediary metabolism. It stimulates peripheral glucose utilization and inhibits gluconeogeneis, thereby reducing hyperglycemia in individuals with diabetes mellitus. It decreases circulating lipid and lipoprotein levels by inhibing lipogenesis and cholesterolgenesis, in patients with disorders of lipoprotein metabolism. DCA facilitates oxidation of lactate and decreases morbidity in lactic acidosis by stimulating the activity of PDH. The drug improves cardiac output and LV mechanical efficiency under conditions of myocardial ischemia or failure, probably by accelerating myocardial metabolism of carbohydrate and lactate as opposed to fat (Stacpoole, 1989). DCA promotes myocardial glucose oxidation at the expense of myocardial fatty acid β-oxidation; however, unlike trimetazidine and ranolazine, DCA stimulates the mitochondrial PDH complex by directly inhibiting the activity of PDH kinase. Experimental studies have demonstrated the ability of DCA to enhance the postischemic recovery of cardiac function in vitro as well as in vivo. An increase in cardiac efficiency, and an improved coupling between glycolysis and glucose oxidation, accompany the cardioprotective effects of DCA (Lopaschuk et al., 2010). DCA may also increase regional lactate removal and restoration of brain function in the cerebral ischemia. DCA appears to inhibit its own metabolism, which may increase the duration of its pharmacologic actions and lead to toxicity. DCA can cause a reversible peripheral neuropathy that may be related to thiamine deficiency and may be ameliorated or prevented with thiamine supplementation. Despite its potential toxicity and limited clinical experience, DCA and its derivatives may be useful in the acute or chronic treatment of several metabolic disorders (Stacpoole, 1989).

5.7.4 Experimental and clinical findings on beneficial effects uses of DCA in cardiovascular diseases

When myocardial carbohydrate oxidation is acutely increased in heart failure patients by activating PDH with intravenous DCA, there is a rapid improvement in LV performance (Sabbah & Stanley, 2002). Clinical experience with DCA is limited; however, in a small clinical trial, DCA increased LV stroke volume and myocardial efficiency, effects accompanied by increased lactate utilization. As the metabolic effects of DCA are similar to those of trimetazidine and ranolazine, it may be relevant in the therapeutic management of angina pectoris; however, its antiischemic efficacy has yet to be established in such a setting (Lopaschuk et al., 2010).

5.8 Perhexiline

Perhexiline has similar metabolic and antianginal effects which are found with inhibition of CPT-I using such as ranolazine (Sabbah & Stanley, 2002).

5.8.1 Structure of perhexiline

Perhexiline is 3 2-(2,2-dicyclohexylethyl) piperidine (Dawson et al., 1986) with following structure (Fig. 8).

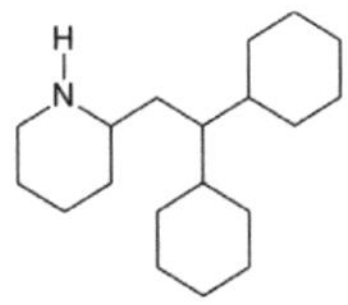

Fig. 8. The chemical structure of perhexiline (http://en.wikipedia.org/wiki/Perhexiline).

5.8.2 Pharmacokinetics of perhexiline

Perhexiline has only ever been available as an oral formulation, thus its bioavailability is unknown. However, it has been reported that in a small group of volunteers receiving 400 mg of perhexiline daily for 14 days, 24 h recoveries of unchanged perhexiline in faeces on days 12, 13 or 14 averaged 7.7% (range 0–32.5%), suggesting good absorption from the gastrointestinal tract. The major determinant of perhexiline clearance appears to be hepatic metabolism, since in humans only approximately 0.1% of a dose is eliminated as unchanged drug in urine. Perhexiline forms two primary monohydroxy (OH) metabolites, cis-OH-perhexiline and trans-OH-perhexiline, which can undergo further secondary metabolism to dihydroxy metabolites, as well as glucuronide conjugates. Formation of the major primary metabolite, cis-OH-perhexiline is catalysed by CYP2D6, and this metabolic pathway is thought to give rise to both the saturability and genetic polymorphism in perhexiline clearance (Sallustio et al., 2002).

5.8.3 Mechanism of action of perhexiline

Although initially designated as a calcium-channel blocker, it has no significant calcium channel blocking activity at therapeutic concentrations. Perhexiline is not negatively inotropic and does not change systemic vascular resistance within therapeutic concentrations and it is well tolerated by patients with combined angina and LV systolic dysfunction. It acts by shifting myocardial substrate utilization from fatty acids to carbohydrates through inhibition of CPT-1 following in increased glucose and lactate utilization (Lee et al., 2004). It seems that, inhibition of CPT-1 then decreasing fatty acid β-oxidation is an effective therapeutic approach in various types of ischemic heart diseases (Lopaschuk et al., 2010).

5.8.4 Experimental and clinical findings on beneficial effects uses of perhexiline in cardiovascular diseases

Perhexiline was developed as a prophylactic antianginal agent approximately 40 years ago. It was initially thought to be a coronary vasodilator, although in fact its vasomotor effects are minimal - later its weak L-type calcium channel blocking effects were thought to underlie its effects. This was inherently implausible, because the observed antianginal effects of perhexiline were extraordinary, with relief of otherwise intractable symptoms in many patients. Despite its antianginal efficacy, perhexiline induced substantial toxicity, which caused a decline in its therapeutic uses from 1980. It was shown that the toxicity of perhexiline was preventable, and that the toxicity were observed in patients in whom plasma perhexiline levels were elevated beyond 600 μg/ml whereas dosage titration to achieve steady-state levels between 150 and 600 μg/ml, serious toxicity was turned away. These findings have permitted a reevaluation of the therapeutic role of perhexiline in severe angina, and an extension to possible therapeutics of other conditions such as heart failure and inoperable aortic stenosis (Horowitz et al., 2010). Of importance is the fact that the hepatic toxicity of perhexeline is due to the inhibition of the hepatic isoform of CPT 1. In vitro studies clearly demonstrate that the cardiac isoform of CPT 1 is more sensitive to inhibition by perhexeline, an effect that allows for the use of dose titration to avoid or limit adverse effects. Several clinical trials have demonstrated the beneficial effects of perhexeline in aortic stenosis, heart failure, and angina pectoris (Lopaschuk et al., 2010).

5.8.5 Adverse effects of perhexiline

Long-term therapy with perhexiline frequently induced both hepatotoxicity and neurotoxicity by phospholipidosis in hepatocytes and Schwann cells with this agent. Other side effects are nausea, dizziness or both, and hypoglycemia in diabetics. These effects were later demonstrated to occur most commonly in patients who are slow hydroxylators, bearers of a genetic variant of the cytochrome P-450 enzyme family. These patients are slow metabolisers of perhexiline due to saturation of hepatic metabolic pathways, which leads to accumulation of the drug and toxicity. The mechanism for toxicity appears to be due to phospholipids accumulation, which is a direct consequence of CPT-1 inhibition. Hence, this is a potential side effect of any drug that inhibits CPT-1, including amiodarone, which exhibits weak CPT-1-inhibitor properties. This is thought to be the mechanism responsible for the peripheral neuropathy and hepatitis occasionally seen with amiodarone use (Lee et al., 2004).

6. Conclusion

Alterations in fatty acid β-oxidation have important implications on cardiac function in both heart failure and IHD. Of importance is that emerging evidence suggests that inhibition of fatty acid β-oxidation may be a useful approach to improve heart function in the setting of obesity, diabetes, heart failure, and IHD. Metabolic agents modulate fatty acid and glucose utilization by the myocardium during I/R to protect the heart from I/R injuries such as arrhythmias. Some of the agents have well-documented antiischemic and antiarrhythmic effects against I/R-induced cardiac arrhythmias.

7. References

Akgun, S.; Tekeli, A.; Kurtkaya, O.; Civelek, A.; Isbir, SC.; Ak, K.; Arsan, S. & Sav, A. (2004). Neuroprotective effects of FK-506, L-carnitine and azathioprine on spinal cord ischemia-reperfusion injury, *European Journal of Cardio-thoracic Surgery,* Vol. 25, No. 1, pp. 105-110.

Al-Majed, AA.; Sayed-Ahmed, MM.; Abdulaziz A.; Al-Yahya, AA.; Aleisa, MA.; Al-Rejaie, SS. & Al-Shabanah, AO. (2006). Propionyl-l-carnitine prevents the progression of cisplatin-induced cardiomyopathy in a carnitine-depleted rat model, *Pharmacological Research*, Vol. 53, pp. 278–286.

Ancerewicz, J.; Migliavacca, E.; Carrupt, PA.; Testa, B.; Brée, F.; Zini, R.; Tillement, JP.; Labidalle, S.; Guyot, D.; Chauvet-Monges, AM.; Crevat, A. & Le Ridant, A. (1998). Structure–Property Relationships of Trimetazidine Derivatives and Model Compounds as Potential Antioxidants, *Free Radical Biology and Medicine*, Vol. 25, No. 1, pp. 113-120.

Arsenian, MA.; New, PS. & Cafasso, CM. (1996). Safety, tolerability, and efficacy of a glucose-insulin-potassium-magnesium-carnitine solution in acute myocardial infarction, *The American Journal of Cardiology*, Vol. 78, No. 4, pp. 477-479.

Aureli, T.; Capuani, G.; Di Cocco, ME.; Ricciolini, R.; Ghirardi, O.; Giuliani, A.; Ramacci, MT. & Miccheli, A. (1994_a). Changes in brain lipid composition during aging: effect of long-term acetyl-L-carnitine treatment, *Q Magn Res Biol Med*, Vol. 1, pp. 47–52.

Aureli, T.; Miccheli, A.; Di Cocco, ME.; Ghirardi, O.; Giuliani, A.; Ramacci, MT. & Conti, F. (1994_b). Effect of acetyl-L-carnitine on recovery of brain phosphorus metabolites and lactic acid level during reperfusion after cerebral ischemia in the rat, *Brain Research*, Vol. 643, pp. 92–99.

Aureli, T.; Miccheli, A.; Ricciolini, R.; Di Cocco, ME.; Ramacci, MT.; Angelucci, L.; Ghirardi, O. & Conti, F. (1990). Aging brain: effect of acetyl-L-carnitine treatment on rat brain energy and phospholipids metabolism, *Brain Research*, Vol. 526, pp. 112–118.

Bach, AC.; Schirardin, H.; Sihr, MO. & Storck, D. (1983). Free and total carnitine in human serum after oral ingestion of L-carnitine, *Diabetes & Metabolism*, Vol. 9, No. 2, pp. 121-124.

Baetz, D.; Bernard, M. Pinet, C. Tamareille, S. Chattou, S. El Banani, H. Coulombe, A. & Feuvray, D. (2003). Different pathways for sodium entry in cardiac cells during ischemia and early reperfusion, *Molecular and Cellular Biochemistry*, Vol. 242, No. 1-2, pp. 115-120.

Barbieri, M.; Carbonin, PU.; Cerbai, E.; Gambassi, G.; Lo Giudice, P.; Masini, L.; Mugelli, A. & Pahor, M. (1991). Lack of correlation between the antiarrhythmic effect of L-propionylcarnitine on reoxygenation-induced arrhythmias and its electrophysiological properties, *British Journal of Pharmacology*, Vol. 102, pp. 73-78.

Barhwala, K.; Singh, BS.; Hotaa, KS.; Jayalakshmia, K. & Ilavazhagan, G. (2007). Acetyl-l-Carnitine ameliorates hypobaric hypoxic impairment and spatial memory deficits in rats, *European Journal of Pharmacology*, Vol. 570, No. 1-3, pp. 97-107.

Bellinghieri, G.; Santoro, D.; Calvani, M.; Mallamace, A. & Savica, V. (2003). Carnitine and hemodialysis, *American Journal of Kidney Diseases*, Vol. 41, No. 3 Suppl 1, pp. S116-122.

Bertomeu-Gonzalez, V.; Bouzas-Mosquera, A. & Kaski, JC. (2006). Role of trimetazidine in management of ischemic cardiomyopathy, *The American Journal of Cardiology*, Vol. 4, No. 98(5A), pp.19J-24J.

Bhandari, B. & Subramanian, L. (2007). Ranolazine, a Partial Fatty Acid Oxidation Inhibitor, its Potential Benefit in Black, CS. (2000). In vivo models of myocardial ischemia and reperfusion injury Application to drug discovery and evaluation, *Journal of Pharmacological and Toxicological Methods*, Vol. 43, pp. 153- 167.

Brass, EP. (2000). Supplemental carnitine and exercise, *The American Journal of Clinical Nutrition,* Vol. 72, No. 2 Suppl, pp. 618S-623S.

Bremer, J. (1990). The role of carnitine in intracellular metabolism. *J Clin Chem Clin Biochem* , Vol. 28, No. 5, pp. 297-301.

Budavari, S. (2001). *The Merck Index* (13), pp. 16.

Burlina, AP.; Sershen, H.; Debler, EA. & Lajtha, A. (1989). Uptake of acetyl-Lcarnitine in the brain. *Neurochemical Research,* Vol. 14, pp. 489–493.

Butterfield, DA. & Lauderback, CM. (2002). Lipid peroxidation and protein oxidation in Alzheimer's disease brain: potential causes and consequences involving amyloid beta-peptide-associated free radical oxidative stress. *Free Radical Biology and Medicine,* Vol. 32, pp. 1050–1060.

Butterfield, DA.; Boyd-Kimball, D. & Castegna, A. (2003). Proteomics in Alzheimer's disease: insights into potential mechanisms of neurodegeneration, *Journal of Neurochemistry,* Vol. 86, pp. 1313–1327.

Cairns, AJ. (2006). Ranolazine: Augmenting the Antianginal Armamentarium, *Journal of the American College of Cardiology,* Vol. 48, No. 3, pp. 576–578.

Calvani, M.; Reda, E. & Arrigoni-Martelli, E. (2000). Regulation by carnitine of myocardial fatty acid and carbohydrate metabolism under normal and pathological conditions, *Basic Research in Cardiology,* Vol. 95, No. 2, pp. 75-83.

Caprioli, A.; Markowska, AL. & Olton, DS. (1995). Acetyl-l-carnitine: chronic treatment improves spatial acquisition in a new environment in aged rats, *Journal of Gerontology. Series A, Biological Sciences and Medical Sciences,* Vol. 50, pp. 232–236.

Cata, JP.; Weng, HR.; Lee, BN.; Reuben, JM. & Dougherty, PM. (2006). Clinical and experimental findings in humans and animals with chemotherapy induced peripheral neuropathy, *Minerva Anesthesiologica* , Vol. 72, pp. 151–169.

Colucci, WJ. & Gandour, RD. (1988). Carnitine acyltransferase: a review of its biology, enzymology and bioorganic chemistry. *Bioorganic Chemistry,* Vol. 16, pp. 307-334.

Corsi, C.; Pollastri, M.; Marrapodi, E.; Leanza, D.; Giordano, S. & D'Iddio, S. (1995). L-Propionylcarnitine Effect on Postexercise and Postischemic Hyperemia in Patients Affected by Peripheral Vascular Disease, *Angiology,* Vol. 46, No. 8, pp.705-713.

Cui, J.; Das, DK.; Bertelli, A. & Tosaki, A. (2003). Effects of L-carnitine and its derivatives on post-ischemic cardiac function, ventricular fibrillation and necrotic and apoptotic cardiomyocyte death in isolated rat hearts, *Molecular and Cellular Biochemistry,* Vol. 254, No. 1-2, pp. 227-234.

David, W. (2000). Encyclopedia of Mind Enhancing Foods, Drugs and Nutritional Substances.1st ed. New York, 26-27.

Dawson, BM.; Katz, H. & Glusker JP. (1986). Perhexiline [2-(2,2-dicyclohexylethyl)piperidine] maleate, *Acta Crystallographica,* C42, pp. 67-71.

De Simone, C.; Tzantzoglou, S.; Famularo, G.; Moretti, S.; Paoletti, F.; Vullo, V. & Delia, S. (1993). High dose L-carnitine improves immunologic and metabolic parameters in AIDS patients, *Immunopharmacology and Immunotoxicology,* Vol. 15, No. 1, pp. 1-12.

Dell, EA.; Iuvone, L.; Calzolari, S. & Geloso, MC. (1997). Effect of acetyl-lcarnitine on hyperactivity and spatial memory deficits of rats exposed to neonatal anoxia. *Neuroscience Letters,* Vol. 223, pp. 201–205.

Dhalla, KA.; Wang, W.; Dow, J.; Shryock, CJ.; Belardinelli, L.; Bhandari, A. & Kloner, AR. (2009). Ranolazine, an antianginal agent, markedly reduces ventricular arrhythmias induced by ischemia and ischemia-reperfusion, *American Journal of Physiology, Heart and Circulation Physiology,* Vol. 297, pp. H1923–H1929.

Di Giacomo, C.; Latteri, F.; Fichera, C.; Sorrenti, V.; Campisi, A.; Castorina, C.; Russo, A.; Pinturo, R. & Vanella, A. (1993). Effect of acetyl-L-carnitine on lipid peroxidation and xanthine oxidase activity in rat skeletal muscle. *Neurochemical Research,* Vol. 18, No. 11, pp. 1157–1162.

Dichloroacetic_acid, June 2011, Available from http://en.wikipedia.org/wiki/Dichloroacetic_acid.

Dougherty, PM.; Cata, JP.; Cordella, JV.; Burton, A. & Weng, HR. (2004). Taxolinduced sensory disturbance is characterized by preferential impairment of myelinated fiber function in cancer patients. *Pain,* Vol. 109, pp. 32–42.

Elanchezhian, RM.; Sakthivel, P.; Geraldine, P. & Thomas A. (2009). The effect of acetyl-L-carnitine on lenticular calpain activity in prevention of selenite-induced cataractogenesis. *Experimental Eye Research,* Vol. 88, pp. 938–944.

Farkas, V.; Bock, I.; Cseko, J. & Sandor, A. (1996). Inhibition of carnitine biosynthesis by valproic acid in rats--the biochemical mechanism of inhibition, *Biochemical Pharmacology,* Vol. 52, No. 9, pp. 1429-1433.

Ferrari, R.; Merli, E.; Cicchitelli, G.; Mele, D.; Fucili, A. & Ceconi, C. (2004). Therapeutic effects of L-carnitine and propionyl-L-carnitine on cardiovascular diseases: a review, *Annals of the New York Academy of Sciences,* Vol. 1033, pp. 79-91.

Flatters, SJL. & Bennett, GJ. (2006). Studies of peripheral sensory nerves in paclitaxel-induced painful peripheral neuropathy. *Pain,* Vol. 122, pp. 245–257.

Ford, DA. (2002). Alterations in myocardial lipid metabolism during myocardial ischemia and reperfusion, *Progress in Lipid Research,* Vol. 41, No. 1, pp. 6-26.

Furlong, JH. (1996). Acetyl-L-carnitine: Metabolism and Applications in Clinical Practice. Alternative Medicine Review, Vol. 1, No. 2, pp 85-93.

Gandhi, C.; Upaganalawar, A. & Balaraman, R. (2009), Protection against in vivo focal myocardial ischemia/reperfusion injury-induced arrhythmias and apoptosis by hesperidin, *Free Radical Research,* Vol. 43, No. 9, pp. 817-827.

Geraldine, P.; Sneha, BB.; Elanchezhian, R.; Ramesh, E.;, Kalavathy, CM.; Kaliamurthy, J. & Thomas, PA. (2006). Prevention of selenite-induced cataractogenesis by acetyl-Lcarnitine: an experimental study, *Experimental Eye Research,* Vol. 83 No. 6, pp. 1340–1349.

Ghirardi, O.; Lo Giudice, P.; Pisano, C.; Vertechy, M.; Bellucci, A.; Vesci, L.; Cundari, S.; Miloso, M.; Rigamonti, LM.; Nicolini, G.; Zanna, C. & Carminati, P. (2005a). Acetyl-L-Carnitine prevents and reverts experimental chronic neurotoxicity induced by oxaliplatin, without altering its antitumor properties, *Anticancer Research,* Vol. 25, pp. 2681–2687.

Ghirardi, O.; Vertechy, M.; Vesci, L.; Canta, A.;Nicolini, G.; Galbiati, S.; Ciogli, C.; Quattrini, G.; Pisano, C.; Cundari, S. & Rigamonti, LM. (2005b). Chemotherapy-induced allodynia: neuroprotective effect of acetyl- L-carnitine, *In Vivo,* Vol. 19, No. 3, pp. 631-637.

Goa, KL. & Brogden, A. (1987). L-carnitine, a preliminary review of its pharmacokinetics, and its therapeutic use in ischaemic cardiac disease and primary and secondary carnitine deficiencies in relationship to its role in fatty acid metabolism, *Drugs,* 34, 1-24.

Gross, CJ.; Henderson, LM. & Savaiano, DA. (1986). Uptake of L-carnitine, D-carnitine and acetyl-L-carnitine by isolated guinea-pig enterocytes. *Biochimica et Biophysica Acta*, Vol. 886, No. 3, pp. 425-433.

Hara, A.; Matsumura, H.; Maruyama, K.; Hashizume, H.; Ushikubi, F. & Abiko, Y. (1999). Ranolazine: an anti-ischemic drug with a novel mechanism of action, *Cardiovascular Drug Reviews*, Vol. 17, No. 1, pp. 58-74.

Hendler, SS. & Rorvik, D. (2001). Acetyl-L-carnitine, L-carnitine. *NIEHS*, Vol. 9, No. 11, pp. 255-259.

Horowitz, JD.; Chirkov, YY.; Kennedy, JA. & Sverdlov, A.L. (2010). Modulation of myocardial metabolism: an emerging therapeutic principle, *Current Opinion in Cardiology*, Vol. 25, pp. 329–334

Hume, RJ & Grant, OA. (2007). Agents Used in Cardiac Arrhythmias, In: *Basic & Clinical Pharmacology*, Katzung, BG.; Masters, BS. & Trevor, JA, pp. 211-235, The McGraw-Hill Companies, USA.

Ilias, I.; Manoli, I.; Blackman, MR.; Gold, PW. & Alesci, S. (2004). L-carnitine and acetyl-L-carnitine in the treatment of complications associated with HIV infection and antiretroviral therapy, *Mitochondrion*, Vol. 4, No. 2-3, pp. 163-168.

Jones, MG.; Goodwin, CS.; Amjad, S. & Chalmers, RA. (2005). Plasma and urinary carnitine and acylcarnitines in chronic fatigue syndrome. *Clinica Chimica Acta* , Vol. 360, pp. 173–177.

Kantor, PF.; Lucien, A.; Kozak, R. & Lopaschuk, GD. (2000). The Antianginal Drug Trimetazidine Shifts Cardiac Energy Metabolism From Fatty Acid Oxidation to Glucose Oxidation by Inhibiting Mitochondrial Long-Chain 3-Ketoacyl Coenzyme A Thiolase, *Circulation Research*, Vol. 86, pp. 580-588.

Kaur, J.; Sharma, D. & Singh, R. (2001). Acetyl-L-carnitine enhances Na(+), K(+)-ATPase glutathione-S-transferase and multiple unit activity and reduces lipid peroxidation and lipofuscin concentration in aged rat brain regions, *Neuroscience*, Vol. 301, No. 1, pp. 1–4.

Kazmi, WH.; Obrador, GT.; Sternberg, M.; Lindberg, J.; Schreiber, B.; Lewis, V. & Pereira, BJ. (2005). Carnitine therapy is associated with decreased hospital utilization among hemodialysis patients, *American Journal of Nephrology*, Vol. 25, No. 2, pp. 106-115.

Kennedy, JA. & Horowitz, JD. (1998). Effect of trimetazidine on carnitine palmitoyltransferase-1 in the rat heart, *Cardiovascular Drugs and Therapy*, Vol. 12, pp. 359-363.

Kerner, J. & Hoppel, C. (1998). Genetic disorders of carnitine metabolism and their nutritional management, *Annual Review of Nutrition*, Vol. 18, pp. 179-206.

Lam, A. & Lopaschuk, DG. (2007). Anti-anginal effects of partial fatty acid oxidation inhibitors, *Current Opinion in Pharmacology*, Vol. 7, No. 2, pp. 179-185.

Lango, R.; Smolenski, RT.; Narkiewicz, M.; Suchorzewska, J. & Lysiak-Szydlowska, W. (2001). Influence of L-carnitine and its derivatives on myocardial metabolism and function in ischemic heart disease and during cardiopulmonary bypass, *Cardiovascular Research*, Vol. 51, No. 1, pp. 21-29.

Lee, L.; Horowitz, J. & Frenneaux, M. (2004). Metabolic manipulation in ischemic heart disease, a novel approach to treatment, *European Heart Journal*, Vol. 25, No. 8, pp. 634-641.

Létienne, R.; Vié, B.; Puech, A.; Vieu, S.; Le Grand, B. & John, WG. (2001). Evidence that ranolazine behaves as a weak β1- and β 2-adrenoceptor antagonist in the rat cardiovascular system, *Naunyn-Schmiedeberg's Archives of Pharmacology*, Vol. 363, pp. 464–471.

Liu, Q.; Docherty, CJ.; Rendell, TCJ.; Clanachan, SA. & Lopaschuk, DG. (2002). High Levels of Fatty Acids Delay the Recovery of Intracellular pH and Cardiac Efficiency in Post-Ischemic Hearts by Inhibiting Glucose Oxidation, *Journal of the American College of Cardiology*, Vol. 39, No. 4, pp. 718 –725.

Liu, J.; Head, E.; Kuratsune, H.; Cotman, CW. & Ames, BN. (2004). Comparison of the effects of L-carnitine and acetyl-L-carnitine on carnitine levels, ambulatory activity, and oxidative stress biomarkers in the brain of old rats. *Annals of the New York Academy of Sciences*, pp. 117-131.

Lombard, KA.; Olson, AL.; Nelson, SE. & Rebouche, CJ. (1989). Carnitine status of lactoovovegetarians and strict vegetarian adults and children. *American Journal of Clinical Nutrition*, Vol. 50, No. 2, pp. 301-306.

Lopaschuk, GD.; Ussher, JR.; Folmes, CDL.; Jaswal, JS. & Stanley, WC. (2010). Myocardial Fatty Acid Metabolism in Health and Disease, *Physiological Reviews*, Vol. 90, pp. 207–258.

LoVecchio, F.; Shriki, J. & Samaddar, R. (2005). L-carnitine was safely administered in the setting of valproate toxicity", *The American Journal of Emergency Medicine*, Vol. 23, No. 3, pp. 321-322.

Lu, RH.; Yang, P.; Remeysen, P.; Saels, A.; Dai, D. & Clerck, DF. (1999). Ischemia-reperfusion-induced arrhythmias in anaesthetized rats: a role of Na^+ and Ca^{2+} influx, *European Journal of Pharmacology*, Vol. 365, pp. 233–239.

Malaguarnera, M.; Gargante, MP.; Cristaldi, E.; Colonna, V.; Messano, M.; Koverech, A.; Neri, S.; Vacante, M.; Cammalleri, L. & Motta, M. (2007). Acetyl L-carnitine (ALC) treatment in elderly patients with fatigue, *Arch Gerontol Geriatr*, Vol. 1728, pp. 1-10 .

Malaguarnera, M.; Gargante, MP.; Cristaldi, E.; Vacante, M.; Risino, C.; Cammalleri, L.; Pennisi, G. & Rampello, L. (2008). Acetyl-L-Carnitine Treatment in Minimal Hepatic Encephalopathy, *Digestive Diseases and Sciences*, Vol. 53, No. 11, pp. 3018-3025.

Marcus, R. & Coulston, AM. (1996). Water-soluble vitamins. *The Pharmacological Basis of Therapeutics*. 9th edition. New York.

Martí Massó, JF.; Martí, I.; Carrera, N.; Poza, JJ. & López, A. (2005). Trimetazidine induces parkinsonism, gait disorders and tremor, *Therapie*, Vol. 60, No. 4, pp. 419-422.

McBride, FB. & White, M. (2003). Ranolazine, A novel metabolic modulator for the treatment of chronic stable angina, *Formulary*, Vol. 38, pp. 461–476.

McCormack, GJ.; Stanley, CW. & Wolff, AA. (1998). Ranolazine: A Novel Metabolic Modulator for the Treatment of Angina, *General Pharmacology*, Vol. 30, No. 5, pp. 639–645.

Milio, G.; Novo, G.; Genova, C.; Almasio, PL.; Novo, S.& Pinto, A. (2009). Pharmacological Treatment of Patients with Chronic Critical Limb Ischemia: L-Propionyl-Carnitine Enhances the Short-Term Effects of PGE-1, *Cardiovascular Drugs and Therapy*, Vol. 23, pp. 301–306.

Mingrone, G. (2004). Carnitine in type 2 diabetes, *Annals of the New York Academy of Sciences*, Vol. 1033, pp. 99-107.

Monti, LD.; Setola, E.; Fragasso, G.; Camisasca, RP.; Lucotti, P.; Galluccio, E.; Origgi, A.; Margonato, A. & Piatti, P. (2006). Metabolic and endothelial effects of trimetazidine on forearm skeletal muscle in patients with type 2 diabetes and ischemic cardiomyopathy, *American Journal of Physiology - Endocrinology and Metabolism*, Vol. 290, pp. E54–E59.

Moretti, S.; Alesse, E.; Di Marzio, L.; Zazzeroni, F.; Ruggeri, B.; Marcellini, S.; Famularo, G.; Steinberg, S.M.; Boschini, A.; Cifone, MG. & De Simone, C. (1998). Effect of L-carnitine on human immunodeficiency virus-1 infection-associated apoptosis: a pilot study, *Blood*, Vol. 91, No. 10, pp. 3817-3824.

Morin, D.; Hauet, T.; Spedding, M. & Tillement, J. (2001). Mitochondria as target for anti-ischemic drugs, *Advanced Drug Delivery Reviews*, Vol. 49, No. 1-2, pp. 151-174.

Movassaghi, M/& Turek, PJ. (2008). The Cost-Effectiveness of Treatments for Male Infertility: Medical Therapy, *Expert Rev Pharmacoecon Outcomes Res*, Vol. 8, No. 2, pp. 197-206.

Moyle, GJ. & Sadler, M. (1998). Peripheral neuropathy with nucleoside antiretrovirals: risk factors, incidence and management, *Drug Saf*, Vol.19, pp. 481-494.

Naguib, Y. (2005). Carnitine: essential fuel for the cellular engine, June 2011, Available from http://www.hnherbs.com/carnitine.pdf

Najafi, M. & Eteraf-Oskouei, T. (2007). Comparison between the effect of Etomoxir and Ranolazine on ischemia-reperfusion induced cardiac arrhythmias in isolated rat heart, *Journal of Babol University of Medical Sciences*, Vol. 9, No. 5, pp. 7-13.

Najafi, M. & Garjani, A., (2005). The effect of L-carnitine on arrhythmias in the ischemic rat heart, *Iranian Journal of Basic Medical Sciences*, Vol. 8, No. 1, pp. 38-44.

Najafi, M.; Garjani, A. & Dustar, Y. (2007). Effects of L-carnitine on cardiac apoptosis in the ischemic–reperfused isolated rat heart, *Iranian Journal of Pharmaceutical sciences*, Vol. 3, No. 1, pp. 19-24..

Najafi, M.; Garjani, A.; Maleki, N. & Eteraf-Oskouei, T. (2008). Antiarrhythmic and Arrhythmogenic Effects of L-Carnitine in Ischemia and Reperfusion, *Bulletin of Experimental Biology and Medicine*, Vol. 146, No. 2, pp. 210- 213.

Najafi, M.; Ghaffary, S. & Shaseb,E. (2010b). Effects of Acetyl-L-Carnitine on Cardiac Arrhythmias and Infarct Size in Ischemic-Reperfused Isolated Rat Heart, *Iranian Journal of Basic Medical Sciences*, Vol. 13, No.1, pp. 216-222.

Najafi, M.; Javidnia, A.; Ghorbani-Haghjo, A.; Mohammadi, S. & Garjani, A. (2010a). Pharmacological Preconditioning with L-carnitine: Relevance to Myocardial Hemodynamic Function and Glycogen and Lactate Content, *Pakistan Journal of Pharmaceutical Sciences*, Vol. 23, No.3, pp. 250-255.

Nnama, H. The side effects of propionyl-l-carnitine, June 2011, Available from http://www.livestrong.com/article/331703-the-side-effects-of-propionyl-l-carnitine.

Pace, S.; Longo, A.; Toon, S.; Rolan, P. & Evans, AM. (2000). Pharmacokinetics of propionyl-l-carnitine in humans: evidence for saturable tubular reabsorption, *British Journal of Clinical Pharmacology*, Vol. 50, No. 5, pp. 441–448.

Paradies, G.; Petrosillo, G.; Gadaleta, MN. & Ruggiero, FM. (1999). The effect of aging and acetyl-L-carnitine on the pyruvatetransport and oxidation in rat heart mitochondria, *FEBS Letter*, Vol. 454, pp. 207-209.

Paradies, G.; Ruggiero, FM.; Petrosillo, G.; Gadaleta, MN. & Quagliariello, E. (1994). Enhanced cytochrome oxidase activity and modification of lipids in heart mitochondria from hyperthyroid rats. *FEBS Letter,* Vol. 350, pp. 213–215.

Parnetti, L.; Gaiti, A. & Mecocci, P. (1992). Pharmacokinetics of IV and oral acetyl-L-carnitine in a multiple dose regimen in patients with senile dementia of Alzheimer type, *European Journal of Clinical Pharmacology,* Vol. 42, pp. 89-93.

Perhexiline, June 2011, Available from http://en.wikipedia.org/wiki/Perhexiline

Poon, HF.; Calabrese, V.; Calvani, M. & Butterfield, DA. (2006). Proteomics analyses of specific protein oxidation and protein expression in aged rat brain and its modulation by L-acetylcarnitine: insights into the mechanisms of action of this proposed therapeutic agent for CNS disorders associated with oxidative stress, *Antioxid Redox Signal,* Vol. 8, pp. 381–394.

Pourkhalili, K.; Hajizadeh, S.; Tiraihi, T.; Akbari, Z.; Esmailidehaj, M.; Bigdeli, M. & Khoshbaten, A. (2009). Ischemia and reperfusion-induced arrhythmias: role of hyperoxic preconditioning, *Journal of Cardiovascular Medicine,* Vol. 10, No. 8, pp. 635–642.

Qureshi, K.; Rao, KV. & Qureshi, IA. (1998). Differential inhibition by hyperamonemia of the electron transport chain enzymes in synaptosomes and nonsynaptic mitochondria in ornithine transcarbamylase-deficient spf mice: restoration by acetyl-L-carnitine, *Neurochemical Research,* Vol. 23, pp. 855–861.

Rebouche, CJ. & Seim, H. (1998). Carnitine metabolism and its regulation in microorganisms and mammals, *Annual Review of Nutrition,* Vol. 18, pp. 39-61.

Rebouche, CJ. (2004). Kinetics, pharmacokinetics, and regulation of L-carnitine and acetyl-L-carnitine metabolism, *Annals of the New York Academy of Sciences,* Vol. 1033, pp. 30-41.

Rebouche, CJ.; Shils, ME.; Shike, M.; Ross, AC.; Caballero, B. & Cousins, RJ. (2006). *Modern Nutrition in Health and Disease,* 10th ed. Philadelphia, 537-544.

Ricciolini, R.; Scalibastri, M.; Sciarroni, AF.; Dottori, S.; Calvani, M.; Lligon˜a-Trulla, L.; Conti, R. & Arduini, A. (1997). The carnitine system and acyl trafficking in CNS, *Cell Mol Clin Asp,* pp. 1071–1076.

Rizzon, P.; Biasco, G. ; Di Biase, M.; Boscia, F. ; Rizzo, U.; Minafra, F.; Bortone, A.; Siliprandi, N.; Procopio, A. & Bagiella, E. (1989). High doses of L-carnitine in acute myocardial infarction: metabolic and anti-arrhythmic effects, *European Heart Journal,* Vol. 10, No. 6, pp. 502-508.

Ronca, F.; Palmieri, L.; Malengo, S. & Bertelli, A. (1994). Effect of L-propionyl carnitine on in-vitro membrane alteration of sickle-cell anemia erythrocytes, *International Journal of Tissue Reactions,* Vol.16, No. 4, pp.187-194.

Rosenthal, RE.; Bogaert, YE. & Fiskum, G. (2005). Delayed therapy of experimental global cerebral ischemia with acetyl-l-carnitine in dogs. *Neuroscience Letters,* Vol. 378, pp. 82–87.

Sabbah, NH. & Stanley, CW. (2002). Partial fatty acid oxidation inhibitors: a potentially new class of drugs for heart failure, *European Journal of Heart Failure,* Vol. 4, pp. 3-6.

Sallustio, BC.; Westley, IS. & Morris RG. (2002). Pharmacokinetics of the antianginal agent perhexiline: relationship between metabolic ratio and steady-state dose, *British Journal of Clinical Pharmacology,* Vol. 54, No. 2, pp. 107–114.

Sambandam, N. & Lopaschuk, GD. (2003). AMP-activated protein kinase (AMPK) control of fatty acid and glucose metabolism in the ischemic heart, *Progress in Lipid Research,* Vol. 42, No. 3, pp. 238-256.

Sayed-Ahmed, MM.; Shouman, AS.; Rezk, MB.; Khalifa, MH.; Osman, MA. & EL-MERZABANI, MM. (2000). Propionyl-l-carnitine as potential protective agent against adriamycin-induced impairment of fatty acid beta-oxidation in isolated heat mitochondria, *Pharmacological Research,* Vol. 41, No. 2, pp. 143-150

Scarpini, E.; Sacilotto, G.; Baron, P.; Cusini, M. & Scarlato, G. (1997). Effect of acetyl-L-carnitine in the treatment of painful peripheral neuropathies in HIV+ patients, *Journal of Peripheral Nerve System,* Vol. 2, pp. 250-252.

Sethia, R.; Dhalla, KS.; Ganguly, PK.; Ferrari, R. & Dhalla, NS. (1999). Beneficial effects of propionyl L-carnitine on sarcolemmal changes in congestive heart failure due to myocardial infarction, *Cardiovascular Research,* Vol. 42, pp. 607–615.

Signorelli, SS.; Pino, LD.; Costa, MP.; Digrandi, D.; Pennisi, G. & Marchese, G. (2001). Efficacy of L-Propionyl Carnitine in the Treatment of Chronic Critical Limb Ischaemia, *Clinical Drug Investigation,* Vol. 21, No. 8, pp. 555-561.

Sima, AF.; Ristic, H.; Andrew, M.; Kamijo, M.; Lattimer, S.; Stevens, M. & Greene, D. (1996). Primary Preventive and Secondary Interventionary Effects of Acetyl-L -Carnitine on Diabetic Neuropathy in the Bio-Breeding Worcester Rat, *Journal of Clinical Investigation,* Vol. 97, No. 8, pp. 1900-1907.

Spagnoli A, Lucca U, Menasce G. (1991).Long-term acetyl-L-carnitine treatment in Alzheimer's disease. *Neurology,* 41, 1726-1732.

Stacpoole, PW. (1989). The pharmacology of dichloroacetate, *Metabolism,* Vol. 38, No. 11, pp. 1124-1144.

Stacpoole, PW.; Henderson, GN.; Yan, Z. & James, MO. (1998). Clinical Pharmacology and Toxicology of Dichloroacetate, *Environmental Health Perspectives,* Vol. 106, No. 4, pp.989-994.

Suleiman, M.S.; Halestrap, AP. & Griffiths, EJ. (2001). Mitochondria: a target for myocardial protection, *Pharmacology & Therapeutics,* Vol. 89, No. 1, pp. 29-46.

Suzuki, Y.; Kamikawa, T. & Yamazaki, N. (1981). Effects of L-carnitine on ventricular arrhythmias in dogs with acute myocardial ischemia and a supplement of excess free fatty acids, *Japanese Circulation Journal,* Vol. 45, No. 5, pp. 552-559.

Sweetman, CS. (2002). Carnitine, in: *Martindale, the complete drug reference,* Pharmaceutical press, 33 rd edition, London, pp. 1356.

Szewczyk, A. & Wojtczak, L. (2002). Mitochondria as a pharmacological target, *Pharmacological Reviews,* Vol. 54, No. 1, pp. 101-127.

Taglialatela, G.; Caprioli, A.; Giuliani, A. & Ghirardi, O. (1996). Spatial memory and NGF levels in aged rats: natural variability and effects of acetyll- carnitine treatment, *Experimental Gerontology,* Vol. 31, pp. 577–587.

Tanaka, R.; Haramura, M.; Tanaka, A. & Hirayama, N. (2005). Structure of Trimetazidine. *Analytical Sciences,* Vol. 21, pp.3x-4x

Tomassini, V.; Pozzilli, C.; Onesti, E.; Pasqualetti, P.; Marinelli, F.; Pisani, A. & Fieschi, C. (2004). Comparison of the effects of acetyl L-carnitine and amantadine for the treatment of fatigue in multiple sclerosis: results of a pilot, randomised, double-blind, crossover trial, *Journal of Neurological Sciences,* Vol. 218, pp. 103–108.

Trimetazidine Tablets, June 2011, Available from

http://www.cipladoc.com/therapeutic/pdf_cipla/trivedon_mr.pdf.
Vermeulen, RC. & Scholte, HR. (2004). Exploratory open label, randomized study of acetyl- and propionylcarnitine in chronic fatigue syndrome, *Psychosomatic Medicine*, Vol. 66, No. 2, pp. 276-282.
Virmani, A.; Gaetani, F. & Binienda, Z. (2005). Effects of metabolic modifiers such as carnitines, coenzyme Q10, and PUFAs against different forms of neurotoxic insults: metabolic inhibitors, MPTP, and methamphetamine, *Annals of the NewYork Academy of Sciences*, Vol. 21053, pp. 183–191.
Wei, A. & Yang, J. (2006). Protective effects of Ping-Lv-Mixture (PLM), a medicinal formula on arrhythmias induced by myocardial ischemia-reperfusion, *Journal of Ethnopharmacology*, Vol. 108, pp. 90–95.
Wiseman, LR. & Brogden, RN. (1998). Propionyl-L-carnitine, *Drugs and Aging*, Vol. 12, No. 3, pp.243-248.
Zacharowski, K.; Blackburn, B. & Thiemermann, C. (2001). Ranolazine, a partial fatty acid oxidation inhibitor, reduces myocardial infarct size and cardiac troponin T release in the rat, *European Journal of Pharmacology*, Vol. 418, pp. 105-110.
Zanelli, SA.; Solenski, NJ.; Rosenthal, RE. & Fiskum, G. (2005). Mechanisms of ischemic neuroprotection by acetyl-L-carnitine, *Annals of the NewYork Academy of Sciences*, Vol. 1053, pp. 153–161.
Zemlji, G.; Vrtove, B. & Bun, M. (2010). Trimetazidine Shortens QTc Interval in Patients with Ischemic Heart Failure, *The Journal of Cardiovascular Pharmacology and Therapeutics*, Vol. 15, No. 1, pp. 31-36.

8

Mechanisms of Ca^{2+}–Triggered Arrhythmias

Simon Sedej and Burkert Pieske
Department of Cardiology, Medical University of Graz
Austria

1. Introduction

The first evidence that altered intracellular Ca^{2+} homeostasis is causally involved in ventricular tachyarrhythmias was revealed by investigations of the pathophysiology of digitalis intoxication (Ferrier et al., 1973; Rosen et al., 1973). More recently, spontaneous Ca^{2+} release from the sarcoplasmic reticulum (SR) through the cardiac ryanodine receptor (RyR2) has been found to play a fundamental role in the generation of lethal arrhythmias. Such arrhythmias occur in both acquired forms of cardiac diseases (e.g., heart failure, atrial fibrillation) and in a number of congenital arrhythmia syndromes associated with mutations of RyR2 or calsequestrin[1], such as cathecholaminergic polymorphic ventricular tachycardia (CPVT[2]). The currently incomplete understanding of the mechanism underlying disrupted Ca^{2+} regulation in arrhythmogenesis in heart failure has led scientists to the consideration that CPVT as a simplified human and experimental model may help to clarify the disruption of Ca^{2+} homeostasis as a substrate for triggered activity (Priori & Napolitano, 2005). Therefore, a better understanding of the similarities and differences between the mechanisms underlying triggered arrhythmias in acquired and inherited cardiac diseases, holds the promise to develop new specific diagnostic and therapeutic approaches for effective treatment of defective ion handling.

In this chapter, we will review common mechanisms that cause the susceptibility to, and initiation of, Ca^{2+}-dependent arrhythmias with a focus on increased SR Ca^{2+} release due to congenital or acquired RyR2 dysfunction and increased SR Ca^{2+} load. Finally, RyR2 stabilizers and Ca^{2+}/calmodulin-dependent protein kinase II (CaMKII) inhibitors as novel therapeutic targets will be discussed.

2. Altered Ca^{2+} homeostasis is an arrhythmogenic substrate

In a normal cardiac myocyte, Ca^{2+} couples electrical activation (action potential) to mechanical activity (contraction and relaxation) through a process referred to as *excitation-contraction coupling*. The cardiac cycle begins with membrane depolarization, which activates L-type voltage-gated Ca^{2+} channels resulting in a Ca^{2+} influx. This small elevation of cytosolic [Ca^{2+}] binds to the RyR2. The RyR2 opens, resulting in a larger Ca^{2+} release from

---

[1] SR Ca^{2+} buffer protein
[2] Induced by emotional stress or physical activity in the absence of structural heart disease

the SR, a phenomenon termed *calcium-induced calcium release* (Endo, 1977). Using confocal microscopy with Ca^{2+}-sensitive dyes, the opening of individual RyR2 clusters can be visualized as brief increases of $[Ca^{2+}]_i$, called Ca^{2+} sparks (Cheng et al., 1993). SR Ca^{2+} release units are normally synchronized to release Ca^{2+} simultaneously. Ca^{2+} release from the SR is the major source of Ca^{2+} required for excitation-contraction coupling. The whole process of Ca^{2+} movement is characterized by a transient increase in intracellular $[Ca^{2+}]$ from 100 nM (resting or diastolic Ca^{2+}) to about 1 μM (systolic Ca^{2+}), which initiates the contraction (Bers, 2001). Relaxation is initiated by the termination of SR Ca^{2+} release, of which mechanisms are complex and rather controversial. These mechanisms include RyR2 adaptation, RyR2 inactivation, SR Ca^{2+} depletion and luminal regulation of the RyR2 (Stern & Cheng, 2004). Ca^{2+} then dissociates from troponin C and is recycled into the SR through phospholamban-regulated SR Ca^{2+}-ATPase (SERCA2a) and removed from the cells via the Na^+/Ca^{2+} exchanger across the sarcolemmal membrane (Bers, 2002). The orchestrated interplay between these Ca^{2+} fluxes within different compartments is a prerequisite for the maintenance of Ca^{2+} homeostasis and ultimately, the heart rhythm. However, spontaneous Ca^{2+} release from the SR (also called Ca^{2+} leak) between two consecutive Ca^{2+} cycles will alter Ca^{2+} homeostasis and generate an arrhythmogenic substrate, which will directly disturb the cardiac rhythm. Abnormal changes in intracellular Ca^{2+} handling may cause contractile dysfunction, subcellular Ca^{2+} alternans and oscillations of the myocyte membrane potential, such as early afterdepolarizations (EADs) and delayed afterdepolarizations (DADs). Both EADs and DADs may evoke a number of triggered arrhythmias (Figure 1) potentially causing sudden cardiac death.

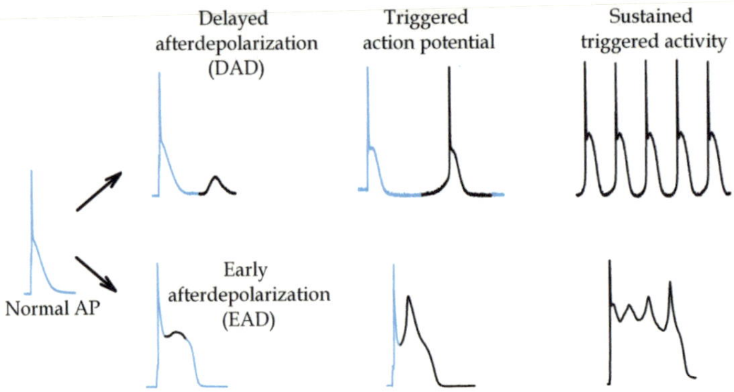

Fig. 1. Delayed (DAD) and early afterdepolarization (EAD) can evoke single or sustained trains of action potentials. Pro-arrhythmogenic and arrhythmic events are coloured black.

3. Triggered activity

The term *triggered activity* was coined to identify and differentiate pro-arrhythmic cellular events triggered by a preceding action potential from spontaneous depolarization of abnormal automaticity. Triggered activity is caused by membrane afterdepolarizations classified into (1) *early afterdepolarizations* (EADs) and (2) *delayed afterdepolarizations* (DADs) (Wit & Rosen, 1983). EADs are abnormal depolarizing oscillations of membrane potential that occur during the plateau or late repolarization of an action potential, while DADs are depolarizing membrane potential oscillations initiated after full repolarization of the triggering action potential (Figure 1). When EAD and DAD reach thresholds of depolarizing currents, new triggering action potentials are generated that may elicit self-sustaining trains of triggered activity (Figure 1). Of the different cell types in the heart, Purkinje cells are particularly prone to initiating afterdepolarizations, suggesting that Ca^{2+}-dependent arrhythmic triggers may arise from the Purkinje fiber network (Boyden et al., 2000; Cerrone et al., 2007). This pro-arrhythmic behaviour is enhanced by disease-causing mutations in the RyR2 and greatly exacerbated by cathecholaminergic stimulation (Kang et al., 2010).

3.1 Role of Ca^{2+} in EADs

Action potential prolongation and slowing of repolarization seem to be crucial determinants in the initiation and facilitation of EADs. Reactivation of the L-type Ca^{2+} channels at potentials within the "Ca^{2+} window current" (Hirano et al., 1992; January & Riddle, 1989), or and re-opening of Na^+ channels (Boutjdir et al., 1994) have been proposed to underlie synchronous changes of $[Ca^{2+}]_i$ and upstroke of EADs. However, the concept that a change in membrane potential during an EAD primarily causes synchronous changes of $[Ca^{2+}]_i$ throughout the cardiac myocyte has been recently re-examined. Under β-adrenergic stimulation, spontaneous SR Ca^{2+} release in the form of propagating Ca^{2+} waves as a result of elevated SR Ca^{2+} content can also occur during the repolarizing phase of the action potential (Volders et al., 1997; Volders et al., 2000). This activates a Na^+/Ca^{2+} exchanger-dependent depolarizing current (NCX), which in an ischemic or failing heart triggers $[Ca^{2+}]_i$ alternans and concomitant sudden changes in action potential duration may give rise to EADs and trigger extrasystoles (Xie et al., 2009). EADs appear to depend on $[Ca^{2+}]_i$, NCX current (Patterson et al., 2006) and CaMKII (Anderson et al., 1998). Increased $[Ca^{2+}]_i$ further enhances L-type Ca^{2+} currents through the activation of CaMKII and is associated with transient inward currents carried by NCX.

More recently, another type of EADs associated with immediate recurrences of atrial fibrillation has been described (Burashnikov & Antzelevitch, 2006; Patterson et al., 2007). These EADs occur at potentials more negative than that of activation of L-type Ca^{2+} current, when the combination of short action potentials (parasympathetic stimulation) and increased SR Ca^{2+} load (sympathetic stimulation) were present. Triggered action potential generates a massive Ca^{2+} release of the Ca^{2+} accumulated in the SR during the pause that exceeds the duration of action potential. Because the action potential is short, the high $[Ca^{2+}]_i$ and the negative membrane potential generate NCX-mediated inward current that produces EADs. The most important hallmark of this type of triggered activity is that late phase 3 EADs are triggered by a massive but essentially *normal* SR Ca^{2+} release. This differs from other types of triggered activity, in which DADs and other EADs occur in conditions of *spontaneous* SR Ca^{2+} release. Normally, EADs occur under bradycardic conditions, whereas DADs are more likely to occur during tachycardia or rapid pacing (reviewed by Schotten et al., 2011).

3.2 Role of Ca^{2+} in DADs

DADs typically result from abnormal increase in $[Ca^{2+}]_i$ during diastole (Figure 2). The principal causes of elevated diastolic $[Ca^{2+}]_i$ and thus, cytosolic $[Ca^{2+}]$ oscillations are (1) *increased SR Ca^{2+} load,* (2) *defective regulation of the RyR2-mediated Ca^{2+} release* or a combination of both. Both alterations increase the spontaneous RyR2 open probability and SR Ca^{2+} leak and cause sufficient cytosolic [Ca^{2+}] elevation associated with regenerative Ca^{2+} wave propagation. Ca^{2+} wave in turn may initiate a depolarizing Ca^{2+}-dependent inward current (I_{ti}). This transient current is largely carried by electrogenic NCX (>90% of I_{ti}) operating in its forward mode; NCX current depolarizes the sarcolemma and generates DADs by extruding 1 Ca^{2+} and taking up 3 Na^+. If the amplitude of a DAD reaches the threshold potential for voltage-gated Na^+ channels, a triggered action potential can result (Figure 1 and 2). This mechanism forms the basis for the typical rate and magnitude dependence of DADs: the faster is the triggering rhythm, the shorter is the interval of the triggered response and the faster are self-sustaining trains of DADs (Katra & Laurita, 2005). In other words, only spontaneous SR Ca^{2+} release events of sufficient magnitude and rate occurring at multiple sites synchronously within the cell will trigger DAD-mediated action potentials (Hoeker et al., 2009). The action potential initiation from a DAD is facilitated in cardiac myocytes from failing hearts, because of the increased expression of NCX and the reduction of repolarizing K^+ currents as a consequence of the electrophysiological remodelling (Tomaselli & Zipes, 2004). This implies that for any given rise in $[Ca^{2+}]_i$, the inward current carried by the NCX will be larger, and the reduction of outwardly directed K^+ currents will amplify the depolarizing effect of a given NCX current.

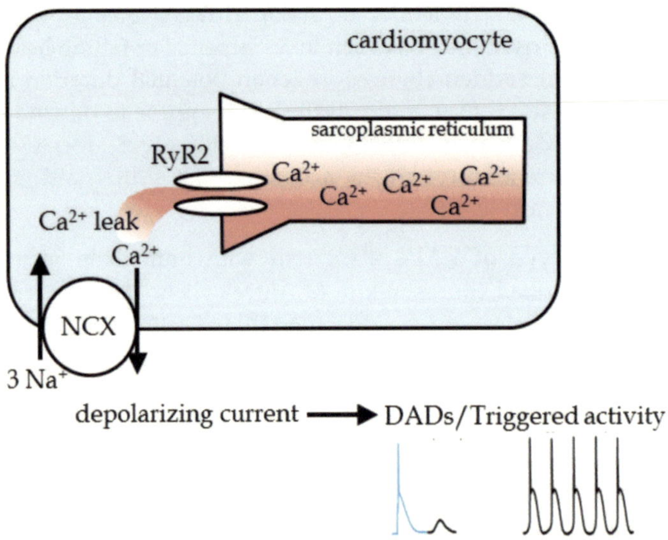

Fig. 2. Simplified electrophysiological mechanism underlying delayed afterdepolarization and triggered activity: spontaneous SR Ca^{2+} release ("Ca^{2+} leak") through dysfunctional RyR2 activates NCX exchange and causes membrane positive oscillations (DADs), which may escalate into triggered action potentials and sustained triggered activity (adapted from Kockskamper & Pieske, 2006).

4. The mechanism of triggered activity in situ

In conditions of increased spontaneous SR Ca^{2+} release, which may trigger DAD-evoked action potentials within a single myocyte, the presence of neighbouring cardiomyocytes *in situ* act as a current sink, which inhibits DAD generation. To produce a triggered beat and overcome the current sink, spontaneous Ca^{2+} oscillations during diastole must occur in multiple neighbouring cells within a fairly narrow time scale. Whereas it is now well accepted that neighbouring cells are the source of spontaneous Ca^{2+} oscillations during diastole (Hoeker et al., 2009; Mulder et al., 1989), the mechanisms underlying triggered activity *in situ* remain elusive. It is unknown whether spontaneous Ca^{2+} oscillations originate from the extracellular space through L-type Ca^{2+} channels, or from SR via RyR2, or perhaps from other sources (e.g. myofilaments). The concept that neighbouring cells collectively share the same susceptibility for Ca^{2+} oscillations proved unlikely, for example, the Ca^{2+} handling properties required for the synchronization of triggered activity between cardiomyocytes vary both from apex to base and transmurally (Katra et al., 2004; Laurita et al., 2003; Prestle et al., 1999). Evidence is emerging that enhanced RyR2 open probability increases the amplitude and temporal synchronisation of spontaneous diastolic Ca^{2+} release, despite decreased cell-to-cell coupling and therefore, increased electrical membrane resistance (Plummer et al., 2011). Since these experiments were conducted on intact hearts, it remains unresolved whether the same mechanism underlies the propagation of triggered action potentials in, for example, non-ischemic failing hearts.

5. Ca^{2+}-induced arrhythmias in heart failure

Heart failure is associated with approximately 50% incidence of sudden cardiac death from ventricular fibrillation (Packer, 1985; Packer et al., 1999). A substantial body of evidence has accumulated demonstrating that *acquired* alterations in Ca^{2+} homeostasis lead to DADs in heart failure (reviewed by Pogwizd et al., 2001). Changes in Ca^{2+} handling, structural and electrophysiological remodelling are thought to account for abnormalities of excitation-contraction coupling and the susceptibility for cardiac arrhythmias, as well as to the reduced contractile force, prolongation of relaxation and the negative force-frequency relationship. The fundamental changes in Ca^{2+} handling that occur with heart failure are (1) increased NCX function resulting in increased removal of Ca^{2+} from the cytosol and larger depolarizing current and (2) the concurrently decreased inward rectifier K^+ current resulting in an even larger depolarisation; (3) reduced SR Ca^{2+} uptake due to decreased SERCA2a expression and reduced phosphorylation of phospholamban, (4) altered regulation of the RyR2 due to increased RyR2 phosphorylation associated with a decreased threshold for SR Ca^{2+} release (Trafford et al., 2000b) and (5) decreased β_1-adrenergic responsiveness, but increased β_2-adrenergic drive, which increases SR Ca^{2+} load (Desantiago et al., 2008). In heart failure, however, Ca^{2+} waves and DADs occur at reduced SR Ca^{2+} content. It is the adrenergic stimulation that is thought to increase SR Ca^{2+} load above the threshold required for triggered activity. Indeed, experimental findings from atrial and ventricular myocytes from failing hearts are consistent with enhanced SR Ca^{2+} loading associated with spontaneous SR Ca^{2+} release. The seemingly conflicting observation is that Ca^{2+}-dependent arrhythmias are more prevalent in heart failure due to enhanced diastolic SR Ca^{2+} release (Pogwizd et al., 2001), despite the decrease of SR Ca^{2+} content (Kubalova et al., 2005). To explain this dichotomy, Sobie et al. (2006) proposed an interesting hypothesis using a mathematical model based on the recent experimental findings. Their model predicts that (1) "rogue RyR2"[3] can operate almost invisibly to produce a fraction of the overall Ca^{2+} leak and (2) coupled gating between clustered RyR2s is disrupted in response to physiologic

[3] (unclustered) RyR2s in the SR membrane that are not part of RyR2 clusters

phosphorylation or excessive phosphorylation of RyR2s in disease states such as heart failure.

Defects in RyR2 regulation may also contribute to triggered activity and arrhythmogenesis in patients with atrial arrhythmias. Atrial fibrillation, the most common human cardiac arrhythmia, occurs in up to 30-40% of patients with heart failure (Cleland et al., 2003). Defects in Ca^{2+} release from the SR during diastole has been reported to be the mechanism underlying greater arrhythmogenic susceptibility in patients with atrial fibrillation (Hove-Madsen et al., 2004; Neef et al., 2010). Generation of transgenic mice harbouring a gain-of-function in the RyR2 has proven to be a valuable tool in unravelling molecular mechanisms causing atrial fibrillation. For instance, in $RyR2^{R176Q+/-}$ mice spontaneous atrial fibrillation was absent at rest but inducible by rapid atrial pacing, which also resulted in increased CaMKII phosphorylation of the RyR2 (Chelu et al., 2009). This implies that Ca^{2+} leak either through phosphorylated or defective RyR2 alone, might not be enough to produce atrial fibrillation. Both increased CaMKII activity and an arrhythmogenic substrate (e.g., RyR2 mutation) are elementary to produce atrial ectopy.

6. SR Ca^{2+} overload - a trigger for spontaneous SR Ca^{2+} release

The amount of Ca^{2+} within the SR is a critical regulator of contraction during normal excitation-contraction coupling. β-adrenergic stimulation, digitalis intoxication, rapid pacing and increased extracellular Ca^{2+} are conditions that increase inotropy by increasing SR Ca^{2+} content. When the amount of Ca^{2+} in the SR excessively increases, a phenomenon known as *SR Ca^{2+} overload* (Trafford et al., 1997; Trafford et al., 2001), a regenerative Ca^{2+} release and arrhythmia may occur. SR Ca^{2+} overload is a consequence of an imbalance between Ca^{2+} influx and efflux. This disequilibrium may evolve from (1) *the reduced Ca^{2+} efflux* (primarily due to increased NCX current in forward mode), (2) *increased SR Ca^{2+} uptake* (due to increased phosphorylation of phospholamban and/or SERCA2a expression), (3) *increased Ca^{2+} influx* across the sarcolemma (primarily due to increased L-type Ca^{2+} current), and (4) *altered SR Ca^{2+} buffering capacity* (due to a calsequestrin mutation). SR Ca^{2+} overload typically results in spontaneous SR Ca^{2+} release via RyR2. As opposed to the "silent" Ca^{2+} leak through rogue (or unclustered) RyR2 (Sobie et al., 2006), the diastolic Ca^{2+} leak via clustered RyR2 can be experimentally visualized as increased Ca^{2+} spark frequency, which, when high enough in a given volume of the cell, can initiate a Ca^{2+} wave. Once the Ca^{2+} wave has been initiated, the propagation of Ca^{2+} wave will largely depend on the amount of SR Ca^{2+} content. The greater the SR Ca^{2+} content, the more likely a Ca^{2+} wave is to propagate (Cheng et al., 1996) and trigger DAD. To distinguish spontaneous Ca^{2+} release due to the elevated SR Ca^{2+} load from depolarisation-initiated Ca^{2+} release, Wayne Chen's group coined the term *store overload-induced Ca^{2+} release* (SOICR) (Jiang et al., 2004). SOICR occurs when the threshold level for Ca^{2+} retention by RyR2 is exceeded. In addition to the SR Ca^{2+} content, the threshold is also determined by the properties of RyR2. For instance, the application of low dose caffeine, which increases the open probability of the RyR2 (Rousseau & Meissner, 1989), decreases the threshold and increases diastolic SR Ca^{2+} leak (Trafford et al., 2000b). On the other hand, tetracaine, which decreases RyR2 opening (Gyorke et al., 1997; Xu et al., 1993), increases threshold and decreases SR Ca^{2+} leak (Overend et al., 1997). Thus, modulation of RyR2 may have a significant impact on the properties of SOICR and therefore on the occurrence of DADs and triggered arrhythmias, while sustained impact on Ca^{2+}-

induced Ca^{2+} release is unlikely. Based on these observations, (Trafford et al., 2000b) proposed the *"SR Ca^{2+} auto-regulation" hypothesis,* which predicts that increased open probability of the RyR2 only transiently enhances spontaneous SR Ca^{2+} release, because of SR luminal Ca^{2+} regulation. Changes in RyR2 activity are compensated for by the SR Ca^{2+} content, implying that increased release reduces the steady-state SR Ca^{2+} content and consequently spontaneous Ca^{2+} release.

7. Arrhythmias triggered by dysfunctional SR Ca^{2+} handling

7.1 Catecholaminergic polymorphic ventricular tachycardia (CPVT)

Abnormalities of intracellular Ca^{2+} regulation caused by dominant mutations in the RyR2 gene (Priori et al., 2001) and by recessive mutations in the calsequestrin gene (Lahat et al., 2001), encoding SR Ca^{2+} binding protein (calsequestrin 2), may account for malignant catecholamine-induced polymorphic ventricular arrhythmias (CPVT) (Priori et al., 2001; Swan et al., 1999). CPVT occurs suddenly and unexpectedly in young and otherwise healthy individuals under emotional stress or physical exercise (e.g. increased catecholaminergic stimulation). Known RyR2 and calsequestrin mutations account for approximately 50-60% and 1-2% of CPVT mutations, respectively (Cerrone et al., 2009). Causes for the remaining CPVT mutations have yet to be identified. Even prior to the linkage of RyR2 mutations and CPVT, the striking similarity between ECG patterns (bidirectional or polymorphic ventricular tachycardia) observed in CPVT patients and digitalis-induced arrhythmias in patients with digitalis-intoxication, led to the hypothesis that arrhythmias in CPVT were most likely initiated by SR Ca^{2+} overload and consequently by DADs and triggered activity (Leenhardt et al., 1995).

7.1.1 RyR2 mutations

Generation of genetically modified mouse models has advanced our understanding of mechanisms of both autosomal-dominant and recessive CPVT. The first CPVT transgenic mouse model with a gain-of-function defect in the RyR2 was generated by the Priori group (Cerrone et al., 2005). The introduction of the $RyR2^{R4496C+/-}$ mutation reliably reproduced the human phenotype. On exposure to isoproterenol (β-adrenergic agonist), this mouse model produced DADs and triggered activity underlying CPVT (Liu et al., 2006). Subsequent studies using other transgenic mouse models (Kannankeril et al., 2006; Lehnart et al., 2008; Uchinoumi et al., 2010) confirmed that RyR2 mutations modify intracellular Ca^{2+} regulation through an increased SR Ca^{2+} leak as a result of increased RyR2 open probability at resting conditions (Jiang et al., 2005). It is this increased SR Ca^{2+} leak that accounts for the increased propensity of DAD-mediated triggered activity. Lowered threshold due to the increased Ca^{2+} sensitivity to luminal and/or cytosolic Ca^{2+} has been attributed for the elevated propensity to arrhythmias in the $RyR2^{R4496C+/-}$ mutant (Fernandez-Velasco et al., 2009; Jiang et al., 2005). The decreased threshold may explain why mice expressing the RyR2 mutation are more likely to develop Ca^{2+} waves and DADs. However, neither mice nor patients with CPVT develop arrhythmias at rest. Faster heart rate and SR Ca^{2+} uptake during β-adrenergic stimulation is the physiological trigger, which increases SR Ca^{2+} load and subsequent Ca^{2+} waves followed by DAD-mediated triggered beats in ventricular cardiomyocytes harbouring RyR2 mutations (Kannankeril et al., 2006; Lehnart et al., 2008; Liu et al., 2006).

This raises the question as to why β-adrenergic stimulation is required to produce CPVT. β-adrenergic stimulation has been reported to produce Ca^{2+} waves by increasing the SR Ca^{2+} content and not by decreasing the threshold for SR Ca^{2+} release (Kashimura et al., 2010). β-adrenergic stimulation even increased the threshold for spontaneous SR Ca^{2+} release independent of SERCA2a activity in both wild-type and $RyR2^{R4496C+/-}$ cardiac myocytes, suggesting the reduced rather than increased arrhythmogenic potential for Ca^{2+}-dependent arrhythmias. This does not exclude the possibility that different RyR2 mutations respond differently to β-adrenergic stimulation, indicating diverse implications on the severity of the phenotype. For instance, it has been reported that the $RyR2^{R2474+/-}$ mutation renders the RyR2 more sensitive to adrenergic stimulation by destabilizing interdomain interaction within RyR2 (Uchinoumi et al., 2010). Such a defect could lower the SR Ca^{2+} threshold, so that enhanced SR Ca^{2+} uptake induced by β-adrenergic stimulation causes the level of free Ca^{2+} to overshoot its lowered SOICR threshold (Priori & Chen, 2011). Importantly, triggered activity in $RyR2^{R4496C+/-}$ cardiomyocytes does occur in the absence of β-adrenergic stimulation, if SR Ca^{2+} content is increased by ouabain, a cardiac glycoside with Na^+/K^+-ATPase inhibiting effect. Ouabain elevates cytosolic [Na^+] and thus, indirectly elevates SR Ca^{2+} load through the reverse mode of NCX and, in contrast to wild-type cardiac myocytes, massively increases the occurrence of DADs and triggered action potentials in $RyR2^{R4496C+/-}$ cardiomyocytes (Sedej et al., 2010). The finding that increased SR Ca^{2+} content (in the absence of catecholamines) suffices to induce arrhythmogenic events in mouse cardiomyocytes with a human CPVT mutation (Sedej et al., 2010), inspired Brette (2010) to give CPVT a new name: *Calcium* polymorphic ventricular tachycardia. Taken together, these findings highlight the importance of SR Ca^{2+} content in the CPVT arrhythmogenesis.

7.1.2 Calsequestrin 2 mutations

The recessive forms of CPVT due to the calsequestrin gene mutation (casq) are found in approximately 1-2% of CPVT patients (Cerrone et al., 2009). Calsequestrin is an intra-SR Ca^{2+} binding protein, which plays a pivotal role in regulating SR Ca^{2+} release by (1) increasing the SR luminal total Ca^{2+} content through its low Ca^{2+} binding affinity, (2) buffering free Ca^{2+} levels in the SR lumen, and (3) regulating SR Ca^{2+} release either through the direct (MacLennan & Chen, 2009) or indirect interaction with RyR2 (calsequestrin-triadin-junction complex) (Gyorke & Terentyev, 2008; Qin et al., 2008). Reduced levels of calsequestrin may result in rapid recovery of SR free Ca^{2+} after each Ca^{2+} release and a potentially higher level of SR free Ca^{2+} during a sudden increase in SR Ca^{2+} loading (e.g., β-adrenergic stimulation). The common hallmark of all calsequestrin-associated CPVT mutations is decreased luminal Ca^{2+} binding and Ca^{2+} buffering resulting in increased luminal free Ca^{2+}, which exceeds the normal threshold for SOICR. In turn, this increases the propensity for SR Ca^{2+} release from the overloaded SR and evokes DADs and triggered activity. Studies on $casq^{-/-}$ null mice and humans showed that calsequestrin is not critical for normal RyR2 regulation under resting conditions, since excitation-contraction coupling appeared normal and arrhythmias were not observed under basal conditions. However, the administration of isoproterenol increased the SR Ca^{2+} leak, which was proportional to the calsequestrin loss, indicating that calsequestrin's primary role is a "molecular brake" that prevents spontaneous Ca^{2+} release at high SR Ca^{2+} load (Chopra et al., 2007). Taken together, calsequestrin-induced CPVT and RyR2-mediated CPVT share a common causal arrhythmogenic mechanism involving disruption of Ca^{2+} homeostasis.

8. Molecular mechanisms underlying increased SR Ca^{2+} leak

At present many aspects of the molecular mechanisms by which RyR2 mutations alter the physiological RyR2 properties in acquired (e.g. heart failure) and congenital triggered arrhythmias (e.g. CPVT) remain controversial. However, an increase in Ca^{2+} leak from the SR via RyR2 is the unifying phenomenon for heart failure and CPVT. The concept that arrhythmias occur due to increased Ca^{2+} sensitivity (and thus, lower threshold) of the RyR2 at luminal or cytosolic sites has emerged.

8.1 Increased sensitivity of RyR2 to luminal or cytosolic Ca^{2+} activation

Spontaneous SR Ca^{2+} release occurs when the SR Ca^{2+} content reaches threshold (Dibb et al., 2007), suggesting that luminal Ca^{2+} concentration affects RyR2 opening and modulates the amount of Ca^{2+} released from the SR during SR Ca^{2+} overload. Indeed, increasing luminal Ca^{2+} elevates RyR2 open probability and increases RyR2 sensitivity to Ca^{2+} leading to spontaneous SR Ca^{2+} release (SOICR) (Fernandez-Velasco et al., 2009; Jiang et al., 2004; Jiang et al., 2005). SR Ca^{2+} release increases in nonlinear accelerating fashion with increasing SR luminal Ca^{2+} concentration (Trafford et al., 2000a). This nonlinear relationship implies that SR Ca^{2+} release is not passively driven by a Ca^{2+} concentration gradient and raises the question, whether other mechanisms beside the luminal SR Ca^{2+} concentration may also trigger RyR2 activity.

Numerous CPVT-linked RyR2 mutations expressed in heterologous cells as well as native cardiomyocytes preferentially sensitize the RyR2 to luminal Ca^{2+} activation (Jiang et al., 2004; Jiang et al., 2005; Jones et al., 2008). Consequently, the threshold luminal Ca^{2+} level required for triggering SOICR is reduced and susceptibility for SOICR increased. However, few RyR2 mutations affects both the response of the RyR2 to cytosolic and luminal Ca^{2+} concentration (Fernandez-Velasco et al., 2009; Jiang et al., 2004; Jones et al., 2008). Despite the increased sensitivity to both cytosolic and luminal Ca^{2+} concentration, Ca^{2+}-induced Ca^{2+} release in cardiomyocytes harbouring CPVT RyR2 mutations is at resting conditions little, if at all, affected (Mohamed et al., 2007). This can be explained by the "SR Ca^{2+} auto-regulation" hypothesis (Trafford et al., 2000a). SR Ca^{2+} content counterbalances defective luminal or cytosolic Ca^{2+} activation of the RyR2. For instance, increased SR Ca^{2+} release due to enhanced luminal or cytosolic Ca^{2+} activation will lead to reduced SR Ca^{2+} load, which will counteract increased Ca^{2+} release propensity from the SR (auto-regulation). Altered Ca^{2+} activation of RyR2 will have only a transient effect on Ca^{2+}-induced Ca^{2+} release under resting conditions and lead to a new steady-state within few heartbeats. In conditions above the critical SR Ca^{2+} load (e.g., emotional stress, physical exercise, β-adrenergic stimulation in heart failure), the "SR Ca^{2+} auto-regulation" fails to prevent cardiomyocytes from SOICR, the trigger of DADs and triggered arrhythmias. Taken together, it is the increase in SR Ca^{2+} content what renders the SR Ca^{2+} leak uncontrolled.

To explain lower threshold for SOICR release, two mechanisms have been proposed and they will be presented below: (1) excessive RyR2 phosphorylation linked with the FKBP12.6 dissociation from the RyR2 complex and (2) weaker interdomain interactions within RyR2.

8.1.1 FKBP12.6 unbinding hypothesis (increased RyR2 phosphorylation)

RyR2 forms a macromolecular complex with numerous proteins on the SR luminal side (e.g., triadin, junctin, calsequestrin) as well as the cytosolic side (e.g., calmodulin, FKBP12.6), just to name a few. In addition, two main kinases are also part of the RyR2 complex involved in RyR2 phosphorylation: protein kinase A (PKA), activated by β-adrenergic stimulation, and CaMKII, activated by increased cytosolic Ca^{2+} turnover (e.g. increased heart rate). These proteins provide different regulatory modalities to control RyR2 open probability. Disruption of critical protein-protein interactions within the RyR2 macromolecular complex may alter the sensitivity of the RyR2 to Ca^{2+} activation. For instance, stabilization of the RyR2 is thought to depend on the 12.6. kDa FK506-binding protein (FKBP12.6 or calstabin 2). This protein prevents aberrant activation of the RyR2 during the diastole. The dissociation of FKBP12.6 from RyR2 as a result of a RyR2 mutation or phosphorylation of RyR2 by PKA during β-adrenergic stimulation has been shown to increase the sensitivity of the RyR2 to cytosolic Ca^{2+} activation (Lehnart et al., 2008; Marx et al., 2000; Wehrens et al., 2003). In other words, RyR2 mutations or the "hyperadrenergic" state as often seen in heart failure make the RyR2 channel leaky and increase the susceptibility for the initiation and propagation of Ca^{2+} waves. These findings led to the paradigm that impaired binding of FKBP12.6 to RyR2 is a common final pathway for arrhythmogenesis in CPVT and heart failure (Wehrens et al., 2003). However, other studies failed to reproduce these findings. Furthermore, in later studies the same CPVT RyR2 mutations showed either no effect on FKBP12.6 binding (George et al., 2003; Jiang et al., 2005; Liu et al., 2006) or even increased binding affinity of FKBP12.6 for the RyR2 (Tiso et al., 2002). Recent evidence even suggests that PKA is not involved in the dissociation of FKBP12.6 from RyR2, thus questioning the causality between RyR2 phosphorylation and FKBP12.6 dissociation (Guo et al., 2010).

8.1.2 Domain unzipping hypothesis (weaker interdomain interaction)

Proper folding of the RyR2 relies on intimate intermolecular interaction between RyR2 domains. These domain interactions are believed to stabilize and maintain the closed state of the RyR2 channel (Ikemoto & Yamamoto, 2000), suggesting a close mechanistic similarity between PKA-mediated FKBP12.6 dissociation and domain-domain interaction within the RyR2 channel (Ikemoto & Yamamoto, 2002). For example, defective RyR2 interdomain interactions (also called domain unzipping) between the N-terminal domain and central domain in the context of RyR2 mutations weaken this interaction and destabilize the closed state of the RyR2 (Ikemoto & Yamamoto, 2000; Tateishi et al., 2009). Weakening of these interdomain interactions occurs transiently on a beat-to-beat basis during excitation-contraction coupling, but permanently in both CPVT-associated RyR2 mutations and in pacing-induced failing hearts (Oda et al., 2005). Destabilisation of the zipped state may alter the sensitivity of RyR2 to luminal or cytosolic Ca^{2+} and contribute to abnormal SR Ca^{2+} leak. Although the majority of the reported CPVT mutation sites are within the N-terminal and central domain, it is possible that "domain unzipping" also affects less conserved regions of RyR2 mutations associated with CPVT. It has been demonstrated that, depending on the location of the RyR2 mutation, a distinct pattern of conformational instability in Ca^{2+} handling and interdomain interaction is introduced. This suggests that the mutational locus may be an important mechanistic determinant of Ca^{2+} release channel dysfunction in arrhythmia and sudden cardiac death (George et al., 2006).

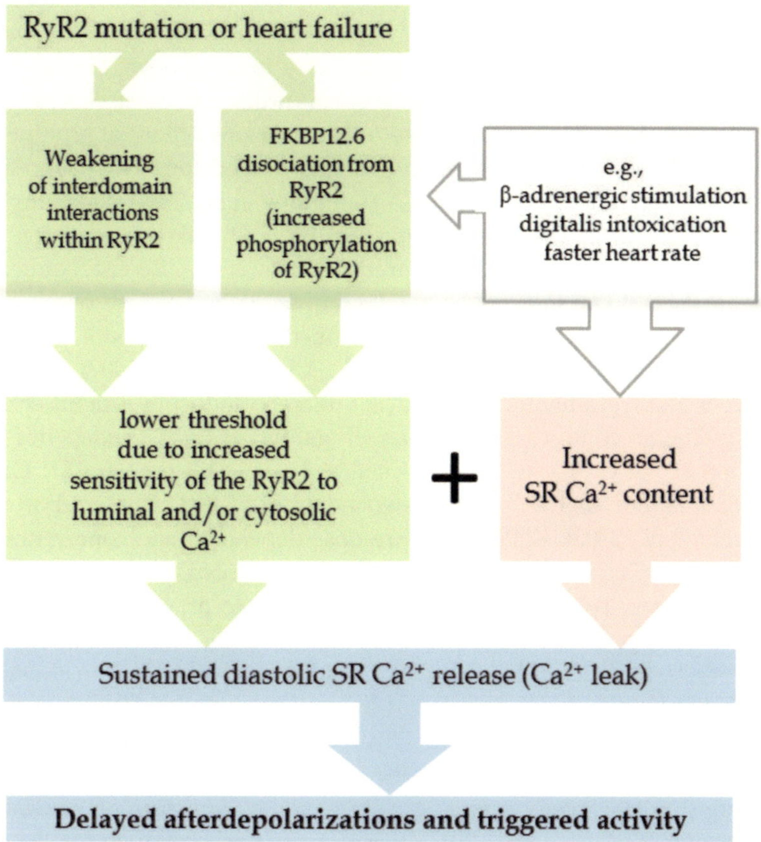

Fig. 3. Hypothetical mechanisms of acquired (e.g. heart failure) and inherited RyR2 dysfunction (e.g. CPVT): (1) *domain unzipping* and (2) *FKBP12.6 unbinding* due to enhanced RyR2 phosphorylation. Both RyR2 aberrations increase the sensitivity of the RyR2 and lower the threshold for SR Ca^{2+} release. The maintenance of increased SR Ca^{2+} load during, for example, β-adrenergic stimulation is considered a major determinant for the sustained spontaneous Ca^{2+} release from the SR and arrhythmogenesis. If SR Ca^{2+} content is normal, a transient diastolic SR Ca^{2+} release will occur.

9. Normalizing RyR2 function prevents triggered arrhythmias

After the discovery that mutations in the RyR2 gene underlie Ca^{2+} homeostasis disturbances associated with CPVT (Laitinen et al., 2001; Priori et al., 2001), important insights into novel and specifically tailored therapies that may target the common pathway underlying CPVT and heart failure have emerged. Recent studies suggest the usage of therapeutic approaches that should combine two actions: (1) *suppression of SR Ca^{2+} overload* and (2) *stabilization of the RyR2 dysfunction* by reducing the RyR2 open probability and thence, increasing the SR threshold. Such therapeutic actions might together effectively prevent RyR2-mediated SR Ca^{2+} leak in CPVT carriers, whereas RyR2 stabilization alone might be sufficient in heart failure patients. A novel class of drugs - RyR2 stabilisers - that has attracted much attention in the past few years and will remain the subject of intensive investigations include K201, dantrolene and flecainide.

9.1 K201 (or JTV-519)

K201 is the 1, 4-benzothiazepine derivative that was initially developed to prevent Ca^{2+} overload-induced myocardial infarction and sudden cardiac cell death (Kaneko et al., 1997). As shown in Table 1, K201 has been reported to have various actions at multiple sites in the cardiomyocyte, including non-specific multi-ion channel blocking effect (Kimura et al., 1999; Nakaya et al., 2000) and inhibition of SERCA (Loughrey et al., 2007). Most important is the finding that K201 stabilizes RyR2 and suppresses SR Ca^{2+} leak by increasing the binding affinity for the FKBP12.6 to RyR2 (Wehrens et al., 2004). Recent studies, however, demonstrated that FKBP12.6 may not be involved in regulation of Ca^{2+} release from the SR, since loss of FKBP12.6 failed to increase RyR2-mediated spontaneous Ca^{2+} release and stress-induced ventricular arrhythmias (Guo et al., 2010; Xiao et al., 2007). K201 binds to the central region of RyR2 (Yamamoto et al., 2008), thereby inducing a rapid conformational change in RyR2 correcting defective channel gating of RyR2 independent of RyR2 phosphorylation (Yano et al., 2003). The closed state of RyR2 prevents SR Ca^{2+} leak and propagation of spontaneous Ca^{2+} waves independent of FKBP12.6 association (Hunt et al., 2007; Yamamoto et al., 2008). K201 effects are dose-dependent and concentrations up to 1 μM ensure RyR2-mediated action (Table 1). K201 prevented ventricular arrhythmias in FKBP12.6-deficient mice (Wehrens et al., 2004), but failed to prevent DADs and ventricular tachycardia induced by isoproterenol and caffeine in a CPVT mouse model carrying a human $RyR2^{R4496C+/-}$ mutation (Liu et al., 2006). On the other hand, pre-treatment with K201 massively reduced triggered activity evoked by ouabain-induced SR Ca^{2+} overload in the $RyR2^{R4496C+/-}$ cardiomyocytes (Sedej et al., 2010). Taken together, it is still unclear whether K201 exerts its antiarrhythmic effects specifically through stabilization of the RyR2 or through synergistic inhibitory actions on sarcolemmal ion currents or by any other additional action(s). Nevertheless, K201 appears a suitable prototype for development of compounds that more specifically target RyR2, such as S107, a more specific RyR2 stabilizer (Lehnart et al., 2008).

9.2 Dantrolene

Emerging evidence suggests that defective interdomain interactions within RyR2 play a key role in abnormal channel gating of RyR2 in failing hearts and RyR2 mutations (Kobayashi et al., 2009; Oda et al., 2005). Therefore, correction of the defective interdomain interaction may represent a new therapeutic strategy against heart failure and possibly cardiac arrhythmia. Dantrolene has been primarily used to treat acute malignant hyperthermia by targeting skeletal muscle RyR1. Recently, dantrolene has been also found to bind to domain 601-620 of RyR2 and reduce abnormal SR Ca^{2+} leak by correcting defective interdomain interaction within RyR2 in pacing-induced heart failure. As a result, DADs and Ca^{2+} spark frequency are reduced (Kobayashi et al., 2005; Kobayashi et al., 2009). Pre-treatment with dantrolene prevents both ventricular arrhythmia induced by either epinephrine or exercise in $RyR2^{R2474S+/-}$ knock-in mouse model for human CPVT (Kobayashi et al., 2010). Dantrolene also improves contractile function in dogs after pacing-induced heart failure (Kobayashi et al., 2009). Importantly, dantrolene has no appreciable effect on normal SR and cardiac function, indicating that dantrolene may be effective for stabilizing RyR2 merely in the unzipped state.

K201 concentration/ duration of intervention	Animal model,origin of cells	In vivo effect	In vitro effect	References
1-10 μM acute	Guinea-pig, Ventricle	no data	Frequency and voltage-dependent inhibition of Na^+, Ca^{2+}, K^+ currents, reduced action potential duration	(Kimura et al., 1999; Kiriyama et al., 2000)
1 μM acute	Guinea-pig, Atrium	inhibition of atrial fibrillation	Inhibition of the muscarinic acetylcholine-receptor operated K current, delayed rectifier K^+ current, prolonged action potential duration	(Nakaya et al., 2000)
1 and 3 μM (2-3 min)	Rabbit, Ventricle	no data	inhibition of RyR2 and SERCA reduced diastolic Ca^{2+} release, reduction of Ca^{2+} wave velocity and frequency, unchanged SR Ca^{2+} content and L-type Ca^{2+}-current, K201 effect FKBP12.6-independent	(Loughrey et al., 2007)
0.5 mg/kg/h (1 week) 1 μM (2h pre-incubation)	Mouse, FKBP12.6$^{+/-}$ Ventricle	No exercise-induced ventricular tachycardia & sudden death	reduced inward transient current (I_{ti}), K201 effect FKBP12.6-dependent	(Lehnart et al., 2006; Wehrens et al., 2004)
0.5 mg/kg/h (1 week) 1 μM and 10 μM (acute)	Mouse, RyR2$^{R4496C+/-}$ Ventricle	CPVT	isoproterenol-induced triggered activity	(Liu et al., 2006)
1 μM (1h pre-incubation)	Mouse, RyR2$^{R4496C+/-}$ Ventricle	no data	reduced ouabain-evoked triggered activity (DAD and triggered AP frequency)	(Sedej et al., 2010)
1-10 μM	Rat, Ventricle HEK-293 cells	no data	no SR Ca^{2+} leak, K201 effect FKBP12.6-independent	(Hunt et al., 2007)
0.5 mg/kg/h (1, 4 weeks) 1 μM (acute)	Dog, HF model, SR vesicles	no data	no SR Ca^{2+} leak, normal PKA phosphorylation, K201 effect FKBP12.6-dependent	(Kohno et al., 2003)
0.3 μM	Dog, HF model, SR vesicles and ventricle	no data	no SR Ca^{2+} leak, reduced Ca^{2+} spark frequency (RyR2 mutations mimicked using synthetic peptides)	(Tateishi et al., 2009)
1 μM	Dog, MI model, Purkinje cells	no data	reduced micro Ca^{2+} waves	(Boyden et al., 2004)
0.5 mg/kg/h (4 weeks)	Dog, HF model, SR vesicles	no data	no SR Ca^{2+} leak, normal PKA phosphorylation, K201 effect FKBP12.6-dependent	(Yano et al., 2003)

Abbreviations: HEK-293= human embryonic kidney cell line 293, HF= heart failure, PKA= protein kinase A, RV= right ventricle, SR= sarcoplasmic reticulum, MI= myocardial infarction

Table 1. K201 effects on triggered activity in different animal models

9.3 Flecainide

In analogy with the local anaesthetic-tetracaine, flecainide is effective in suppressing spontaneous SR Ca^{2+} release by directly inhibiting RyR2 activity in mice and in humans with calsequestrin-associated CPVT (Watanabe et al., 2009) and murine Purkinje cells harbouring $RyR2^{R4496C+/-}$ mutation (Kang et al., 2010). This effect has been attributed to the reduced duration of channel openings without affecting closed channel duration and net spark-mediated Ca^{2+} leak (Hilliard et al., 2010). Thus, flecainide directly targets the molecular defect responsible for arrhythmogenic Ca^{2+} waves that trigger exercise- and catecholamine-induced polymorphic ventricular arrhythmias. In combination with flecainide's Na^{+}-channel inhibition, which reduces the rate of triggered activity, flecainide seems to be a safe and effective therapy in the majority of CPVT patients who suffer from exercise-induced ventricular arrhythmias (van der Werf et al., 2011). Given the rare onset of CPVT episodes and different causality of fatal arrhythmias (exercise-independent), further long-term follow-up clinical studies are required to justify the use of flecainide in preventing fatal arrhythmias in CPVT patients. Collectively, blocking the RyR2 open state has emerged as a new promising therapeutic strategy to prevent Ca^{2+} wave propagation during diastole.

9.4 CaMKII inhibition

In heart failure, the expression and activity of CaMKII are increased (Hoch et al., 1999; Kirchhefer et al., 1999). Chronic activation of CaMKII phosphorylates common Ca^{2+} regulatory proteins with PKA, including L-type voltage-gated Ca^{2+} channels, phospholamban and RyR2 (Ji et al., 2003). The increased L-type Ca^{2+} current may facilitate Ca^{2+} window currents (Dzhura et al., 2000) and trigger EADs, whereas CaMKII phosphorylation of RyR2 increases the sensitivity to Ca^{2+}-dependent activation and the frequency of Ca^{2+} sparks (Guo et al., 2006). Such effects may enhance diastolic SR Ca^{2+} release and trigger DADs, despite reduced SR Ca^{2+} content (Chelu et al., 2009; Maier et al., 2003; Wu et al., 2002). A CaMKII inhibitor, KN-93, effectively blocks both EADs (Anderson et al., 1998) and DADs resulting from enhanced diastolic SR Ca^{2+} leak and Ca^{2+} waves in an arrhythmogenic rabbit model of non-ischemic heart failure (Ai et al., 2005; Curran et al., 2010).

CaMKII activation and Ca^{2+} handling abnormalities have been reported to play a major role in the vicious cycle of arrhythmogenesis promotion and mechanical dysfunction that characterizes electrical storm[4] . Infusion of a calmodulin antagonist W-7 to a rabbit model of electrical storm reduces CaMKII hyperphosphorylation, suppresses ventricular tachycardia or fibrillation, and rescues left ventricular dysfunction (Tsuji et al., 2011).

CaMKII activity also increases during exercise in healthy individuals and may play a role in CPVT (Kemi et al., 2005; Rose & Hargreaves, 2003). Genetic overexpression of CaMKII in a CPVT mouse model with a gain-of-function RyR2 mutation (R4496C) causes increased diastolic SR Ca^{2+} leak, DADs and fatal ventricular arrhythmias (Dybkova et al., 2011), whereas acute CaMKII inhibition in the same CPVT mouse model prevents arrhythmias (Liu et al., 2011). Acute CaMKII inhibition has also been proven to be beneficial in treating atrial arrhythmias induced by rapid pacing in CPVT mice with another RyR2 mutation (R176Q). These mice showed increased susceptibility to atrial fibrillation induction due to CaMKII-mediated increase in RyR2-dependent Ca^{2+} leak (Chelu et al., 2009). Consistent with

[4] defined as 3 or more episodes of ventricular tachycardia or fibrillation in a 24-hour period

these findings, CaMKII inhibition completely reverses the effects of overexpressed miR-1[5] (also in the presence of β-adrenergic activation), a small muscle-specific noncoding microRNA, which increases the diastolic SR Ca^{2+} leak and reduces SR Ca^{2+} content (Terentyev et al., 2009).

It is important to distinguish the specificity of the CaMKII-dependent targets contributing to arrhythmias from other CaMKII-dependent physiological pathways. However, it is becoming increasingly clear that CaMKII inhibitors reduce RyR2 sensitivity to Ca^{2+} and thereby, restore the threshold for spontaneous SR Ca^{2+} release to a normal or even higher level. Taken together, confirming these findings with pharmacologic targeting of RyR2 in conjunction with selected CaMKII signalling might be a promising target for the treatment of cardiac arrhythmias, such as heart failure, CPVT and electrical storms.

10. Conclusion

Since the discovery that mutations in the RyR2 gene underlie Ca^{2+} homeostasis disturbances associated with CPVT, important new insights have been obtained into the molecular mechanisms underlying Ca^{2+}-triggered atrial and ventricular arrhythmias. Increased sensitivity of the RyR2 and lowered threshold for the spontaneous SR Ca^{2+} leak have emerged as causal arrhythmogenic mechanisms linking acquired and congenital arrhythmias in patients with heart failure and CPVT, respectively. The emerging evidence that inhibition of CaMKII reduces RyR2 sensitivity to Ca^{2+} and restores the threshold for spontaneous SR Ca^{2+} release has paved the way to move from bench to bedside. Selected targeting of RyR2 in conjunction with CaMKII signalling might be a promising target for the treatment of Ca^{2+}-triggered arrhythmias.

11. Acknowledgement

The authors cordially thank Dr. William E. Louch for critical proofreading of the chapter and valuable suggestions. This work was supported by the State of Styria grant (Land Steiermark).

12. References

Ai, X., Curran, J.W., Shannon, T.R., Bers, D.M. & Pogwizd, S.M. (2005). Ca2+/calmodulin-dependent protein kinase modulates cardiac ryanodine receptor phosphorylation and sarcoplasmic reticulum Ca2+ leak in heart failure. *Circulation research*, Vol. 97, No. 12, pp. 1314-1322, 1524-4571; 0009-7330

Anderson, M.E., Braun, A.P., Wu, Y., Lu, T., Wu, Y., Schulman, H. & Sung, R.J. (1998). KN-93, an inhibitor of multifunctional Ca++/calmodulin-dependent protein kinase, decreases early afterdepolarizations in rabbit heart. *The Journal of pharmacology and experimental therapeutics*, Vol. 287, No. 3, pp. 996-1006, 0022-3565; 0022-3565

Bers, D.M. (2002). Cardiac excitation-contraction coupling. *Nature*, Vol. 415, No. 6868, pp. 198-205, 0028-0836; 0028-0836

Bers, D.M. (2001). *Excitation-contraction coupling and cardiac contractile force*, Kluwer Academic Press, Dordrecht, Netherlands

[5] miR-1 is upregulated in heart failure (Thum et al., 2007)

Boutjdir, M., Restivo, M., Wei, Y., Stergiopoulos, K. & el-Sherif, N. (1994). Early afterdepolarization formation in cardiac myocytes: analysis of phase plane patterns, action potential, and membrane currents. *Journal of cardiovascular electrophysiology*, Vol. 5, No. 7, pp. 609-620, 1045-3873; 1045-3873

Boyden, P.A., Dun, W., Barbhaiya, C. & Ter Keurs, H.E. (2004). 2APB- and JTV519(K201)-sensitive micro Ca2+ waves in arrhythmogenic Purkinje cells that survive in infarcted canine heart. *Heart rhythm : the official journal of the Heart Rhythm Society*, Vol. 1, No. 2, pp. 218-226, 1547-5271; 1547-5271

Boyden, P.A., Pu, J., Pinto, J. & Keurs, H.E. (2000). Ca(2+) transients and Ca(2+) waves in purkinje cells : role in action potential initiation. *Circulation research*, Vol. 86, No. 4, pp. 448-455, 1524-4571; 0009-7330

Brette, F. (2010). Calcium polymorphic ventricular tachycardia: a new name for CPVT?. *Cardiovascular research*, Vol. 87, No. 1, pp. 10-11, 1755-3245; 0008-6363

Burashnikov, A. & Antzelevitch, C. (2006). Late-phase 3 EAD. A unique mechanism contributing to initiation of atrial fibrillation. *Pacing and clinical electrophysiology : PACE*, Vol. 29, No. 3, pp. 290-295, 0147-8389; 0147-8389

Cerrone, M., Napolitano, C. & Priori, S.G. (2009). Catecholaminergic polymorphic ventricular tachycardia: A paradigm to understand mechanisms of arrhythmias associated to impaired Ca(2+) regulation. *Heart rhythm : the official journal of the Heart Rhythm Society*, Vol. 6, No. 11, pp. 1652-1659, 1556-3871; 1547-5271

Cerrone, M., Noujaim, S.F., Tolkacheva, E.G., Talkachou, A., O'Connell, R., Berenfeld, O., Anumonwo, J., Pandit, S.V., Vikstrom, K., Napolitano, C., Priori, S.G. & Jalife, J. (2007). Arrhythmogenic mechanisms in a mouse model of catecholaminergic polymorphic ventricular tachycardia. *Circulation research*, Vol. 101, No. 10, pp. 1039-1048, 1524-4571; 0009-7330

Cerrone, M., Colombi, B., Santoro, M., di Barletta, M.R., Scelsi, M., Villani, L., Napolitano, C. & Priori, S.G. (2005). Bidirectional ventricular tachycardia and fibrillation elicited in a knock-in mouse model carrier of a mutation in the cardiac ryanodine receptor. *Circulation research*, Vol. 96, No. 10, pp. e77-82, 1524-4571; 0009-7330

Chelu, M.G., Sarma, S., Sood, S., Wang, S., van Oort, R.J., Skapura, D.G., Li, N., Santonastasi, M., Muller, F.U., Schmitz, W., Schotten, U., Anderson, M.E., Valderrabano, M., Dobrev, D. & Wehrens, X.H. (2009). Calmodulin kinase II-mediated sarcoplasmic reticulum Ca2+ leak promotes atrial fibrillation in mice. *The Journal of clinical investigation*, Vol. 119, No. 7, pp. 1940-1951, 1558-8238; 0021-9738

Cheng, H., Lederer, M.R., Lederer, W.J. & Cannell, M.B. (1996). Calcium sparks and [Ca2+]i waves in cardiac myocytes. *The American Journal of Physiology*, Vol. 270, No. 1 Pt 1, pp. C148-59, 0002-9513; 0002-9513

Cheng, H., Lederer, W.J. & Cannell, M.B. (1993). Calcium sparks: elementary events underlying excitation-contraction coupling in heart muscle. *Science (New York, N.Y.)*, Vol. 262, No. 5134, pp. 740-744, 0036-8075; 0036-8075

Chopra, N., Kannankeril, P.J., Yang, T., Hlaing, T., Holinstat, I., Ettensohn, K., Pfeifer, K., Akin, B., Jones, L.R., Franzini-Armstrong, C. & Knollmann, B.C. (2007). Modest reductions of cardiac calsequestrin increase sarcoplasmic reticulum Ca2+ leak independent of luminal Ca2+ and trigger ventricular arrhythmias in mice. *Circulation research*, Vol. 101, No. 6, pp. 617-626, 1524-4571; 0009-7330

Cleland, J.G., Swedberg, K., Follath, F., Komajda, M., Cohen-Solal, A., Aguilar, J.C., Dietz, R., Gavazzi, A., Hobbs, R., Korewicki, J., Madeira, H.C., Moiseyev, V.S., Preda, I., van Gilst, W.H., Widimsky, J., Freemantle, N., Eastaugh, J., Mason, J. & Study Group on Diagnosis of the Working Group on Heart Failure of the European Society of Cardiology. (2003). The EuroHeart Failure survey programme-- a survey on the quality of care among patients with heart failure in Europe. Part 1: patient characteristics and diagnosis. *European heart journal*, Vol. 24, No. 5, pp. 442-463, 0195-668X; 0195-668X

Curran, J., Brown, K.H., Santiago, D.J., Pogwizd, S., Bers, D.M. & Shannon, T.R. (2010). Spontaneous Ca waves in ventricular myocytes from failing hearts depend on Ca(2+)-calmodulin-dependent protein kinase II. *Journal of Molecular and Cellular Cardiology*, Vol. 49, No. 1, pp. 25-32, 1095-8584; 0022-2828

Desantiago, J., Ai, X., Islam, M., Acuna, G., Ziolo, M.T., Bers, D.M. & Pogwizd, S.M. (2008). Arrhythmogenic effects of beta2-adrenergic stimulation in the failing heart are attributable to enhanced sarcoplasmic reticulum Ca load. *Circulation research*, Vol. 102, No. 11, pp. 1389-1397, 1524-4571; 0009-7330

Dibb, K.M., Eisner, D.A. & Trafford, A.W. (2007). Regulation of systolic [Ca2+]i and cellular Ca2+ flux balance in rat ventricular myocytes by SR Ca2+, L-type Ca2+ current and diastolic [Ca2+]i. *The Journal of physiology*, Vol. 585, No. Pt 2, pp. 579-592, 0022-3751; 0022-3751

Dybkova, N., Sedej, S., Napolitano, C., Neef, S., Rokita, A.G., Hunlich, M., Brown, J.H., Kockskamper, J., Priori, S.G., Pieske, B. & Maier, L.S. (2011). Overexpression of CaMKIIdeltac in RyR2R4496C+/- knock-in mice leads to altered intracellular Ca2+ handling and increased mortality. *Journal of the American College of Cardiology*, Vol. 57, No. 4, pp. 469-479, 1558-3597; 0735-1097

Dzhura, I., Wu, Y., Colbran, R.J., Balser, J.R. & Anderson, M.E. (2000). Calmodulin kinase determines calcium-dependent facilitation of L-type calcium channels. *Nature cell biology*, Vol. 2, No. 3, pp. 173-177, 1465-7392; 1465-7392

Endo, M. (1977). Calcium release from the sarcoplasmic reticulum. *Physiological Reviews*, Vol. 57, No. 1, pp. 71-108, 0031-9333; 0031-9333

Fernandez-Velasco, M., Rueda, A., Rizzi, N., Benitah, J.P., Colombi, B., Napolitano, C., Priori, S.G., Richard, S. & Gomez, A.M. (2009). Increased Ca2+ sensitivity of the ryanodine receptor mutant RyR2R4496C underlies catecholaminergic polymorphic ventricular tachycardia. *Circulation research*, Vol. 104, No. 2, pp. 201-9, 12p following 209, 1524-4571; 0009-7330

Ferrier, G.R., Saunders, J.H. & Mendez, C. (1973). A cellular mechanism for the generation of ventricular arrhythmias by acetylstrophanthidin. *Circulation research*, Vol. 32, No. 5, pp. 600-609, 0009-7330; 0009-7330

George, C.H., Jundi, H., Walters, N., Thomas, N.L., West, R.R. & Lai, F.A. (2006). Arrhythmogenic mutation-linked defects in ryanodine receptor autoregulation reveal a novel mechanism of Ca2+ release channel dysfunction. *Circulation research*, Vol. 98, No. 1, pp. 88-97, 1524-4571; 0009-7330

George, C.H., Higgs, G.V. & Lai, F.A. (2003). Ryanodine receptor mutations associated with stress-induced ventricular tachycardia mediate increased calcium release in stimulated cardiomyocytes. *Circulation research*, Vol. 93, No. 6, pp. 531-540, 1524-4571; 0009-7330

Guo, T., Cornea, R.L., Huke, S., Camors, E., Yang, Y., Picht, E., Fruen, B.R. & Bers, D.M. (2010). Kinetics of FKBP12.6 binding to ryanodine receptors in permeabilized cardiac myocytes and effects on Ca sparks. *Circulation research*, Vol. 106, No. 11, pp. 1743-1752, 1524-4571; 0009-7330

Guo, T., Zhang, T., Mestril, R. & Bers, D.M. (2006). Ca2+/Calmodulin-dependent protein kinase II phosphorylation of ryanodine receptor does affect calcium sparks in mouse ventricular myocytes. *Circulation research*, Vol. 99, No. 4, pp. 398-406, 1524-4571; 0009-7330

Gyorke, S. & Terentyev, D. (2008). Modulation of ryanodine receptor by luminal calcium and accessory proteins in health and cardiac disease. *Cardiovascular research*, Vol. 77, No. 2, pp. 245-255, 0008-6363; 0008-6363

Gyorke, S., Lukyanenko, V. & Gyorke, I. (1997). Dual effects of tetracaine on spontaneous calcium release in rat ventricular myocytes. *The Journal of physiology*, Vol. 500 (Pt 2), No. Pt 2, pp. 297-309, 0022-3751; 0022-3751

Hilliard, F.A., Steele, D.S., Laver, D., Yang, Z., Le Marchand, S.J., Chopra, N., Piston, D.W., Huke, S. & Knollmann, B.C. (2010). Flecainide inhibits arrhythmogenic Ca2+ waves by open state block of ryanodine receptor Ca2+ release channels and reduction of Ca2+ spark mass. *Journal of Molecular and Cellular Cardiology*, Vol. 48, No. 2, pp. 293-301, 1095-8584; 0022-2828

Hirano, Y., Moscucci, A. & January, C.T. (1992). Direct measurement of L-type Ca2+ window current in heart cells. *Circulation research*, Vol. 70, No. 3, pp. 445-455, 0009-7330; 0009-7330

Hoch, B., Meyer, R., Hetzer, R., Krause, E.G. & Karczewski, P. (1999). Identification and expression of delta-isoforms of the multifunctional Ca2+/calmodulin-dependent protein kinase in failing and nonfailing human myocardium. *Circulation research*, Vol. 84, No. 6, pp. 713-721, 0009-7330; 0009-7330

Hoeker, G.S., Katra, R.P., Wilson, L.D., Plummer, B.N. & Laurita, K.R. (2009). Spontaneous calcium release in tissue from the failing canine heart. *American journal of physiology.Heart and circulatory physiology*, Vol. 297, No. 4, pp. H1235-42, 1522-1539; 0363-6135

Hove-Madsen, L., Llach, A., Bayes-Genis, A., Roura, S., Rodriguez Font, E., Aris, A. & Cinca, J. (2004). Atrial fibrillation is associated with increased spontaneous calcium release from the sarcoplasmic reticulum in human atrial myocytes. *Circulation*, Vol. 110, No. 11, pp. 1358-1363, 1524-4539; 0009-7322

Hunt, D.J., Jones, P.P., Wang, R., Chen, W., Bolstad, J., Chen, K., Shimoni, Y. & Chen, S.R. (2007). K201 (JTV519) suppresses spontaneous Ca2+ release and [3H]ryanodine binding to RyR2 irrespective of FKBP12.6 association. *The Biochemical journal*, Vol. 404, No. 3, pp. 431-438, 1470-8728; 0264-6021

Ikemoto, N. & Yamamoto, T. (2002). Regulation of calcium release by interdomain interaction within ryanodine receptors. *Frontiers in bioscience : a journal and virtual library*, Vol. 7, pp. d671-83, 1093-4715; 1093-4715

Ikemoto, N. & Yamamoto, T. (2000). Postulated role of inter-domain interaction within the ryanodine receptor in Ca(2+) channel regulation. *Trends in cardiovascular medicine*, Vol. 10, No. 7, pp. 310-316, 1050-1738; 1050-1738

January, C.T. & Riddle, J.M. (1989). Early afterdepolarizations: mechanism of induction and block. A role for L-type Ca2+ current. *Circulation research*, Vol. 64, No. 5, pp. 977-990, 0009-7330; 0009-7330

Ji, Y., Li, B., Reed, T.D., Lorenz, J.N., Kaetzel, M.A. & Dedman, J.R. (2003). Targeted inhibition of Ca2+/calmodulin-dependent protein kinase II in cardiac longitudinal sarcoplasmic reticulum results in decreased phospholamban phosphorylation at threonine 17. *The Journal of biological chemistry*, Vol. 278, No. 27, pp. 25063-25071, 0021-9258; 0021-9258

Jiang, D., Wang, R., Xiao, B., Kong, H., Hunt, D.J., Choi, P., Zhang, L. & Chen, S.R. (2005). Enhanced store overload-induced Ca2+ release and channel sensitivity to luminal Ca2+ activation are common defects of RyR2 mutations linked to ventricular tachycardia and sudden death. *Circulation research*, Vol. 97, No. 11, pp. 1173-1181, 1524-4571; 0009-7330

Jiang, D., Xiao, B., Yang, D., Wang, R., Choi, P., Zhang, L., Cheng, H. & Chen, S.R. (2004). RyR2 mutations linked to ventricular tachycardia and sudden death reduce the threshold for store-overload-induced Ca2+ release (SOICR). *Proceedings of the National Academy of Sciences of the United States of America*, Vol. 101, No. 35, pp. 13062-13067, 0027-8424; 0027-8424

Jones, P.P., Jiang, D., Bolstad, J., Hunt, D.J., Zhang, L., Demaurex, N. & Chen, S.R. (2008). Endoplasmic reticulum Ca2+ measurements reveal that the cardiac ryanodine receptor mutations linked to cardiac arrhythmia and sudden death alter the threshold for store-overload-induced Ca2+ release. *The Biochemical journal*, Vol. 412, No. 1, pp. 171-178, 1470-8728; 0264-6021

Kaneko, N., Ago, H., Matsuda, R., Inagaki, E. & Miyano, M. (1997). Crystal structure of annexin V with its ligand K-201 as a calcium channel activity inhibitor. *Journal of Molecular Biology*, Vol. 274, No. 1, pp. 16-20, 0022-2836; 0022-2836

Kang, G., Giovannone, S.F., Liu, N., Liu, F.Y., Zhang, J., Priori, S.G. & Fishman, G.I. (2010). Purkinje cells from RyR2 mutant mice are highly arrhythmogenic but responsive to targeted therapy. *Circulation research*, Vol. 107, No. 4, pp. 512-519, 1524-4571; 0009-7330

Kannankeril, P.J., Mitchell, B.M., Goonasekera, S.A., Chelu, M.G., Zhang, W., Sood, S., Kearney, D.L., Danila, C.I., De Biasi, M., Wehrens, X.H., Pautler, R.G., Roden, D.M., Taffet, G.E., Dirksen, R.T., Anderson, M.E. & Hamilton, S.L. (2006). Mice with the R176Q cardiac ryanodine receptor mutation exhibit catecholamine-induced ventricular tachycardia and cardiomyopathy. *Proceedings of the National Academy of Sciences of the United States of America*, Vol. 103, No. 32, pp. 12179-12184, 0027-8424; 0027-8424

Kashimura, T., Briston, S.J., Trafford, A.W., Napolitano, C., Priori, S.G., Eisner, D.A. & Venetucci, L.A. (2010). In the RyR2(R4496C) mouse model of CPVT, beta-adrenergic stimulation induces Ca waves by increasing SR Ca content and not by decreasing the threshold for Ca waves. *Circulation research*, Vol. 107, No. 12, pp. 1483-1489, 1524-4571; 0009-7330

Katra, R.P. & Laurita, K.R. (2005). Cellular mechanism of calcium-mediated triggered activity in the heart. *Circulation research*, Vol. 96, No. 5, pp. 535-542, 1524-4571; 0009-7330

Katra, R.P., Pruvot, E. & Laurita, K.R. (2004). Intracellular calcium handling heterogeneities in intact guinea pig hearts. *American journal of physiology.Heart and circulatory physiology*, Vol. 286, No. 2, pp. H648-56, 0363-6135; 0363-6135

Kemi, O.J., Haram, P.M., Loennechen, J.P., Osnes, J.B., Skomedal, T., Wisloff, U. & Ellingsen, O. (2005). Moderate vs. high exercise intensity: differential effects on aerobic fitness, cardiomyocyte contractility, and endothelial function. *Cardiovascular research*, Vol. 67, No. 1, pp. 161-172, 0008-6363; 0008-6363

Kimura, J., Kawahara, M., Sakai, E., Yatabe, J. & Nakanishi, H. (1999). Effects of a novel cardioprotective drug, JTV-519, on membrane currents of guinea pig ventricular myocytes. *Japanese journal of pharmacology*, Vol. 79, No. 3, pp. 275-281, 0021-5198; 0021-5198

Kirchhefer, U., Schmitz, W., Scholz, H. & Neumann, J. (1999). Activity of cAMP-dependent protein kinase and Ca2+/calmodulin-dependent protein kinase in failing and nonfailing human hearts. *Cardiovascular research*, Vol. 42, No. 1, pp. 254-261, 0008-6363; 0008-6363

Kiriyama, K., Kiyosue, T., Wang, J.C., Dohi, K. & Arita, M. (2000). Effects of JTV-519, a novel anti-ischaemic drug, on the delayed rectifier K+ current in guinea-pig ventricular myocytes. *Naunyn-Schmiedeberg's archives of pharmacology*, Vol. 361, No. 6, pp. 646-653, 0028-1298; 0028-1298

Kobayashi, S., Yano, M., Uchinoumi, H., Suetomi, T., Susa, T., Ono, M., Xu, X., Tateishi, H., Oda, T., Okuda, S., Doi, M., Yamamoto, T. & Matsuzaki, M. (2010). Dantrolene, a therapeutic agent for malignant hyperthermia, inhibits catecholaminergic polymorphic ventricular tachycardia in a RyR2(R2474S/+) knock-in mouse model. *Circulation journal : official journal of the Japanese Circulation Society*, Vol. 74, No. 12, pp. 2579-2584, 1347-4820; 1346-9843

Kobayashi, S., Yano, M., Suetomi, T., Ono, M., Tateishi, H., Mochizuki, M., Xu, X., Uchinoumi, H., Okuda, S., Yamamoto, T., Koseki, N., Kyushiki, H., Ikemoto, N. & Matsuzaki, M. (2009). Dantrolene, a therapeutic agent for malignant hyperthermia, markedly improves the function of failing cardiomyocytes by stabilizing interdomain interactions within the ryanodine receptor. *Journal of the American College of Cardiology*, Vol. 53, No. 21, pp. 1993-2005, 1558-3597; 0735-1097

Kobayashi, S., Bannister, M.L., Gangopadhyay, J.P., Hamada, T., Parness, J. & Ikemoto, N. (2005). Dantrolene stabilizes domain interactions within the ryanodine receptor. *The Journal of biological chemistry*, Vol. 280, No. 8, pp. 6580-6587, 0021-9258; 0021-9258

Kockskamper, J. & Pieske, B. (2006). Phosphorylation of the cardiac ryanodine receptor by Ca2+/calmodulin-dependent protein kinase II: the dominating twin of protein kinase A?. *Circulation research*, Vol. 99, No. 4, pp. 333-335, 1524-4571; 0009-7330

Kohno, M., Yano, M., Kobayashi, S., Doi, M., Oda, T., Tokuhisa, T., Okuda, S., Ohkusa, T., Kohno, M. & Matsuzaki, M. (2003). A new cardioprotective agent, JTV519, improves defective channel gating of ryanodine receptor in heart failure. *American journal of physiology.Heart and circulatory physiology*, Vol. 284, No. 3, pp. H1035-42, 0363-6135; 0363-6135

Kubalova, Z., Terentyev, D., Viatchenko-Karpinski, S., Nishijima, Y., Gyorke, I., Terentyeva, R., da Cunha, D.N., Sridhar, A., Feldman, D.S., Hamlin, R.L., Carnes, C.A. & Gyorke, S. (2005). Abnormal intrastore calcium signaling in chronic heart failure.

Proceedings of the National Academy of Sciences of the United States of America, Vol. 102, No. 39, pp. 14104-14109, 0027-8424; 0027-8424

Lahat, H., Pras, E., Olender, T., Avidan, N., Ben-Asher, E., Man, O., Levy-Nissenbaum, E., Khoury, A., Lorber, A., Goldman, B., Lancet, D. & Eldar, M. (2001). A missense mutation in a highly conserved region of CASQ2 is associated with autosomal recessive catecholamine-induced polymorphic ventricular tachycardia in Bedouin families from Israel. *American Journal of Human Genetics*, Vol. 69, No. 6, pp. 1378-1384, 0002-9297; 0002-9297

Laitinen, P.J., Brown, K.M., Piippo, K., Swan, H., Devaney, J.M., Brahmbhatt, B., Donarum, E.A., Marino, M., Tiso, N., Viitasalo, M., Toivonen, L., Stephan, D.A. & Kontula, K. (2001). Mutations of the cardiac ryanodine receptor (RyR2) gene in familial polymorphic ventricular tachycardia. *Circulation*, Vol. 103, No. 4, pp. 485-490, 1524-4539; 0009-7322

Laurita, K.R., Katra, R., Wible, B., Wan, X. & Koo, M.H. (2003). Transmural heterogeneity of calcium handling in canine. *Circulation research*, Vol. 92, No. 6, pp. 668-675, 1524-4571; 0009-7330

Leenhardt, A., Lucet, V., Denjoy, I., Grau, F., Ngoc, D.D. & Coumel, P. (1995). Catecholaminergic polymorphic ventricular tachycardia in children. A 7-year follow-up of 21 patients. *Circulation*, Vol. 91, No. 5, pp. 1512-1519, 0009-7322; 0009-7322

Lehnart, S.E., Mongillo, M., Bellinger, A., Lindegger, N., Chen, B.X., Hsueh, W., Reiken, S., Wronska, A., Drew, L.J., Ward, C.W., Lederer, W.J., Kass, R.S., Morley, G. & Marks, A.R. (2008). Leaky Ca2+ release channel/ryanodine receptor 2 causes seizures and sudden cardiac death in mice. *The Journal of clinical investigation*, Vol. 118, No. 6, pp. 2230-2245, 0021-9738; 0021-9738

Lehnart, S.E., Terrenoire, C., Reiken, S., Wehrens, X.H., Song, L.S., Tillman, E.J., Mancarella, S., Coromilas, J., Lederer, W.J., Kass, R.S. & Marks, A.R. (2006). Stabilization of cardiac ryanodine receptor prevents intracellular calcium leak and arrhythmias. *Proceedings of the National Academy of Sciences of the United States of America*, Vol. 103, No. 20, pp. 7906-7910, 0027-8424; 0027-8424

Liu, N., Ruan, Y., Denegri, M., Bachetti, T., Li, Y., Colombi, B., Napolitano, C., Coetzee, W.A. & Priori, S.G. (2011). Calmodulin kinase II inhibition prevents arrhythmias in RyR2(R4496C+/-) mice with catecholaminergic polymorphic ventricular tachycardia. *Journal of Molecular and Cellular Cardiology*, Vol. 50, No. 1, pp. 214-222, 1095-8584; 0022-2828

Liu, N., Colombi, B., Memmi, M., Zissimopoulos, S., Rizzi, N., Negri, S., Imbriani, M., Napolitano, C., Lai, F.A. & Priori, S.G. (2006). Arrhythmogenesis in catecholaminergic polymorphic ventricular tachycardia: insights from a RyR2 R4496C knock-in mouse model. *Circulation research*, Vol. 99, No. 3, pp. 292-298, 1524-4571; 0009-7330

Loughrey, C.M., Otani, N., Seidler, T., Craig, M.A., Matsuda, R., Kaneko, N. & Smith, G.L. (2007). K201 modulates excitation-contraction coupling and spontaneous Ca2+ release in normal adult rabbit ventricular cardiomyocytes. *Cardiovascular research*, Vol. 76, No. 2, pp. 236-246, 0008-6363; 0008-6363

MacLennan, D.H. & Chen, S.R. (2009). Store overload-induced Ca2+ release as a triggering mechanism for CPVT and MH episodes caused by mutations in RYR and CASQ genes. *The Journal of physiology*, Vol. 587, No. Pt 13, pp. 3113-3115, 1469-7793; 0022-3751

Maier, L.S., Zhang, T., Chen, L., DeSantiago, J., Brown, J.H. & Bers, D.M. (2003). Transgenic CaMKIIdeltaC overexpression uniquely alters cardiac myocyte Ca2+ handling: reduced SR Ca2+ load and activated SR Ca2+ release. *Circulation research*, Vol. 92, No. 8, pp. 904-911, 1524-4571; 0009-7330

Marx, S.O., Reiken, S., Hisamatsu, Y., Jayaraman, T., Burkhoff, D., Rosemblit, N. & Marks, A.R. (2000). PKA phosphorylation dissociates FKBP12.6 from the calcium release channel (ryanodine receptor): defective regulation in failing hearts. *Cell*, Vol. 101, No. 4, pp. 365-376, 0092-8674; 0092-8674

Mohamed, U., Napolitano, C. & Priori, S.G. (2007). Molecular and electrophysiological bases of catecholaminergic polymorphic ventricular tachycardia. *Journal of cardiovascular electrophysiology*, Vol. 18, No. 7, pp. 791-797, 1540-8167; 1045-3873

Mulder, B.J., de Tombe, P.P. & ter Keurs, H.E. (1989). Spontaneous and propagated contractions in rat cardiac trabeculae. *The Journal of general physiology*, Vol. 93, No. 5, pp. 943-961, 0022-1295; 0022-1295

Nakaya, H., Furusawa, Y., Ogura, T., Tamagawa, M. & Uemura, H. (2000). Inhibitory effects of JTV-519, a novel cardioprotective drug, on potassium currents and experimental atrial fibrillation in guinea-pig hearts. *British journal of pharmacology*, Vol. 131, No. 7, pp. 1363-1372, 0007-1188; 0007-1188

Neef, S., Dybkova, N., Sossalla, S., Ort, K.R., Fluschnik, N., Neumann, K., Seipelt, R., Schondube, F.A., Hasenfuss, G. & Maier, L.S. (2010). CaMKII-dependent diastolic SR Ca2+ leak and elevated diastolic Ca2+ levels in right atrial myocardium of patients with atrial fibrillation. *Circulation research*, Vol. 106, No. 6, pp. 1134-1144, 1524-4571; 0009-7330

Oda, T., Yano, M., Yamamoto, T., Tokuhisa, T., Okuda, S., Doi, M., Ohkusa, T., Ikeda, Y., Kobayashi, S., Ikemoto, N. & Matsuzaki, M. (2005). Defective regulation of interdomain interactions within the ryanodine receptor plays a key role in the pathogenesis of heart failure. *Circulation*, Vol. 111, No. 25, pp. 3400-3410, 1524-4539; 0009-7322

Overend, C.L., Eisner, D.A. & O'Neill, S.C. (1997). The effect of tetracaine on spontaneous Ca2+ release and sarcoplasmic reticulum calcium content in rat ventricular myocytes. *The Journal of physiology*, Vol. 502 (Pt 3), No. Pt 3, pp. 471-479, 0022-3751; 0022-3751

Packer, M., Poole-Wilson, P.A., Armstrong, P.W., Cleland, J.G., Horowitz, J.D., Massie, B.M., Ryden, L., Thygesen, K. & Uretsky, B.F. (1999). Comparative effects of low and high doses of the angiotensin-converting enzyme inhibitor, lisinopril, on morbidity and mortality in chronic heart failure. ATLAS Study Group. *Circulation*, Vol. 100, No. 23, pp. 2312-2318, 0009-7322; 0009-7322

Packer, M. (1985). Sudden unexpected death in patients with congestive heart failure: a second frontier. *Circulation*, Vol. 72, No. 4, pp. 681-685, 0009-7322; 0009-7322

Patterson, E., Jackman, W.M., Beckman, K.J., Lazzara, R., Lockwood, D., Scherlag, B.J., Wu, R. & Po, S. (2007). Spontaneous pulmonary vein firing in man: relationship to tachycardia-pause early afterdepolarizations and triggered arrhythmia in canine pulmonary veins in vitro. *Journal of cardiovascular electrophysiology*, Vol. 18, No. 10, pp. 1067-1075, 1540-8167; 1045-3873

Patterson, E., Lazzara, R., Szabo, B., Liu, H., Tang, D., Li, Y.H., Scherlag, B.J. & Po, S.S. (2006). Sodium-calcium exchange initiated by the Ca2+ transient: an arrhythmia trigger within pulmonary veins. *Journal of the American College of Cardiology*, Vol. 47, No. 6, pp. 1196-1206, 1558-3597; 0735-1097

Plummer, B.N., Cutler, M.J., Wan, X. & Laurita, K.R. (2011). Spontaneous calcium oscillations during diastole in the whole heart: the influence of ryanodine reception function and gap junction coupling. *American journal of physiology.Heart and circulatory physiology*, Vol. 300, No. 5, pp. H1822-8, 1522-1539; 0363-6135

Pogwizd, S.M., Schlotthauer, K., Li, L., Yuan, W. & Bers, D.M. (2001). Arrhythmogenesis and contractile dysfunction in heart failure: Roles of sodium-calcium exchange, inward rectifier potassium current, and residual beta-adrenergic responsiveness. *Circulation research*, Vol. 88, No. 11, pp. 1159-1167, 1524-4571; 0009-7330

Prestle, J., Dieterich, S., Preuss, M., Bieligk, U. & Hasenfuss, G. (1999). Heterogeneous transmural gene expression of calcium-handling proteins and natriuretic peptides in the failing human heart. *Cardiovascular research*, Vol. 43, No. 2, pp. 323-331, 0008-6363; 0008-6363

Priori, S.G. & Chen, S.R. (2011). Inherited dysfunction of sarcoplasmic reticulum Ca2+ handling and arrhythmogenesis. *Circulation research*, Vol. 108, No. 7, pp. 871-883, 1524-4571; 0009-7330

Priori, S.G. & Napolitano, C. (2005). Cardiac and skeletal muscle disorders caused by mutations in the intracellular Ca2+ release channels. *The Journal of clinical investigation*, Vol. 115, No. 8, pp. 2033-2038, 0021-9738; 0021-9738

Priori, S.G., Napolitano, C., Tiso, N., Memmi, M., Vignati, G., Bloise, R., Sorrentino, V. & Danieli, G.A. (2001). Mutations in the cardiac ryanodine receptor gene (hRyR2) underlie catecholaminergic polymorphic ventricular tachycardia. *Circulation*, Vol. 103, No. 2, pp. 196-200, 0009-7322; 0009-7322

Qin, J., Valle, G., Nani, A., Nori, A., Rizzi, N., Priori, S.G., Volpe, P. & Fill, M. (2008). Luminal Ca2+ regulation of single cardiac ryanodine receptors: insights provided by calsequestrin and its mutants. *The Journal of general physiology*, Vol. 131, No. 4, pp. 325-334, 1540-7748; 0022-1295

Rose, A.J. & Hargreaves, M. (2003). Exercise increases Ca2+-calmodulin-dependent protein kinase II activity in human skeletal muscle. *The Journal of physiology*, Vol. 553, No. Pt 1, pp. 303-309, 0022-3751; 0022-3751

Rosen, M.R., Gelband, H., Merker, C. & Hoffman, B.F. (1973). Mechanisms of digitalis toxicity. Effects of ouabain on phase four of canine Purkinje fiber transmembrane potentials. *Circulation*, Vol. 47, No. 4, pp. 681-689, 0009-7322; 0009-7322

Rousseau, E. & Meissner, G. (1989). Single cardiac sarcoplasmic reticulum Ca2+-release channel: activation by caffeine. *The American Journal of Physiology*, Vol. 256, No. 2 Pt 2, pp. H328-33, 0002-9513; 0002-9513

Schotten, U., Verheule, S., Kirchhof, P. & Goette, A. (2011). Pathophysiological mechanisms of atrial fibrillation: a translational appraisal. *Physiological Reviews*, Vol. 91, No. 1, pp. 265-325, 1522-1210; 0031-9333

Sedej, S., Heinzel, F.R., Walther, S., Dybkova, N., Wakula, P., Groborz, J., Gronau, P., Maier, L.S., Vos, M.A., Lai, F.A., Napolitano, C., Priori, S.G., Kockskamper, J. & Pieske, B. (2010). Na+-dependent SR Ca2+ overload induces arrhythmogenic events in mouse cardiomyocytes with a human CPVT mutation. *Cardiovascular research*, Vol. 87, No. 1, pp. 50-59, 1755-3245; 0008-6363

Sobie, E.A., Guatimosim, S., Gomez-Viquez, L., Song, L.S., Hartmann, H., Saleet Jafri, M. & Lederer, W.J. (2006). The Ca 2+ leak paradox and rogue ryanodine receptors: SR Ca 2+ efflux theory and practice. *Progress in biophysics and molecular biology*, Vol. 90, No. 1-3, pp. 172-185, 0079-6107; 0079-6107

Stern, M.D. & Cheng, H. (2004). Putting out the fire: what terminates calcium-induced calcium release in cardiac muscle?. *Cell calcium*, Vol. 35, No. 6, pp. 591-601, 0143-4160; 0143-4160

Swan, H., Piippo, K., Viitasalo, M., Heikkila, P., Paavonen, T., Kainulainen, K., Kere, J., Keto, P., Kontula, K. & Toivonen, L. (1999). Arrhythmic disorder mapped to chromosome 1q42-q43 causes malignant polymorphic ventricular tachycardia in structurally normal hearts. *Journal of the American College of Cardiology*, Vol. 34, No. 7, pp. 2035-2042, 0735-1097; 0735-1097

Tateishi, H., Yano, M., Mochizuki, M., Suetomi, T., Ono, M., Xu, X., Uchinoumi, H., Okuda, S., Oda, T., Kobayashi, S., Yamamoto, T., Ikeda, Y., Ohkusa, T., Ikemoto, N. & Matsuzaki, M. (2009). Defective domain-domain interactions within the ryanodine receptor as a critical cause of diastolic Ca2+ leak in failing hearts. *Cardiovascular research*, Vol. 81, No. 3, pp. 536-545, 1755-3245; 0008-6363

Terentyev, D., Belevych, A.E., Terentyeva, R., Martin, M.M., Malana, G.E., Kuhn, D.E., Abdellatif, M., Feldman, D.S., Elton, T.S. & Gyorke, S. (2009). miR-1 overexpression enhances Ca(2+) release and promotes cardiac arrhythmogenesis by targeting PP2A regulatory subunit B56alpha and causing CaMKII-dependent hyperphosphorylation of RyR2. *Circulation research*, Vol. 104, No. 4, pp. 514-521, 1524-4571; 0009-7330

Thum, T., Galuppo, P., Wolf, C., Fiedler, J., Kneitz, S., van Laake, L.W., Doevendans, P.A., Mummery, C.L., Borlak, J., Haverich, A., Gross, C., Engelhardt, S., Ertl, G. & Bauersachs, J. (2007). MicroRNAs in the human heart: a clue to fetal gene reprogramming in heart failure. *Circulation*, Vol. 116, No. 3, pp. 258-267, 1524-4539; 0009-7322

Tiso, N., Salamon, M., Bagattin, A., Danieli, G.A., Argenton, F. & Bortolussi, M. (2002). The binding of the RyR2 calcium channel to its gating protein FKBP12.6 is oppositely affected by ARVD2 and VTSIP mutations. *Biochemical and biophysical research communications*, Vol. 299, No. 4, pp. 594-598, 0006-291X; 0006-291X

Tomaselli, G.F. & Zipes, D.P. (2004). What causes sudden death in heart failure?. *Circulation research*, Vol. 95, No. 8, pp. 754-763, 1524-4571; 0009-7330

Trafford, A.W., Diaz, M.E. & Eisner, D.A. (2001). Coordinated control of cell Ca(2+) loading and triggered release from the sarcoplasmic reticulum underlies the rapid inotropic response to increased L-type Ca(2+) current. *Circulation research*, Vol. 88, No. 2, pp. 195-201, 1524-4571; 0009-7330

Trafford, A.W., Diaz, M.E., Sibbring, G.C. & Eisner, D.A. (2000a). Modulation of CICR has no maintained effect on systolic Ca2+: simultaneous measurements of sarcoplasmic reticulum and sarcolemmal Ca2+ fluxes in rat ventricular myocytes. *The Journal of physiology*, Vol. 522 Pt 2, pp. 259-270, 0022-3751; 0022-3751

Trafford, A.W., Sibbring, G.C., Diaz, M.E. & Eisner, D.A. (2000b). The effects of low concentrations of caffeine on spontaneous Ca release in isolated rat ventricular myocytes. *Cell calcium*, Vol. 28, No. 4, pp. 269-276, 0143-4160; 0143-4160

Trafford, A.W., Diaz, M.E., Negretti, N. & Eisner, D.A. (1997). Enhanced Ca2+ current and decreased Ca2+ efflux restore sarcoplasmic reticulum Ca2+ content after depletion. *Circulation research*, Vol. 81, No. 4, pp. 477-484, 0009-7330; 0009-7330

Tsuji, Y., Hojo, M., Voigt, N., El-Armouche, A., Inden, Y., Murohara, T., Dobrev, D., Nattel, S., Kodama, I. & Kamiya, K. (2011). Ca2+-related signaling and protein phosphorylation abnormalities play central roles in a new experimental model of electrical storm. *Circulation*, Vol. 123, No. 20, pp. 2192-2203, 1524-4539; 0009-7322

Uchinoumi, H., Yano, M., Suetomi, T., Ono, M., Xu, X., Tateishi, H., Oda, T., Okuda, S., Doi, M., Kobayashi, S., Yamamoto, T., Ikeda, Y., Ohkusa, T., Ikemoto, N. & Matsuzaki, M. (2010). Catecholaminergic polymorphic ventricular tachycardia is caused by mutation-linked defective conformational regulation of the ryanodine receptor. *Circulation research*, Vol. 106, No. 8, pp. 1413-1424, 1524-4571; 0009-7330

van der Werf, C., Kannankeril, P.J., Sacher, F., Krahn, A.D., Viskin, S., Leenhardt, A., Shimizu, W., Sumitomo, N., Fish, F.A., Bhuiyan, Z.A., Willems, A.R., van der Veen, M.J., Watanabe, H., Laborderie, J., Haissaguerre, M., Knollmann, B.C. & Wilde, A.A. (2011). Flecainide therapy reduces exercise-induced ventricular arrhythmias in patients with catecholaminergic polymorphic ventricular tachycardia. *Journal of the American College of Cardiology*, Vol. 57, No. 22, pp. 2244-2254, 1558-3597; 0735-1097

Volders, P.G., Vos, M.A., Szabo, B., Sipido, K.R., de Groot, S.H., Gorgels, A.P., Wellens, H.J. & Lazzara, R. (2000). Progress in the understanding of cardiac early afterdepolarizations and torsades de pointes: time to revise current concepts. *Cardiovascular research*, Vol. 46, No. 3, pp. 376-392, 0008-6363; 0008-6363

Volders, P.G., Kulcsar, A., Vos, M.A., Sipido, K.R., Wellens, H.J., Lazzara, R. & Szabo, B. (1997). Similarities between early and delayed afterdepolarizations induced by isoproterenol in canine ventricular myocytes. *Cardiovascular research*, Vol. 34, No. 2, pp. 348-359, 0008-6363; 0008-6363

Watanabe, H., Chopra, N., Laver, D., Hwang, H.S., Davies, S.S., Roach, D.E., Duff, H.J., Roden, D.M., Wilde, A.A. & Knollmann, B.C. (2009). Flecainide prevents catecholaminergic polymorphic ventricular tachycardia in mice and humans. *Nature medicine*, Vol. 15, No. 4, pp. 380-383, 1546-170X; 1078-8956

Wehrens, X.H., Lehnart, S.E., Reiken, S.R., Deng, S.X., Vest, J.A., Cervantes, D., Coromilas, J., Landry, D.W. & Marks, A.R. (2004). Protection from cardiac arrhythmia through ryanodine receptor-stabilizing protein calstabin2. *Science (New York, N.Y.)*, Vol. 304, No. 5668, pp. 292-296, 1095-9203; 0036-8075

Wehrens, X.H., Lehnart, S.E., Huang, F., Vest, J.A., Reiken, S.R., Mohler, P.J., Sun, J., Guatimosim, S., Song, L.S., Rosemblit, N., D'Armiento, J.M., Napolitano, C., Memmi, M., Priori, S.G., Lederer, W.J. & Marks, A.R. (2003). FKBP12.6 deficiency and defective calcium release channel (ryanodine receptor) function linked to exercise-induced sudden cardiac death. *Cell*, Vol. 113, No. 7, pp. 829-840, 0092-8674; 0092-8674

Wit, A.L. & Rosen, M.R. (1983). Pathophysiologic mechanisms of cardiac arrhythmias. *American Heart Journal*, Vol. 106, No. 4 Pt 2, pp. 798-811, 0002-8703; 0002-8703

Wu, Y., Temple, J., Zhang, R., Dzhura, I., Zhang, W., Trimble, R., Roden, D.M., Passier, R., Olson, E.N., Colbran, R.J. & Anderson, M.E. (2002). Calmodulin kinase II and arrhythmias in a mouse model of cardiac hypertrophy. *Circulation*, Vol. 106, No. 10, pp. 1288-1293, 1524-4539; 0009-7322

Xiao, J., Tian, X., Jones, P.P., Bolstad, J., Kong, H., Wang, R., Zhang, L., Duff, H.J., Gillis, A.M., Fleischer, S., Kotlikoff, M., Copello, J.A. & Chen, S.R. (2007). Removal of FKBP12.6 does not alter the conductance and activation of the cardiac ryanodine receptor or the susceptibility to stress-induced ventricular arrhythmias. *The Journal of biological chemistry*, Vol. 282, No. 48, pp. 34828-34838, 0021-9258; 0021-9258

Xie, Y., Garfinkel, A., Weiss, J.N. & Qu, Z. (2009). Cardiac alternans induced by fibroblast-myocyte coupling: mechanistic insights from computational models. *American journal of physiology.Heart and circulatory physiology*, Vol. 297, No. 2, pp. H775-84, 1522-1539; 0363-6135

Xu, L., Jones, R. & Meissner, G. (1993). Effects of local anesthetics on single channel behavior of skeletal muscle calcium release channel. *The Journal of general physiology*, Vol. 101, No. 2, pp. 207-233, 0022-1295; 0022-1295

Yamamoto, T., Yano, M., Xu, X., Uchinoumi, H., Tateishi, H., Mochizuki, M., Oda, T., Kobayashi, S., Ikemoto, N. & Matsuzaki, M. (2008). Identification of target domains of the cardiac ryanodine receptor to correct channel disorder in failing hearts. *Circulation*, Vol. 117, No. 6, pp. 762-772, 1524-4539; 0009-7322

Yano, M., Kobayashi, S., Kohno, M., Doi, M., Tokuhisa, T., Okuda, S., Suetsugu, M., Hisaoka, T., Obayashi, M., Ohkusa, T., Kohno, M. & Matsuzaki, M. (2003). FKBP12.6-mediated stabilization of calcium-release channel (ryanodine receptor) as a novel therapeutic strategy against heart failure. *Circulation*, Vol. 107, No. 3, pp. 477-484, 1524-4539; 0009-7322

9

Heart Rate Variability: An Index of the Brain–Heart Interaction

Ingrid Tonhajzerova[1], Igor Ondrejka[2], Zuzana Turianikova[1], Kamil Javorka[1], Andrea Calkovska[1] and Michal Javorka[1]

[1]*Department of Physiology,*
[2]*Psychiatric Clinic, Jessenius Faculty of Medicine, Martin, Comenius University, Slovak Republic*

1. Introduction

The autonomic nervous system plays an important role in a wide range of visceral-somatic and mental diseases. Cardiac parameters, particularly heart rate as a physiological measure, are extremely sensitive to autonomic influences. Normally, the activities of the sympathetic and parasympathetic branches of the autonomic nervous system are in dynamic balance indicating healthy and flexible physiological system. The autonomic imbalance - low parasympathetic activity and/or sympathetic overactivity resulting in tachycardia - is common to a broad range of maladaptive conditions and it is associated with the increased risk of cardiovascular adverse outcomes (Friedman, 2007; Porges, 2007; Thayer & Sternberg, 2006).

Heart rate is a widely used and easily determinable measure of cardiac rhythm. In many previous investigations, high heart rate has shown to be associated with increased risk of cardiovascular mortality (Shaper et al., 1993). Reunanen et al. (2000) referred to close association between tachycardia and mortality (from cardiovascular as well as noncardiovascular reasons) in a large adult population study. Thus, high heart rate is considered as a simple significant nonspecific predictor of mortality; and the average heart rate could be used as an important indicator of the organism complex state.

Heart rate control is determined by dynamic interaction of acceleratory sympathetic nervous system activation, and deceleratory parasympathetic nervous system activity resulting in rhythmical oscillations - heart rate variability. Its analysis should represent a noninvasive window into cardiac chronotropic regulation providing then important information about central-peripheral interaction. During this decade the pathomechanisms by which central nervous system modulates cardiac autonomic control in various mental disorders as well as the potential links between emotional/cognitive processes and cardiac activity have drawn increasing interest.

This chapter will be focused on the essential questions related to the heart-brain interaction indexed by the heart rate variability: 1. What is its physiological and psychophysiological background? 2. What methods exist in the heart rate variability analysis? 3. What is the clinical implication of the stated methods especially in children and adolescents suffering from mental disorders?

2. Heart rate and its variability – a link between the brain and the heart

Average-mean value of the heart rate results from a rather complex interplay. Its value is determined by intrinsic activity as well as the joint modifications of the parasympathetic and sympathetic neurons terminating at sinoatrial node. Importantly, when both cardiac vagal and sympathetic inputs are pharmacologically blocked (e.g. atropine plus propranolol as „double blockade"), intrinsic heart rate (IHR) is higher than the normal resting heart rate; therefore, vagal inhibitory influence is dominant. Additionally, like normal resting heart rate the IHR declines with age and its value is calculated according to the mathematical formula: IHR= 118,1-(0,57 x age) (Jose & Collison , 1970).

2.1 Parasympathetic and sympathetic regulation of the heart rate

Parasympathetic innervation of the heart by vagus nerve originates in neurons localized in nucleus ambiguus, dorsal vagal nucleus and in the region between these nuclei (Taylor et al., 1999 and others). Acetylcholine, released by postganglionic parasympathetic terminals at the sinoatrial node, slows the rate of sinoatrial node depolarization and discharge by binding to muscarinic cholinergic receptors and activating a transmembrane potassium channels associated with funny-channels inhibition.

In contrast, sympathetic nerves originate in cervical and stellate ganglia and neurons of these ganglia are under control of sympathetic preganglionic neurons located in intermediolateral nucleus of spinal cord thoracic segments (Kawashima, 2005 and others). Noradrenaline is released by sympathetic terminals on the sinoatrial node and accelerates the sinoatrial node rhythm via $\beta1/\beta2$ receptors-mediated second messenger cascade of intracellular signals and activating of funny-channels. In addition to these classic neurotransmitter actions, the chronotropic state of the heart can be modulated by a variety of neuropeptides, such as neuropeptide Y, that appear to be colocalized with conventional neurotransmitters in autonomic terminals (Kukanova & Mravec, 2006; Shine et al., 1994). Interactions between neurons within intracardiac ganglia together with interconnections between individual anatomical and functional elements form the basis for complex nervous network of the heart, also called „heart brain" (Randall, 2000). Thus, this complex intracardiac nervous system together with dominant extracardiac autonomic activity provides modulation of heart activity on both physiological and pathological conditions (Armour, 1999).

Uijtdehaage & Thayer (2000) have elaborated the problem of accentuated antagonism in the control of human heart rate. Based on animal studies that indicate the accelerative effects of the sympathetic nervous system on heart rate highly depending on the background of vagal activity, the authors used an evaluation of respiratory sinus arrhythmia as an index of cardial vagal modulation and left ventricular ejection time as a sympathetic chronotropic index. They found that sympathetic heart rate effects were substantially smaller with high levels of vagal tone than with low background vagal activity. Furthermore, vagal effects became progressively stronger despite the increasing background sympathetic activity, demonstrating the predominance of parasympathetic control of the heart rate. This finding implies that changes in cardiac activity resulting from changes in sympathetic control cannot be interpreted accurately unless concurrent vagal activity is taken into account, as well (Uijtdehaage & Thayer, 2000).

2.2 The concept of sympathovagal balance

As above mentioned, the cardiac neural control is mediated mainly via sympathetic-parasympathetic interactions interconnected from central nervous system to postganglionic endings. In most physiological conditions, the activation of either sympathetic or vagal outflow is accompanied by the inhibition of the other suggesting the concept of sympathovagal balance (Malliani, 2000, as cited in Montano et al., 2009). This reciprocal organization seems instrumental to the fact that sympathetic excitation and simultaneous vagal inhibition, or vice versa, are both presumed to contribute to the increase or decrease of cardiac activity required for various situations. Thus, the autonomic balance oscillates from rest, when homeostatic negative feedback reflexes predominate, to excitatory states (*e.g.* emotion), when central excitatory mechanisms, possibly reinforced by peripheral positive feedback reflexes, are instrumental to the enhanced cardiac performance (Malliani et al., 1991). This continual dynamic excitatory-inhibitory interaction leads to heart rate instantaneous oscillations - heart rate variability (Fig. 1). The heart rate variability then reflects complex and sophisticated cardiac neural chronotropic control as well as an ability of the end-organ (heart) in response to regulatory effects (Calkovska and Javorka, 2008).

Just like the driver of a car can modify the number of rotations per minute of the automobile engine according to the needs for speed and acceleration, heart rate immediately adapts to the basic needs of the body (Aubert & Ramaekers, 1999). This continuous brisk heart rate adaptability is expressed by its beat-to-beat changes - heart rate variability.

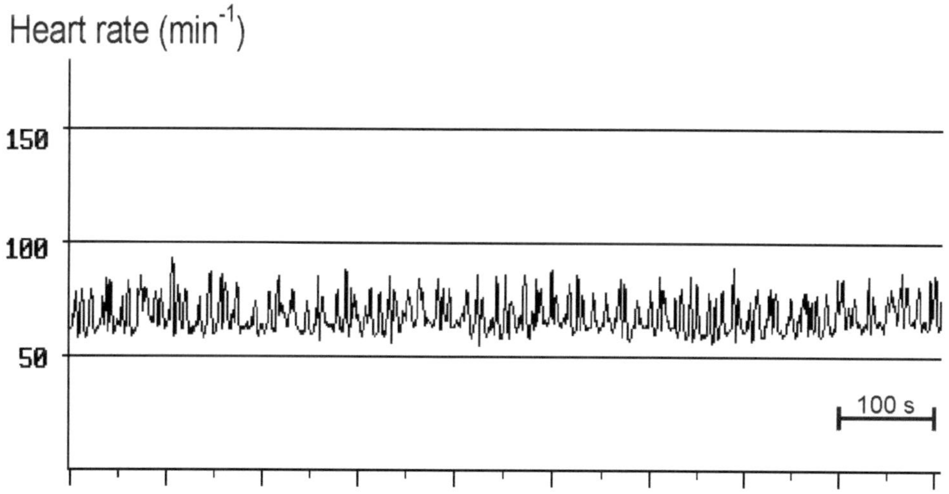

Fig. 1. The recording of the beat-to-beat heart rate oscillations in young healthy subject (modified by Javorka et al., 2011)

On the other hand, Paton et al. (2005) presented interesting review regarding the pattern of sympathetic/parasympathetic balance (as analogy to the Chinese philosophy of yin and yang). Unlike the conventional picture of reciprocal control of cardiac vagal and sympathetic nervous activity, as seen during a baroreceptor reflex, many other reactions involve simultaneous co-activation of both autonomic limbs. Thus, vagal activity may enhance sympathetically mediated tachycardia, or can by itself produce a paradoxical vagally mediated tachycardia. A plausible mechanism for this synergistic interaction includes possible activation of chromaffin or small intensely fluorescent cells in the cardiac ganglia. These cells have abundant vagal innervation and include vesicles containing catecholamines (Levy, 1971). Thus, the paradoxical vagally mediated tachycardia could be due to release of catecholamines from these vesicles contained within the intrinsic cardiac neurones (Horackova et al., 1996, 1999). Moreover, alternative mechanisms might include the releasing of the several neuropeptides as co-transmitters from vagal nerve fibers (e.g. neuropeptide Y) or participation of some sympathetic efferent axons from cardiac vagal nerve (Cheng et al., 1997 and others).

Proper functioning of the sympathetic-parasympathetic dynamic balance at rest as well as in response to various internal/external stimuli is important for organism flexibility, adaptability and health. In contrast, the autonomic imbalance, in which one branch of the autonomic nervous system dominates over the other, is associated with a lack of dynamic flexibility and health. Therefore, the autonomic imbalance typically with sympathetic overactivity associated with parasympathetic hypoactivation, indexed by low heart rate variability, could represent potential pathomechanism leading to increased risk of cardiovascular adverse outcomes and all-cause mortality (Task Force, 1996). In the elderly, some studies showed that higher heart rate variability is stronger indicator of cardiac mortality than decreased heart rate variability. Further studies are needed to confirm these findings and to elucidate their physiologic meaning (de Bruyne et al., 1999).

Modern conceptions based on complexity theory hold with the assumption that organism stability, adaptability, and health are maintaned through a dynamic relationship among system elements; in this case, the sympathetic and parasympathetic branches of the ANS (Thayer & Lane, 2000). That is, patterns of organized variability, rather than static levels, are preserved in the face of constantly changing environmental demands. For example, in healthy individuals, average heart rate is greater during the day (higher sympathetic activity), when energy demands are higher, than at night (higher parasympathetic activity), when energy demands are lower. The system has a different energy minimum for daytime and for nightime. Because the system operates „far from equlibrium", it constantly searches for local energy minima to reduce the energy requirement of the organism. Consequently, optimal system functioning is achieved via lability and variability in its component processes, whereas rigid regularity is associated with mortality, morbidity and ill health (Ellis & Thayer, 2010).

Final common pathway of the central-peripheral heart rate control should be indexed by heart rate variability; therefore, this point is discussed in the following section.

2.3 Heart-brain interaction indexed by heart rate variability

In 1865 Claude Bernard delivered a lecture at the Sorbonne on the physiology of the heart and its connections with the brain (Bernard, 1867; as cited in Thayer & Lane, 2009). His work denoted the first step to systematically investigate the connections between the heart and the brain (Thayer & Lane, 2009).

The studies concerning the brain-heart connection emphasize the modulation of the cardiac activity by the cortex; thus, an extensive research has been directed to identify the pathway by which this neurocardiac control is achieved (Friedman, 2007; Montano et al., 2009; Thayer & Brosschot, 2005; Thayer & Lane, 2009). Benarroch (1993) has described the central autonomic network as an integrated component of an internal regulation system through which the brain controls visceromotor, neuroendocrinne, and behavioural responses that are critical for goal-directed behaviour and adaptability. Structural components of the central autonomic network are found at the level of the forebrain (anterior cingulate; insular and ventromedial prefrontal cortices; central nucles of the amygdala; paraventricular and related nuclei of the hypothalamus), midbrain (periaquaductal gray matter), and hindbrain (parabrachial nucleus, nucleus of the solitary tract, nucleus ambiguus, ventrolateral and ventromedial medulla, medullary tegmental field). The interplay of sympathetic and parasympathetic (vagal) outputs of the central autonomic network through sinoatrial node produces the complex beat-to-beat heart rate variability indicating a healthy and adaptive organism (Thayer & Lane, 2000). Importantly, the output of the central autonomic network is under tonic inhibitory control via GABAergic neurons in the nucleus of the solitary tract. Furthermore, cardiac autonomic afferents send impulses back to the central autonomic network. Then, the heart rate variability can index central autonomic network output, and likewise reflects visceral feedback to the network (Friedman, 2007; Thayer & Lane, 2000).

The importance of the inhibitory processes related to heart rate vagal control leading to complex beat-to-beat heart rate oscillations as a sign of health was emphasized by some research groups (Friedman, 2007; Thayer & Lane, 2000, 2009 etc.). Thayer (2006) in an excellent review implies that the inhibitory nature of cardiac control can be exhibited at different levels - from peripheral end-organ (heart) to the neural structures that serve to link the prefrontal cortex with heart rate variability. The central autonomic network, characterized by the reciprocally interconnected neural structures, allows the prefrontal cortex to exert an inhibitory influence on subcortical structures associated with defensive behavior and thus allows the organism to flexibly regulate its behavior in response to changing environmental demands (Thayer, 2006). For example, the amygdala, which has outputs to autonomic as well as other regulatory systems, and becomes active during threat/uncertainty, is under tonic inhibitory control from the prefrontal cortex. Thus, under conditions of the threat, the prefrontal cortex becomes hypoactive which is associated with disinhibition of sympathoexcitatory circuits. Importantly, proper functioning of inhibitory processes is vital to the preservation of the integrity of the system and therefore is vital to health. In contrast, the psychopathological states such as anxiety or depression are associated with prefrontal hypoactivity resulting in disruption of the inhibitory control (Thayer, 2006; Thayer & Lane, 2009).

Since heart rate variability originates predominantly from oscillations in vagal neural traffic, mediated by rapid changes in acetylcholine, beat-to-beat analysis of the heart rate time series (discussed in the following section in details) can provide important information about dominant inhibitory parasympathetic component in the heart rate regulation (sympathetic cardiac influence is too slow to produce rapid beat-to-beat changes because of norepinephrine kinetics). Specifically, a series of studies using neuroimaging have provided evidence that activity of the prefrontal cortex is associated with cardiac vagal function evaluated by heart rate variability analysis (Lane et al., 2009). For example, Ahs et al. (2009) concluded that vagal modulation of the heart is associated with activity in striatal as well as medial and lateral prefrontal areas in patients with social phobia. Another study reported the correlations in the superior prefrontal cortex, the dorsolateral prefrontal and parietal cortices activities with parasympathetic-linked cardiac control indexed by the heart rate variability spectral analysis (Lane et al., 2009). Similarly, Napadow et al. (2008) demonstrated correlations between heart rate variability and the activity in the hypothalamus, cerebellum, parabrachial nucleus/locus coeruleus, periaqueductal gray, amygdala, hippocampus, thalamus and prefrontal, insular and temporal cortices. As such, these objective and sensitive methods confirm the fact that the heart rate variability serves to index central-peripheral autonomic nervous system integration, and consequently, is a psychophysiological marker for adaptive environmental engagement (Porges, 1995, 2009).

3. Heart rate variability: Analysis and clinical implications

Heart rate variability is a physiological phenomenon and its assessment can provide useful information about cardiac autonomic regulatory mechanisms. From the clinical point of view, our research is focused on the application of the heart rate variability analysis using traditional (linear) and novel nonlinear methods, particularly in children and adolescents suffering from mental disorders. Since impaired cardiac neural regulation is associated with increased risk of cardiovascular morbidity, our original findings (presented in the following sections) underscore the importance of future research regarding the autonomic neurocardiac integrity in mental disorders already in children and adolescents.

3.1 Heart rate variability – linear analysis

Heart rate variability is traditionally quantified by linear methods - time and frequency (spectral) domain analysis - providing the information about the heart rate variability magnitude and frequencies (Task Force, 1996). The short-term heart rate variability spectral analysis allows to isolate the faster high frequency respiratory-coupled influences on the heart rate variability (HF-HRV: 0.15-0.4 Hz) from slower sources of the heart rate variability (LF-HRV: 0.04-0.15 Hz). It seems that the oscillations in cardiac sympathetic nerve activity make a minor contribution to the heart rate oscillations at low-frequency component (LF-HRV); and these oscillations are derived mainly from a baroreflex, vagally mediated response to blood pressure Mayer waves (Elghozi & Julien, 2007). In contrast, the high-frequency cardiac rhythms are mediated primarily by vagal innervation of the sinoatrial node reflecting the respiratory sinus arrhythmia - physiological phenomenon characterized by the heart rate increases during inspiration and decreases during expiration. The respiratory sinus arrhythmia mechanisms include central medullary generator, reflexes from the lungs, baroreflexes, chemoreflexes, as well as local mechanisms (stretching of the sinoatrial node etc.). Respiratory sinus arrhythmia is mediated predominantly by fluctuations of vagal cardiac nerve efferent traffic originating in the nucleus ambiguus and therefore provides a noninvasive index of cardiac vagal regulation (Berntson et al., 1997; Yasuma et al., 2004). As interpreted by Porges in his polyvagal theory (1995, 2009), the nucleus ambiguus is considered as an origin of the more recently developed „smart" vagus to facilitate the complex emotion responses and social behaviour. Two sources of structural evidence link respiratory sinus arrhythmia to emotion. Efferent fibers from the nucleus ambiguus innervate the larynx, an important structure for communication of emotional state through vocalization (Porges, 1995). Also, the nucleus ambiguus fibers are believed to terminate in the source nuclei of the facial and trigeminal nerves, which facilitate the emotion behaviours of facial expression and vocalization. Recently, along with structural evidence, empirical studies relating respiratory sinus arrhythmia to emotion in humans have accumulated (Frazier et al., 2004). Therefore, the respiratory sinus arrhythmia should be considered as an index of both cardiac vagal and emotional regulation.

Our studies analyzed the respiratory sinus arrhythmia changes using the heart rate variability spectral analysis at the high-frequency band in children and adolescents suffering from selected mental disorders (depressive disorder, attention deficit/hyperactivity disorder). Our original results (published by Tonhajzerova et al., 2009a,b, 2010) will be discussed in the last chapter section.

3.2 Heart rate variability – nonlinear analysis

The physiological cardiac control mechanisms integrated from subcellular to systemic levels operate over multiple time scales. This perpetual control results in the complex oscillations of the heart rate - the measured output signal is characterized by great complexity (Javorka et al., 2011). Recently, nonlinear methods measuring qualitative characteristic of the cardiac time series - i.e. complexity, and other system dynamic features have been shown to be more suitable for a detailed description of heart rate autonomic control system (Javorka et al., 2009; Porta et al., 2009).

Moreover, the central autonomic network, resulting in complex beat-to-beat heart rate variability, has many features of a nonlinear dynamical system: reciprocally interconnected components with the function of positive/negative feedback interactions; a presence of a parallel, distributed pathways which are important to a given response (e.g. the modification of the heart rate by various combinations of sympathetic and parasympathetic activity), including other pathways such as circulating hormones (see Friedman, 2007; Thayer & Lane, 2000). From this point of view, the more complex oscillations mean the more complex and healthier regulation indicating better adaptability of the underlying system. Contrary, different diseases are often associated with the reduced heart rate control network complexity indicating insufficient heart rate adaptation to different requirements. Therefore, the loss of complexity was proposed as a general feature of pathological dynamics (see Baumert et al., 2004).

The quantifying of the heart rate variability by linear methods is not sufficient to characterize the complex dynamics of cardiac time series modulation. Therefore, the new parameters quantifying additional information embedded in the heart rate variability signal were developed. However, the application of traditionally used nonlinear methods (e.g. correlation dimension, largest Lyapunov exponent) is limited to long stationary signals - a condition that is only rarely met in physiology (Schreiber, 1999). Then, new methods with applicability to real biological signals are continuously developed to quantify new aspects of short quasistationarity heart rate variability signal with the potential to reveal subtle changes in cardiovascular control system (Aubert & Ramaekers, 1999).

In the case of heart rate variability analysis, entropy measures are therefore used to quantify the complexity of heart rate fluctuations. Firstly, the complexity analysis of heart rate variability was performed by calculation of Approximate Entropy (ApEn) (Pincus, 1995). An improved version of ApEn is a measure of Sample Entropy (SampEn) which quantifies the irregularity and unpredictability of a time series (see Richman & Mooman, 2000). Since heart rate time series under healthy conditions have a complex spatial and temporal structure with correlations on multiple scales, single-scale based traditional entropy measures, including SampEn, fail to account for the multiple time scales inherent in the physiologic systems dynamics. A meaningful measure of the complexity should take into account multiple time scales. Costa et al. (2002) introduced a new method called Multiscale Entropy Analysis to calculate entropy over multiple scales. Multiscale Entropy Analysis describes the complexity for various time scales of fluctuations within the analysed signal.

In our study (Tonhajzerova et al., 2010), we used novel nonlinear method - symbolic dynamics. Symbolic dynamics is a suitable method for the quantification of cardiac time series complexity indepedent of its magnitude and a potentially promising tool for short-term heart rate variability assessment (Guzzetti et al., 2005; Voss et al., 2009). The symbolic dynamics concept allows a simplified description of the system dynamics with a limited set of symbols. Consecutive values of heart rate time series/their differences are encoded according to some transformation rules into a few symbols of a certain alphabet. Subsequently, the dynamics of that symbol string are quantified, providing information about various qualitative aspects of heart dynamics. Then, in our study the following parameters from the resulting symbolic time series were evaluated: *normalized complexity index (NCI)* - computed as a measure of the amount of information (corrected for short-term time series) carried by the L-th sample when the previous L-1 samples are known. NCI is a measure of the complexity of pattern distribution. It ranges from zero (maximum regularity) to one (maximum complexity). The larger the NCI, the more complex and less regular the time series. Our interest was focused on the evaluation of the patterns with two like variations (2LV, the three symbols form an ascending or descending ramp) and the rates of occurence of this pattern was indicated as 2LV%. This parameter could be considered as a marker of vagal activity (Porta et al., 2006).

Recently, the application of novel nonlinear methods is associated with increased interest (Bär et al., 2007; Baumert et al., 2009). Our findings (published by Tonhajzerova et al., 2010) will be outlined in the following section.

3.3 Clinical implications of the heart rate variability analysis

Despite the heart rate variability traditional (linear) analysis - extensively utilized in clinical practice, the application of new nonlinear methods is rare, in particular in children and adolescents suffering from mental disorders. Since the childhood and adolescent age-period is important concerning the brain-heart interaction, our findings (presented below) underscore importance of this problem emphasizing the interdisciplinary approach.

3.3.1 Depressive disorder

Mean heart rate: The findings regarding average value of the heart rate in depressive disorder are controversial. We found significantly higher heart rate in adolescent girls suffering from major depression compared to controls (Tonhajzerova et al., 2009b, 2010). In contrast, other authors found no significant differences in heart rate between depressive adolescents and controls (Henje Blom et al., 2010). Interestingly, Clark & Watson (1991) introduced the tripartite model, in which anxiety, not depression, is associated with physiological hyperarousal reflecting in autonomic hyperactivity and heart rate modifications. Heart rate could be taken as a measure of arousal; the higher heart rate, the higher the arousal level (Greaves-Lord et al. 2007). These authors found higher heart rate in major depression pointing towards relatively high arousal in depression as well as in anxiety. Thus, the idea of hyperarousal in anxiety and not in depression is too simple to reflect more complex reality (Greaves-Lord et al., 2007).

Heart rate variability: Impaired autonomic neural regulation of the heart, characterized by increased sympathetic and/or reduced vagal modulation, is likely an important contributor to the cardiac adverse outcomes associated with major depression (for reviews, see Brown et al., 2009; Carney & Freedland, 2009). Although reduced cardiac vagal modulation is a common finding in adult patients with depression (Kikuchi et al., 2009; Udupa et al., 2007), other studies reported unchanged parasympathetic activity (Bär et al., 2004). It seems that the heart rate variability analysis may contribute to early diagnosis of latent and clinically asymptomatic symptoms of a potential cardiac neural dysregulation associated with depression. However, the adolescence is important age-period regarding the depressive disorder. In early adolescence there is a marked increase in depressive symptoms (Galambos et al., 2004), which have a high expectation to continue into early adult life and adulthood (Lewinsohn et al., 1994; Weissman et al., 1999). Chapman et al. (2010) firstly demonstrated an association between neurocognitive regulation and parasympathetic control of the heart (evaluated by respiratory sinus arrhythmia) in children and adolescents. Thus, the heart and mind may be coordinated in order to facilitate adaptive functioning. It is important to note that the adolescence could be a critical and vulnerable age period due to developmental and brain maturational changes (Thayer et al., 2009; Yang et al., 2007). This makes early adolescence as interesting period for studying the depression because of neurobiological as well as psychological maturation (Bosch et al., 2009).

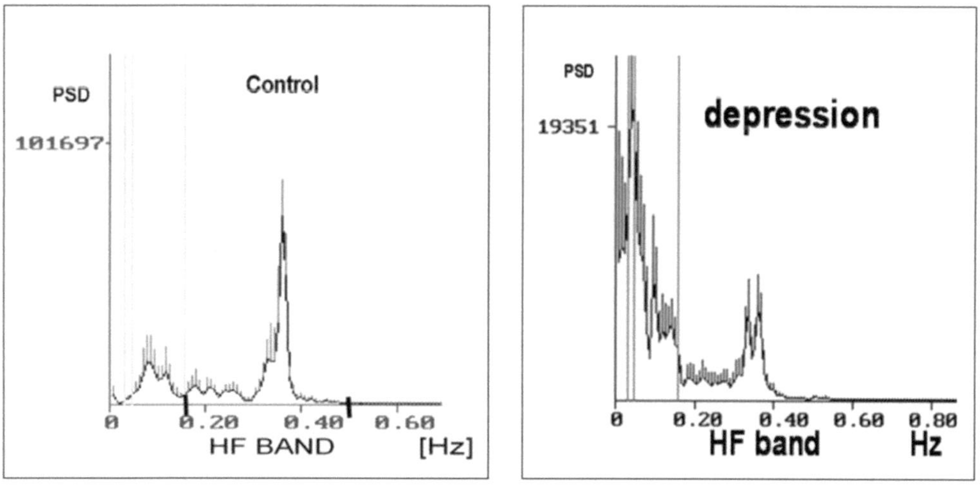

Fig. 2. Graphic protocol of heart rate variability spectral analysis in healthy subject (left) and depressive patient (right) HF – high-frequency band reflecting respiratory sinus arrhythmia. Reduced high-frequency oscillations refer to lower respiratory sinus arrhythmia indicating impaired cardiac vagal control in the patient with major depression. PSD - power spectral density (ms^2/Hz) (modified by Tonhajzerova et al., 2011).

From this point of view, our original findings revealed reduced cardiac time series magnitude indicating impaired neurocardiac regulation already in girls with major depression before treatment (Fig. 2). Interestingly, we found lower complexity of the cardiac time series in a supine position and standing position in the same major depression group (Tonhajzerova et al., 2010). Reduced complexity in heart rate time series is believed to result from a lessened ability of regulatory subsystems to interact (Porta et al., 2007) resulting in maladaptation of physiological system. These findings indicate impaired complex neurocardiac heart rate control in the adolescent girls with major depression before treatment (Tonhajzerova et al., 2010).

Potential mechanisms: The mechanisms of cardiac neural regulation impairment in major depression are still discussed. Thus, it is important to refer to the inhibitory processes described in above-mentioned sections: the prefrontal cortex and its abnormalities (*e.g.* prefrontal hypoactivity) could play a critical role in cardiac autonomic dysregulation associated with major depression because of the failure of the prefrontal cortex to inhibit the amygdala as a region regulating cardiovascular and autonomic responses (Thayer & Lane, 2009). Moreover, other factors participating on abnormal neurocardiac modulation could involve behavioral or lifestyle factors associated with major depression, *e.g.* lack of physical activity. This association is questionable: Uusitalo et al. (2004) found that low-intensity regular exercise training did not prevent heart rate variability from decreasing. Additionally, depressive disorder often overlaps with anxiety. Trait anxiety may moderate the relationship between cardiac vagal regulation and depression, with which anxiety is often associated. For example, low vagal heart rate control was found only in high-anxious subset of the depressive patients (Watkins et al., 1999). In this regard, the reduced vagal modulation of the heart in depression could represent a chronic, consolidated anxiety-related response to everyday aggravations (Berntson et al., 2004).

3.3.2 Attention deficit/hyperactivity disorder (ADHD)

Mean heart rate: Despite the internalizing disorders, the externalizing disorders (ADHD/oppositional defiant disorder-ODD/conduct disorders-CD) are characterized by autonomic underarousal including lower heart rate (Beauchaine, 2001). Generally, low heart rate is considered as a biological marker for externalizing disorders spectrum (see review Ortiz & Raine, 2004), and other authors suggest that low heart rate is a marker of resilience to the effects of environmental challenges in early adolescence (Oldehinkel et al., 2008). The other authors found a tendency towards higher heart rate level in the comorbid ADHD group (ADHD+ODD/CD) in comparison with the heart rate level of the ADHD group (van Lang et al., 2007). These authors suggest that a potential dominance of the parasympathetic activity over the sympathetic nervous system could be more prominent in children with ADHD than in patients with comorbid ODD/CD. Interestingly, the other study revealed tachycardia in children with ADHD in comparison with controls; importantly, this tachycardia was observed during day and night. Nocturnal tachycardia in this group could not be explained by nocturnal activity levels or comorbid externalizing/internalizing problems (Imeraj et al., 2011). These conclusions are consistent with our findings of tachycardia in the children suffering from ADHD-combined type (Tonhajzerova et al., 2009a). The question related to heart rate and ADHD without comorbidities is still discussed.

Heart rate variability: Regarding the autonomic nervous system changes in externalizing psychopathology, each branch can function somewhat indepedently of the other, therefore, inferences concerning sympathetic or parasympathetic activation based on mean heart rate alone are questionable (Berntson et al., 1994). For example, Mezzacappa et al. (1997) reported lower heart rate and reduced respiratory sinus arrhythmia (as an index of cardiac vagal modulation) in the antisocial group in comparison with controls indicating concurrent sympathetic and parasympathetic dysregulation. Crowell et al. (2006) compared autonomic profiles of preschool children with ADHD and ODD with controls using heart rate variability spectral analysis at high frequency as an index of respiratory linked-cardiac vagal control. Children with ADHD and ODD were not significantly different in baseline respiratory sinus arrhythmia, but authors referred to a potential impaired cardiac vagal regulation in later age-period related to emotion dysregulation and lability. Our original findings indicated tachycardia associated with decreased cardiac vagal modulation in a supine position as well as during active orthostatic test in boys with ADHD (Tonhajzerova et al., 2009a). Beauchaine (2001) referred to reduced respiratory sinus arrhythmia, indicating altered cardiac vagal control, as a potential marker of the dysregulated emotional states. It seems that emotional maturation should represent an important factor connected to parasympathetic-linked cardiac activity; thus, it is questionable whether our findings are related to the features of the ADHD (*e.g.* emotional immaturity) or the reflection of subclinical abnormal dynamic activation of the autonomic nervous system in response to posture change in children with ADHD (Tonhajzerova et al., 2009a).

Potential mechanisms: As internalizing disorders, the deficit in frontal functioning connected to limbic system and consequent alteration of baroreflex function as well as the modifications in a network of brain regions are proposed in the ADHD-linked cardiac neural dysregulation (Borger et al., 1999). Additionally, we assume that the study of the relevant neurotransmitter's systems, genetic and other factors will be important for a better understanding of ADHD and cardiac autonomic dysregulation in children with ADHD.

4. Conclusion

Although a lack of sensitive heart rate autonomic control likely reflects impaired cardiac nervous system regulation, the sophisticated brain-heart interactions are incompletely understood. Importantly, cardiac neural dysregulation is associated with the increased risk of cardiovascular morbidity. This chapter tried to summarize the importance of the identifying of neurocardiac control changes reflecting in complex heart rate time series variability, as an index of the central-peripheral interactions, using conventional (linear) as well as nonconventional (nonlinear) methods. Our findings revealed decreased magnitude and complexity of heart rate time series indicating altered neurocardiac regulation in children and adolescents suffering from selected mental disorders (ADHD, major depression) without pharmacotherapy (Tonhajzerova et al., 2009a,b; Tonhajzerova et al., 2010). From the point of clinical utilization, the heart rate variability analysis by both traditional and novel methods might provide important insight into complex cardiac autonomic regulation in children and adolescents with mental disorders. Further research on cardiac autonomic function in ADHD, major depression and other mental disorders is necessary.

5. Acknowledgment

This work was supported by European Center of Excellence for Perinatologic Research No. 26220120036 (CEPVII), co-financed from EU sources, VEGA No.1/0033/11 and 1/0073/09.

6. References

Ahs, F., Sollers, J.J. 3rd, Furmark, T., Frederikson, M. & Thayer, J.F. (2009). High-frequency heart rate variability and cortico-striatal activity in men and women with social phobia. *Neuroimage*, Vol. 47, No. 3, (Epub: June 2009), pp. 815-820, ISSN 10538119

Armour, J.A. (1999). Myocardial ischemia and the cardiac nervous system. *Cardiovascular Research*, Vol. 41, No.1, pp. 41-54, ISSN 0008-6363

Aubert, A.E. & Ramaekers, D. (1999). Neurocardiology: the benefits of irregularity. The basics of methodology, physiology and current clinical applications. *Acta Cardiologica*, Vol. 54, No. 3, pp. 107-120, ISSN 1783-8363

Bär, K.J., Boettger, M.K., Koschke, M., Schulz, S., Chokka, P., Yeragani, V.K. & Voss A. (2007). Non-linear complexity measures of heart rate variability in acute schizophrenia. *Clinical Neurophysiology*, Vol.118, No. 9, pp. 2009-2015, ISSN 1388-2457.

Bär, K.J., Greiner, W., Jochum, T., Friedrich, M., Wagner, G. & Sauer, H. (2004). The influence of major depression and its treatment on heart rate variability and pupillary light reflex parameters. *Journal of Affective Disorders*, Vol. 82, No. 2, pp. 245-252. ISSN 0165-0327.

Baumert, M., Baier, Vm Haueksen J., Wessel, N., Meyersfeldt, U., Schirdewan, A. & Voss, A. (2004). Forecasting of life threating arrhythmias using the compression entropy of heart rate. *Methods of Information in Medicine*, Vol. 43, No.2, pp. 202-206, ISSN 0026-1270.

Baumert, M., Lambert, G.W., Dawood, T., Lambert, E.A., Esler, M.D., McGrane, M., Barton, D., Sanders, P. & Nalivaiko, E. (2009). Short-term heart rate variability and cardiac norepinephrine spillover in patients with depression and panic disorder. *American Journal of Physiology - Heart Circulation Physiology*, Vol. 297, (Epub: June 2009), pp. H674-H679, ISSN 0363-6135

Beauchaine, T. (2001). Vagal tone, development, and Gray´s motivational theory: Toward an integrated model of autonomic nervous system functioning in psychopathology. *Developmental Psychopathology*, Vol. 13, No.2, pp. 183-214. ISSN 0954-5794

Benarroch, E.E. (1993). The central autonomic network: functional organization, dysfunction, and perspective. *Mayo Clinic Proceedings*, Vol. 68, No. 10, pp. 988-1001, ISSN 0025-6196.

Berntson, G.G. & Cacioppo, J.T. (2004). Heart rate variability: Stress and psychiatric conditions. In: *Dynamic electrocardiography*. A.J. Camm, M. Malik (Eds.), pp. 56-63, Futura, New York. ISBN-10: 1405119608.

Berntson, G.G., Bigger, J.T., Eckberg, D.L., Grossman, P., Kaufmann, P.G., Malik, M., Nagaraja, H.N., Porges, S.W., Saul, J.P., Stone, P.H. & van der Molen, M.W. (1997). Heart rate variability: Origins, methods, and interpretive caveats. *Psychophysiology*, Vol. 34, No. 6, pp. 623-648, ISSN 0048-5772.

Berntson, G.G., Cacioppo, J.T., Binkley, P.F., Uchino, B.N., Quigley, K.S. & Fieldstone, A. (1994). Autonomic cardiac control. III. Psychological stress and cardiac response in autonomic space as revealed by pharmacological blockades. *Psychophysiology,* Vol. 31, No. 6, pp. 162-171, ISSN 0048-5772.

Börger, N., van der Meere J., Ronner, A., Alberts, E., Geuze, R. & Bogte, H. (1999). Heart rate variability and sustained attention in ADHD children - attention deficit-hyperactivity disorder. *Journal of Abnormal Child Psychology,* Vol. 27, No. 1, pp. 25-33. ISSN 0091-0627

Bosch, N.M., Riese, H., Ormel, J., Verhulst, F. & Oldehinkel, J.A. (2009). Stressful life events and depressive symptoms in young adolescents: modulation by respiratory sinus arrhythmia? The TRAILS study. *Biological Psychology,* Vol. 81, No. 1, pp. 40-47, (January 2009), ISSN 0301-0511.

Brown, A.D.H., Barton, D.A. & Lambert, G.W. (2009). Cardiovascular abnormalities in patients with major depressive disorder. *CNS Drugs,* Vol. 23, No. 7, pp. 583-602, (Epub: January 2009), ISSN 1172-7047.

Calkovska, A. & Javorka, K. Neural regulation of the heart and heart rate variability. In: *Heart rate variability – mechanisms, evaluation and clinical utilization,* Javorka K., (Ed.), Osveta, pp. 16-19, ISBN 978-80-8063-269-4, Martin, Slovak Republic (in Slovak language).

Carney, R.M. & Freedland, K.E. (2009). Depression and heart rate variability in patients with coronary heart disease. *Cleveland Clinic Journal of Medicine,* Vol. 76, Suppl. (2), S13-S17, ISSN 0891-1150.

Chapman, H.A., Woltering, S., Lamm, C. & Lewis, M.D. (2010). Hearts and minds: Coordination of neurocognitive and cardiovascular regulation in children and adolescents. *Biological Psychology,* Vol. 84, No. 2, (Epub: March 2010), pp. 296-303, ISSN 0301-0511.

Cheng, Z., Powley, T.L., Schwaber, J.S. & Doyle, I.F. (1997). Vagal afferent innervation of the atria of the rat heart reconstructed with confocal microscopy. *Journal of Comparative Neurology,* Vol. 381, No. 1, pp. 1-17, ISSN 1096-9861.

Clark, L.A. & Watson, D. (1991). Tripartite model of anxiety and depression: psychometric evidence and taxonomic implications. *Journal of Abnormal Psychology,* Vol. 100, No.3, pp. 316-336, ISSN 0091-0627.

Costa, M., Goldberger, A.L. & Peng, C.K. (2002). Multiscale entropy analysis of complex physiologic time series. *Physical Review Letters,* Vol. 89, No.6, pp. 068102, (Epub: July, 2002), ISSN 0031-9007.

Crowell, S.E., Beauchaine, T.P., Gatzke-Kopp, L., Sylvers, P., Mead, H. & Chipman-Chacon, J. (2006). Autonomic correlates of attention-deficit/hyperactivity disorder and oppositional defiant disorder in preschool children. *Journal of Abnormal Psychology,* Vol. 115, No.1, pp. 174-178, ISSN 0091-0627.

de Bruyne, M.C., Kors, J.A., Hoes, A.W., Klootwijk, P., Dekker, J.M., Hofman, A., van Bemmel, J.H. & Grobbee, D.E. (1999). Both decreased and increased heart rate variability on the standard 10-second electrocardiogram predict cardiac mortality in the elderly: the Rotterdam Study. *American Journal of Epidemiology,* Vol. 150, No. 12, pp. 1282-1288, ISSN 0002-9262.

Elghozi, J.L. & Julien, C. (2007). Sympathetic control of short-term heart rate variability and its pharmacological modulation. *Fundamental Clinical Pharmacology,* Vol. 21, No. 4, pp. 337-347, ISSN 07673981.

Ellis, R.J. & Thayer, J.F. (2010). Music and autonomic nervous system (dys)function. *Music Perception*, Vol. 27, No. 4, pp. 317-326, ISSN 0730-7829.

Frazier, T.W., Strauss, M.E. & Steinhauer, S.R. (2004). Respiratory sinus arrhythmia as an index of emotional response in young adults. *Psychophysiology*, Vol. 41, No. 1, pp. 75-83, ISSN 0048-5772.

Friedman, B.H. (2007). An autonomic flexibility-neurovisceral integration model of anxiety and cardiac vagal tone. *Biological Psychology*, Vol. 74, No. 2, (Epub: October 2006), pp. 185-199, ISSN 0301-0511.

Galambos, N.L., Leadbeater, B.J. & Barker, E.T. (2004). Gender differences and risk factor for depression in adolescence: a 4-year longitudinal study. *International Journal of Behavioral Development*, Vol. 28, pp. 16-25, ISSN 0165-0254.

Greaves-Lord, K., Ferdinand, R.F., Sondeijker, F.E., Dietrich, A., Oldehinkel, A.J., Rosmalen, J.G., Ormel, J. & Verhulst, F.C. (2007). Testing the tripartite model in young adolescents: is hyperarousal specific for anxiety and not depression? *Journal of Affective Disorders*, Vol. 102, No. 1-3, (Epub: January 2007), pp. 55-63, ISSN 0165-0327.

Guzzetti, S., Borroni, E., Garbelli, P.E., Ceriani, E., Bella, P.D., Montano, N., Cogliati, C., Somers, V.K., Malliani, A. & Porta, A. (2005). Symbolic dynamics of heart rate variability. A probe to investigate cardiac autonomic modulation. *Circulation*, Vol. 112, No. 4, (Epub: July 2005), pp. 465-470, ISSN 0009-7322.

Henje Blom, E.H., Olsson, E.M., Serlachius, E., Ericson, M. & Ingvar, M. (2010). Heart rate variability (HRV) in adolescent females with anxiety disorders and major depressive disorder. *Acta Paediatrica*, Vol. 99, No. 4, pp. 604-611, (Epub: January 2010), ISSN 0803-5253.

Horackova, M., Armour, J.A. & Byczko, Z. (1999). Distribution of intrinsic cardiac neurons in whole-mount guinea pig atria identified by multiple neurochemical coding. A confocal microscope study. *Cell Tissue Research*, Vol. 297, No. 3, pp. 409-421, ISSN 0302-766X.

Horackova, M., Croll, R.P., Hopkins, D.A., Losier, A.M. & Armour, J.A. (1996). Morphological and immunohistochemical properties of primary long-term cultures of adult guinea-pig ventricular cardiomyocytes with peripheral cardiac neurons. *Tissue Cell*, Vol. 28, No. 4, pp. 411-425, ISSN 0040-8166.

Imeraj, L., Antrop, I., Roeyers, H., Deschepper, E., Bal, S. & Deboutte, D. (2011). Diurnal variations in arousal: a naturalistic heart rate study in children with ADHD. *European Child and Adolescent Psychiatry*, Retrieved from doi:10.1007/s00787-011-0188-y. ISSN 1018-8827.

Javorka, M., Tonhajzerova, I., Turianikova, Z., Chladekova, L., Javorka, K. & Calkovska, A. (2011). Quantification of nonlinear features in cardiovascular signals. *Acta Medica Martiniana*, Vol. 11, Suppl 1, pp. 31-40, ISSN 1335-8421.

Javorka, M., Turianikova, Z., Tonhajzerova, I., Javorka, K. & Baumert, M. (2009). The effects of orthostasis on recurrence quantification analysis of heart rate and blood pressure dynamics. *Physiological Measurement*, Vol. 30, No. 1, (Epub: November 2008), pp. 29-41 ISSN 0967-3334.

Jose, A.D. & Collison, D. (1970). The normal range and determinants of the intrinsic heart rate in man. *Cardiovascular Research*, Vol. 4, No. 2, pp. 160-167, ISSN 1755-3245.

Kawashima, T. (2005). The autonomic nervous system of the human heart with special reference to its origin, course, and peripheral distribution. *Anatomical Embryology,* Vol. 209, No. 6, pp. 425-438, ISSN 0340-2061.

Kikuchi, M., Hanaoka, A., Kidani, T., Remijn, G.B., Minabe, Y., Munesue, T. & Koshino, Y. (2009). Heart rate variability in drug-naive patients with panic disorder and major depressive disorder. *Progress in Neuropsychopharmacology and Biological Psychiatry,* Vol. 33, No. 8, (Epub: August 2009), pp. 1474-1478, ISSN 0278-5846.

Kukanova, B. & Mravec, B. (2006). Complex intracardiac nervous system. Bratislavske Lekarske Listy, Vol. 107, No. 3, pp. 45-51. ISSN 1336-0345.

Lane, R.D., McRae, K., Reiman, E.M., Chen, K., Ahern, G.L. & Thayer, J.F. (2009). Neural correlates of heart rate variability during emotion. *Neuroimagine,* Vol. 44, No. 1, (Epub: August 2009), pp. 213-222, ISSN 10538119

Levy, M.N. (1971). Sympathetic-parasympathetic interactions in the heart. *Circulation Research,* Vol. 29, No. 5, pp. 437-445, ISSN 0009-7330.

Lewinsohn, P.M., Clarke, G.N., Seeley, J.R. & Rohde, P. (1994). Major depression in community adolescents: age of onset, episode duration, and time to recurrence. *Journal of the American Academy of Child & Adolescent Psychiatry,* Vol. 33, No. 6, pp. 809-818, ISSN 0890-8567.

Malliani, A., Pagani, M., Lombardi, F. & Cerutti, S. (1991). Cardiovascular neural regulation explored in the frequency domain. *Circulation,* Vol. 84, No. 2, pp. 482-492, ISSN 0009-7322.

Mezzacappa, E., Tremblay, R.E., Kindlon, D., Saul, J.P., Arseneault, L., Seguin, J., Pihl, R.O. & Earls, F. (1997). Anxiety, antisocial behavior, and heart rate regulation in adolescent males. *Journal of Child Psychology and Psychiatry,* Vol. 38, No. 4, pp. 457-469, ISSN 0021-9630.

Montano, N., Porta, A., Cogliati, Ch., Constantino, G., Tobaldini, E., Casali, K.R. & Iellamo, F. (2009). Heart rate variability explored in the frequency domain: A tool to investigate the link between heart and behavior. *Neuroscience and Biobehavioral Reviews,* Vol. 33, No.2, (Epub: July 2008), pp. 71-80, ISSN 0149-7634.

Napadow, V., Dhond, R., Conti, G., Makris, N., Brown, E.N. & Barbieri, R. (2008). Brain correlates of autonomic modulation: combining heart rate variability with fMRI. *Neuroimagine,* Vol. 42, No. 1, (Epub: April 2008), pp. 169-177, ISSN 10538119.

Oldehinkel, A.J., Verhulst, F.C. & Ormel, J. (2008). Low heart rate: a marker of stress resilience. The TRAILS Study. *Biological Psychiatry,* Vol. 63, No. 12, (Epub: February 2008), pp. 1141-1146, ISSN 0006-3223.

Ortiz, J. & Raine, A. (2004). Heart rate level and antisocial behavior in children and adolescents: a meta-analysis. *Journal of the American Academy of Child & Adolescent Psychiatry,* Vol. 43, No. 2, pp. 154-162, ISSN 0890-8567.

Paton, J.F.R., Boscan, P., Pickering, A.E. & Nalivaiko, E. (2005). The yin and yang of cardiac autonomic control: Vago-sympathetic interactions revisited. *Brain Research Reviews,* Vol. 49, No. 3, (Epub: April 2005), pp. 555-565, ISSN 0165-0173.

Pincus S. (1995). Approximate Entropy (ApEn) as a complexity measure. *Chaos* Vol. 5, No. 1, pp. 110-117, ISSN 1054-1500.

Porges, S.W. (1995). Orienting in a defensive world: Mammalian modification of our evolutionary heritage. A polyvagal theory. *Psychophysiology,* Vol. 32, No. 4, pp. 301-318, ISSN 0048-5772.

Porges, S.W. (2007). The polyvagal perspective. *Biological Psychology,* Vol. 74, No. 2, (Epub: October 2006), pp. 116-143, ISSN 0301-0511.

Porges, S.W. (2009). The polyvagal theory: new insights into adaptive reactions of the autonomic nervous system. *Cleveland Clinic Journal of Medicine,* Vol. 76, Suppl. 2, pp. 86-90, ISSN 0891-1150

Porta, A., Daddio, G., Bassani, T., Maestri, R. & Pinna, G.D. (2009). Assessment of cardiovascular regulation through irreversibility analysis of heart period variability: a 24 hours Holter study in healthy and chronic heart failure populations. *Philosophical Transactions of the Royal Society A Mathematical, Physical & Engineering Sciences,* Vol. 367, No. 1892, pp. 1359-1375, ISSN 1364-503X.

Porta, A., Gnecchi-Ruscone, T., Tobaldini, E., Guzzetti, S., Furlan, R., Malliani, A, & Montano, N. (2006). Symbolic analysis of short-term heart period variability during graded head-up tilt. *Computers in Cardiology,* Vol. 33, pp.109-112, ISSN 0276-6574.

Porta, A., Guzzetti, S., Furlan, R., Gnecchi-Ruscone, T., Montano, N. & Malliani, A. (2007). Complexity and nonlinearity in short-term heart rate variability: comparison of methods based on local nonlinear prediction. *IEEE Transactions on Biomedical Engineering,* Vol. 54, No. 1, pp. 94-106, ISSN 0018-9294.

Randall, D.C. (2000). Towards and understanding of the function of the intrinsic cardiac ganglia. *Journal of Physiology,* Vol. 528, No. (Pt 3), pp. 406, ISSN 0022-3751.

Reunanen, A., Krjalainen, J., Ristola, P,, Heliovaara, M., Knekt, P. & Aromaa, A. (2000). Heart rate and mortality. *Journal of Internal Medicine,* Vol. 247, No. 2, pp. 211-239, ISSN 1365-2796.

Richman, S. & Moorman, J.R. (2000). Physiological time-series analysis using approximate entropy and sample entropy. *American Journal of Physiology-Heart and Circulatory Physiology,* Vol. 278, No. 6, pp. H2039-H2049, ISSN 0363-6135.

Schreiber, T. (1999). Interdisciplinary application of nonlinear time series methods. *Physics Reports,* Vol. 308, No. 1, pp. 1-64, ISSN 0370-1573.

Shaper, A.G., Wannamethee, G., Maclarlane, P.W. & Walker, M. (1993). Heart rate, ischemic heart disease, and sudden cardiac death in middle-aged British men. *British Heart Journal,* Vol. 70, No. 1, pp. 49-55, ISSN 0007-0769

Shine, J., Potter, E.K., Biden, T., Selbie, L.A. & Herzog, H. (1994). Neuropeptide Y and regulation of the cardiovascular system. *Journal of Hypertension Suppl,* Vol. 12, No. 10, pp. S41-S45, ISSN 0263-6352

Task Force of the European Society of Cardiology and the North American Society of Pacing and Electrophysiology. (1996). Heart rate variability. Standards of measurement, physiological interpretation, and clinical use. *Circulation,* Vol. 93, No. 5, 1043-1065, ISSN 0009-7322

Taylor, E.W., Jordan, D. & Coote, J.H. (1999). Central control of the cardiovascular and respiratory systems and their interactions in vertebrates. *Physiological Reviews,* Vol. 79, No. 3, pp. 855-916, ISSN 003-9333.

Thayer, J.F. & Brosschot, J.F. (2005). Psychosomatics and psychopathology: looking up and down from the brain. *Psychoneuroendocrinology,* Vol. 30, No. 10, pp. 1050-1058, ISSN 0300-4530.

Thayer, J.F. & Lane, R.D. (2000). A model of neurovisceral integration in emotion regulation and dysregulation. *Journal of Affective Disorders,* Vol. 61, No. 3, pp. 201-216, ISSN 0165-0327.

Thayer, J.F. & Lane, R.D. (2009). Claude Bernard and the heart-brain connection: Further elaboration of a model of neurovisceral integration. *Neuroscience and Biobehavioral Reviews*, Vol. 33, No. 2, pp. 81-88, ISSN 0149-7634.

Thayer, J.F. & Sternberg, E. (2006). Beyond Heart Rate Variability. Vagal Regulation of Allostatic Systems. *Annals of the New York Academy of Sciences,* Vol. 1088, pp. 361-372, (Epub: September 2008), ISSN 0077-8923

Thayer, J.F. (2006). The importance of inhibition central and peripheral manifestations of nonlinear inhibitory processes in neural systems. *Dose Response* , Vol. 4, No. 1, (Epub: August 2008), pp. 2-21, ISSN 1559-3258.

Thayer, J.F., Sollers, III J.J., Labiner, D.M., Weinand, M., Herring, A.M., Lane, R.D. & Ahern GL. (2009). Age-related differences in prefrontal control of heart rate in humans: A pharmacological blockade study. *Internal Journal of Psychophysiology*, Vol. 72, No. 1, pp. 81-88, ISSN 0167-8760.

Tonhajzerova, I., Ondrejka, I., Adamik, P., Hruby, R., Javorka, M., Trunkvalterova, Z., Mokra, D., & Javorka K. (2009a). Changes in the cardiac autonomic regulation in children with attention deficit hyperactivity disorder (ADHD). *Indian Journal of Medical Research*, Vol. 130, No. 1, pp. 44-50, ISSN 0019-5359.

Tonhajzerova, I., Ondrejka, I., Javorka, K., Calkovska, A. & Javorka, M. (2011). Cardiac vagal control in depression and attention deficit/hyperactivity disorder. *Acta Medica Martiniana,* Vol. 11, Suppl 1, pp. 46-51, ISSN 1335-8421

Tonhajzerova, I., Ondrejka, I., Javorka, K., Turianikova, Z., Farsky, I. & Javorka, M. (2010). Cardiac autonomic regulation is impaired in girls with major depression. *Progress in Neuropsychopharmacology and Biological Psychiatry*, Vol. 34, No. 4, (Epub: February 2010), pp. 613-618, ISSN 0278-5846.

Tonhajzerova, I., Ondrejka, I., Javorka, M., Adamik, P., Turianikova, Z., Kerna, V., Javorka, K. & Calkovska, A. (2009b). Respiratory sinus arrhythmia is reduced in adolescent major depressive disorder. *European Journal of Medical Research*, Vol. 14, Suppl. 4, pp. 280-283, ISSN 0949-2321.

Udupa, K., Sathyaprabha, T.N., Thirthalli, J., Kishore, K.R., Lavekar, G.S., Raju, T.R. & Gangadhar, B.N. (2007). Alteration of cardiac autonomic functions in patients with major depression: A study using heart rate variability measures. *Journal of Affective Disorders,* Vol. 100, No.1-3, (Epub: May 2008), pp. 137-141, ISSN 0165-0327.

Uijtdehaage, S.H. & Thayer, J.F. (2000). Accentuated antagonism in the control of human heart rate. *Clinical Autonomic Research,* Vol. 10, No. 3, pp. 107-110, ISSN 0959-9851.

Uusitalo, A.L., Laitinen, T., Vaisanen, S.B., Lansimies, E. & Rauramaa, R. (2004). Physical training and heart rate and blood pressure variability: a 5-yr randomized trial. *American Journal of Physiology-Heart and Circulatory Physiology,* Vol. 286, No. 5, (Epub: January 2004), pp. H1821-H1826, ISSN 0363-6135.

van Lang, N.D., Tulen, J.H., Kallen, V.L., Rosbergen, B., Dieleman, G. & Ferdinand, R.F. (2007). Autonomic reactivity in clinically referred children attention-deficit/hyperactivity disorder versus anxiety disorder. *European Journal of Child and Adolescent Psychiatry,* Vol. 16, No. 2, (Epub: September 2006), pp. 71-78, ISSN 0936-6075.

Voss, A., Schulz, S., Schroeder, R., Baumert, M. & Caminal, P. (2009). Methods derived from nonlinear dynamics for analysing heart rate variability. *Philosophical Transactions A Mathematical, Physical, and Engineering Sciences,* Vol. 367, No. 1887, pp. 277-296, ISSN 1364-503X.

Watkins, I.I., Grossman, P., Krishnan, R. & Blumenthal, J.A. (1999). Anxiety reduces baroreflex cardiac control in older adults with major depression. *Psychosomatic Medicine,* Vol. 61, No.3, pp. 334-340, ISSN 0033-3174.

Weissman, M.M., Wolk, S. & Wickramaratne, P. (1999). Children with prepubertal major depressive disorder and anxietygrown up. *Archives of General Psychiatry,* Vol. 56, No. 9, pp. 794-801, ISSN 0003-990X.

Yang, T.T., Simmons, A.N., Matthews, S.C., Tapert, S.F., Bischoff-Grethe, A., Frank, G.K.W., Arce, E. & Paulus, M.P. (2007). Increased amygdala activation is related to heart rate during emotion processing in adolescent subjects. *Neuroscience Letters,* Vol. 428, No.2-3, pp. 109-114, ISSN 0304-3940.

Yasuma, F. & Hayano, J. (2004). Respiratory sinus arrhythmia: why does the heartbeat synchronize with respiratory rhythm? *Chest,* Vol. 125, No. 2, pp. 683-690, ISSN 0012-3692.